"OASIS has long been a tremendous resource for family members and professionals. The authors have thoughtfully organized a massive amount of critical information into a comprehensive and valuable guide. Every family and professional should have a copy of this book." —**Dr. Cathy Pratt**, board of directors, Autism Society of America

"Barbara L. Kirby and Patricia Romanowski Bashe have provided the community of Asperger Syndrome with more than a rainbow's end of gold. They've opened a treasure chest brimming with understanding and support." —**Liane Holliday Willey, Ed.D.**, author of *Pretending to Be Normal: Living with Asperger's Syndrome* and *Asperger Syndrome in the Family: Redefining Normal*

"If someone were to ask me to suggest the most useful resource about AS, I would not hesitate for an instant: *The OASIS Guide to Asperger Syndrome*. This is a must-read book for parents, educators, and individuals with AS alike." —**Brenda Smith Myles, Ph.D.**, author of *Asperger Syndrome and Difficult Moments: Practical Solutions for Tantrums, Rage, and Meltdowns*

"This inspiring book offers sound advice, comforting support, and remarkable insights with clarity of purpose, profound honesty, and depth of meaning. It's destined to become a classic in its genre." —**Diane Twachtman-Cullen, Ph.D.**, executive director, Autism and Developmental Disabilities Consultation Center

"Rarely does one find such a wealth of quality information all between the same two covers. This book has important work to do, and it is more than up to the task." —**Carol Gray**, director, Gray Center for Social Learning and Understanding

"Incredible! *The OASIS Guide to Asperger Syndrome* contains tremendous advice, tips, and practical solutions to manage the confusion of special ed and Asperger Syndrome. The new parent and seasoned veteran should read the guide cover to cover. It is excellent." —**Peter W. D. Wright, Esq.**, coauthor of *Wrightslaw: Special Education Law* and owner of wrightslaw.com

THE
OASIS GUIDE
TO
ASPERGER
SYNDROME

COMPLETELY REVISED AND UPDATED

• • •

Advice, Support, Insight,
and Inspiration

PATRICIA ROMANOWSKI BASHE, M.S.Ed.
AND BARBARA L. KIRBY,

Founder of the OASIS Asperger Web site

Forewords by SIMON BARON-COHEN, PH.D.,
and TONY ATTWOOD, PH.D.

 CROWN PUBLISHERS   NEW YORK

AUTHORS' NOTE

No book, including this one, can ever substitute for the care of an M.D. or other health professional. One of the points we've emphasized in these pages is the relative scarcity of long-term information on Asperger Syndrome and the treatments and interventions for it. We therefore believe it's especially important to share this book with your doctor and all other persons who will be helping you and your child. The best, most effective approach to Asperger Syndrome is a team approach, and your doctor is an essential member of that team.

A note on resources: Because Web sites and their contents get moved, redesigned, and rearranged, we cannot always provide the URL for specific papers or pages. In most cases you will be able to find a particular document by searching from a Web site's main or home page, or by running a search engine search by the piece's title.

Grateful acknowledgment is made for the following previously published material:

The *DSM-IV-TR* criteria for Asperger's Disorder, reprinted with permission from the *Diagnostic and Statistical Manual of Mental Disorders, Fourth Edition, Text Revision.* Copyright © 2000 American Psychiatric Association. Reprinted by permission of the American Psychiatric Association.

The Australian Scale for Asperger's Syndrome, by Tony Attwood and M. S. Garnett, from *Asperger's Syndrome: A Guide for Parents and Professionals.* Copyright © 1998 Tony Attwood. Reprinted by permission of Tony Attwood.

Excerpt from "The Social Story Kit," from *The New Social Story Book,* by Carol Gray. Copyright © Future Horizons. Reprinted by permission of Future Horizons.

Published in the United States by Crown Publishers, an imprint of the Crown Publishing Group, a division of Random House, Inc., New York.
www.crownpublishing.com

CROWN is a trademark and the Crown colophon is a registered trademark of Random House, Inc.

Originally published in a different form by Crown Publishers, a division of Random House, Inc., in 2001.

Library of Congress Cataloging-in-Publication Data
Bashe, Patricia Romanowski.
   The oasis guide to asperger syndrome : advice, support, insights, and inspiration / Patricia Romanowski Bashe and Barbara L. Kirby.
   Includes bibliographical references and index.
   1. Asperger's syndrome. 2. Autism in children. I. Kirby, Barbara L. II. Title.
RC553.A88.B375   2001
618.92'8982—dc21   2001028369

Printed in the United States of America

Design by Susan Hood

ISBN 1-4000-8152-1

10 9 8 7 6 5 4 3 2 1

First Revised Edition

For Justin Eric Romanowski Bashe—still and always my brightest star, my greatest joy, my favorite friend, my loving boy—this is for you. Love, Sweetie Mom

To the four men in my life: my sons Josh, Ben, and Nick, and my husband, Kirby. You teach me every day the true meaning of unconditional love.

CONTENTS

FOREWORD

by Simon Baron-Cohen, Ph.D.

Barbara Kirby and Patty Romanowski Bashe have given a special gift to families with a child with Asperger Syndrome (AS). They have written a book that communicates directly, from parent to parent. Its tone speaks from the heart, and Barbara and Patty are uniquely positioned to write such a book, having run OASIS for many years.

Parents of children newly diagnosed with AS seek out and find huge relief in discovering OASIS. Packed with information and practical advice, the OASIS Web site and support message boards make parents feel they are not alone, that their child is not the only child developing in this way, and that there are lots of things that they as parents can do to support their special child.

This book speaks from the mind as much as the heart. It covers what is known, in a clear summary of the medical and educational evidence. It is a book that professionals—and especially teachers—will find very useful.

AS is one of those unusual conditions that is a mix of both disability and, at times, talent. It is very easy to misrepresent AS by focusing on just one of these two aspects, but Barbara and Patty avoid this pitfall. They don't shy away from the disabling aspects and in typical fashion meet this challenge head-on, with a wealth of down-to-earth advice, including legal, psychological, and educational.

But equally they emphasize that the special needs of children with AS can involve a different learning style, one that can lead to areas of strength and talent. Examples include a remarkable focus of attention on favorite topics, an ability to pick out detail and remember detail where it fits into a special interest, and at times even a precocious development in some areas (e.g., hyperlexia).

I hope parents find this book supportive. To my mind, that is the overriding message that comes through this book—that people with AS and their families are not alone and can help one another as well as be helped by people who make the effort to understand their difference. And that AS is not just about needing help; it is also about being given the space to be different. In the right environment, people with AS can make remarkably valuable contributions.

May 2004

FOREWORD to the First Edition

by Tony Attwood, Ph.D.

If you have a child with Asperger Syndrome, this is the book for you. Patty Romanowski Bashe and Barb Kirby know the issues faced by parents and, using an analysis of hundreds of thousands of Internet messages and discussions on the OASIS Web site, have written *The OASIS Guide to Asperger Syndrome*. Why have there been so many messages? Although Asperger Syndrome was originally considered to be a rare developmental disorder, recent studies have established that it is much more common than was first thought. It is now recognized that in a town of ten thousand people, there will be around thirty whose pattern of abilities are consistent with a diagnosis of Asperger Syndrome. However, less than half of these unusual individuals will have received a formal diagnosis.

Part One, "Asperger Syndrome," explains our current knowledge of the nature of Asperger Syndrome from the perspective of clinicians and families. The key characteristics are explained using practical language rather than scientific terminology. Where there is limited academic knowledge, the authors have constructed questionnaires for parents. They have collated invaluable information from hundreds of respondents to provide greater understanding in areas such as special interests and sensitivity to certain sensory experiences. The section on the impact of the diagnosis on parents is particularly valuable to clinicians. Parents and professionals both will benefit from the information on dual diagnosis, especially the characteristics associated with attention deficit disorder. While the diagnosis may end a parent's nomadic wandering for an explanation and provide relief that the cause is not due to faulty parenting, the next issue is, what do we do now to help my son or daughter?

Part Two, "Taking Control," explains how parents can gain access to information, support, and treatment for their child. This section is almost a parents' encyclopedia. The authors know the questions raised by parents and families and provide answers that are informed, objective, and reasonable. They review the current range of interventions and therapies, and parents and teachers will be especially interested in the strategies to improve social understanding. Parents have many questions about the value of medication, and the authors have provided a guide to the relevant issues and benefits. As the book is written by two parents and is to be read by parents, the text includes information on the role of parents within the multidisciplinary team, recognizing that they are experts on their child. There is also information on the responsibilities of various government agencies and relevant legislation. This section is basically a guide to the system and how to survive and thrive.

Part Three considers aspects of the whole child, their social and emotional world, life at school, and growing up. If parents feel confused, anxious, and alone, this book will provide clear explanations, reassurance, and a sense of fellowship. I recommend that this book be read by parents immediately after the diagnosis and consulted before subsequent meetings with professionals. It was written by two experts on Asperger Syndrome for prospective experts: parents.

March 2001

THE OASIS GUIDE
TO ASPERGER SYNDROME

COMPLETELY REVISED AND UPDATED

INTRODUCTION

by Barbara L. Kirby

Our son was eight years old in 1993 when we first heard the term *Asperger Syndrome*. We hadn't heard it from any of the score of professionals we had turned to for help throughout the years when we wondered and worried about his particular difficulties and differences. Instead, a friend who knew something about autism had the courage to hand us a copy of a relatively new publication, *Autism and Asperger Syndrome* by Uta Frith, and say, "Please read this. It reminds me of your son."

When I put down the book, I knew I had found an explanation that finally made sense. It helped me to understand that what was happening to my son and to our family wasn't his fault or the fault of my parenting—as so many people, professionals, friends, and family members had so hurtfully suggested. He was not a "bad" child and we were not "bad" parents.

I would like to say that when I finally learned the news, I hit the ground running. But that would be a lie. What really happened is I hit the ground with a huge splat. I can't ever remember being so frightened. My son, whom I loved more than anything in the world, had a problem that could not be fixed even if I would only relax, stop hovering, discipline him properly, stop trying to be his friend and act like a mother, pay more attention, pay less attention, spank

1

him—or follow any of the other "helpful" suggestions offered to me by well-meaning professionals, family, and friends. Certainly none of them ever suggested that my son's problems stemmed from a neurological disorder about which no more than a handful of people around the world knew anything.

Though I'll never forget the pain of those comments, I've learned that there was nothing in my advisors' personal experience that could have allowed them to understand that my son's behaviors were anything other than the result of incompetence—ours at parenting and his at being a "good" boy. They simply did not know. As I soon learned, there was a world of "experts" out there who knew just about as much. Or as little.

You would think that finding a name for our son's behaviors would translate into finding some help and answers. But you would be wrong. Our son's doctor had never heard of Asperger Syndrome, neither the library nor the bookstore had a book on it, the local autism group had "heard" of it but did not have any information, and when I called local hospitals, they told me that the condition was rare and they had never seen a child with the diagnosis. How was this possible?

The realization that we were alone with this disorder, diagnosis, whatever it was, induced a level of fear and frustration that after all these years I still cannot explain. Perhaps it's something only another parent in exactly the same position can understand. Even today, when I open up the OASIS message board and see a post titled "Help! Just Got DX," I feel that ache inside, as if the world had ended. And for most of us, for a day, a week, a year, it feels that way. But it also goes on.

In 1994, about six months after we'd first heard the term, the American Psychiatric Association officially listed Asperger Syndrome in the *Diagnostic and Statistical Manual of Mental Disorders, Fourth Edition* (*DSM-IV*), its diagnostic bible. Doctors agreed that AS was the best diagnostic "fit" for our son. Still, they had no idea what we should do. Once again, we were alone. Six months later we arranged for our son to have a full psychoeducational evaluation; the psychologist suspected Asperger Syndrome. Three months after that, an appointment with a pediatric neurologist confirmed the diagnosis. However, the most any of these professionals could offer were vague, general suggestions and a pat on the back with a reminder that it was not our fault.

My son's teachers were more than willing to help, but they were also in the dark. After all, they weren't trained to deal with students like him. Looking back, I am amazed at how hard they worked at understanding and supporting my son. Still, I cried—and I continued to cry for a very, very long time.

One evening, on a whim, I decided to sign on to America Online, then a relatively new service. I knew nothing about our new home computer, and about all I could do with it was play solitaire and Tetris. I'd never heard of e-mail, I didn't know what a Web site was, and the Internet was someplace much too "scary" for a nontechnical stay-at-home mom like me.

After signing on, I found my way to the disability forums and posted messages asking if anyone had heard of Asperger Syndrome. Within a day, I'd received a message from a woman named Judy, who told me that she had a son who was diagnosed with AS and that I was not alone. One other mother, one other child in the world. I was overjoyed! I spent literally the next two days reading through message boards, leaving messages, and sending and answering e-mail. Finally! I'd found a few other families who understood.

Over the next several months, I was invited to join a small e-mail group for parents of children with a variety of pervasive developmental disorders. At the same time, I met another mother online, and we began collecting names of other AS families, with the goal of convincing AOL that there were enough interested people to open a chat room specifically for Asperger Syndrome. After several months, the AS families formed their own group. We shared what few resources were available at the time. Most important, we shared support and understanding.

In the fall of 1995, I approached the University of Delaware, where my husband is a faculty member, to ask if they would be willing to donate server space so I could automate the e-mail list. They generously agreed to do so and offered me space on their server for the list and for a Web page. I was thrilled—and terrified. I had no idea how to make a Web page, and at that time there were no programs that automatically formatted Web sites. Fortunately, Ted Whaley, who is the parent of a child diagnosed with hyperlexia and who had set up a Web site for the AHA (American Hyperlexia Association), came to the rescue. With his guidance and a copy of *HTML for Dummies,* the Asperger Syndrome Resources Web site was launched in December 1995. It was renamed OASIS (Online Asperger Syndrome Information and Support) several months later, in 1996.

OASIS and the new e-mail group (as-support) quickly became the central meeting place for families whose children were diagnosed with Asperger Syndrome. Any information on AS and related diagnoses, including conferences, parenting ideas, support services, educational resources, and laws, were shared among members and eventually placed on the Web site. By 1998, I'd added a public message board forum and in the summer of 1999 opened the private and moderated OASIS message board and chat room support forum.

The further you delve into the world of autism, the more you are struck by the fact that virtually every organization, research project, support group, piece of legislation, program, and innovation was created by or initially financed by parents of children with autism. It is the parents of children with AS and related disorders and the individuals with autism spectrum diagnoses who have led the way. Today, thanks in no small part to the Internet, parents of AS children and adults with AS are building local and national support networks throughout the country and the world. And in the process, they are changing what it means to have AS and autism.

Patty Romanowski Bashe is one of those parents destined to make a difference. Seeking support and information, she found her way to OASIS in 1998, shortly after her own son was diagnosed. In the summer of 1999, she e-mailed me with an idea: Would I like to write a book about Asperger Syndrome for parents? The more we talked and wrote, the clearer our mission became. This book does not duplicate OASIS, but it is very much a child of the Web site's parent-centered, parent-empowering approach. Parents need a guidebook to this new world. We wanted it to combine state-of-the-art knowledge with the timeless wisdom of other parents. We wanted to make sure no parent ever felt alone, and so we gathered the information we hope will help you enlighten those who care and intimidate those who have yet to "get it." We paid special attention to those subjects about which parents continue to ask the most questions or about which there seems to be the most confusion. We were blessed to have the cooperation and guidance of leading experts, and we were encouraged and supported by the OASIS community. As a gesture of thanks, we made this book heavy enough to make a big, scary noise when slammed down on tables at school district meetings when no one seems to understand.

When this book was first published in November 2001, I began this piece where my own story began. As I write this, my son is on his way to college. A lot has happened in the years in between then and now, since our first edition and this. OASIS has grown, with a message board that includes more than five thousand active members and with Web site visits of more than 3 million. Patty received her M.S.Ed. in special education of individuals with autism, became a certified teacher, and has taught children on the spectrum in both a small private school and through early intervention.

THE OASIS SURVEYS

Through our OASIS surveys, which were conducted in 2000, we found out about those questions that are deemed "too small" for the experts: How does having a child with AS affect a marriage? What percentage of children with AS have Individualized Education Plans (IEPs)? What is the noise that most bothers children with AS? What percentage of other parents have made special trips to replace or purchase an item related to their child's special interest? (The answer is about 90 percent, so you really aren't crazy—or at least you are not alone.)

What medical specialty had the best track record for getting the diagnosis right the first time? How long did parents wait between learning of their child's AS and telling their child about it? We found no studies, so we created our own surveys and posted them through Zoomerang, an online survey service that OASIS members linked to from the Web site. We are not professional pollsters and we would be the last to claim the results were scientific. However, we do believe that once we reached a certain number of responses—and some of our surveys drew well over five hundred— we could make some valid observations. This is particularly true when you consider that most of the scientific and academic literature concerns very small numbers.

Please let us know your thoughts. You can contact us through the OASIS Web site: http://www.udel.edu/bkirby/asperger or http://www.aspergersyndrome.org.

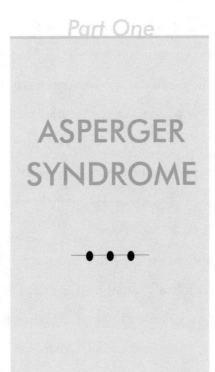

Part One

ASPERGER SYNDROME

BEHIND every diagnosis of Asperger Syndrome there is usually a story. It may be a long, painful tale spanning years and featuring an ever-changing cast of doctors, specialists, teachers, and schools. There were tests that showed "nothing," treatments and interventions that never seemed to work, and other diagnoses that failed to stick. For some fortunate families, it may be a short, relatively happy tale of the right child at the right place with the right doctor. Either way, the diagnosis signals a new direction.

There are many different ways to look at AS. Some consider AS a devastating disability, while others accept it as a gift. Some view persons with AS with pity, because they are outside the mainstream, while many believe that individuals with AS are part of a distinct and positive culture. Understanding Asperger Syndrome goes far beyond knowing the medical diagnostic criteria. It requires careful consideration of how we as parents, educators, and others who know these children and society at large view individuals with disabilities. Understanding a person with Asperger Syndrome also demands that we look carefully and honestly at what it means to be "normal" or "typical."

As we live with AS, most of us find that our thinking about it changes and evolves into a philosophy that guides us and our loved ones. Some feel it important to teach our children how to blend in and not define themselves by their AS. Others are more comfortable teaching their children to accept themselves as they are while showing them how to negotiate the sometimes–foreign culture of what some of us call "Neurotypical Land." (We prefer the term *neurotypical* to the less clearly defined *normal*.) We cannot presume to advise anyone on the "best" way to approach this. We do hope to give you the information and the tools you need to develop the perspective that best serves you, your child, and your family.

Chapter 1

WHAT IS ASPERGER SYNDROME?

W<small>HAT</small> is Asperger Syndrome? Technically, you can identify AS by the symptoms, behaviors, and deficits that constitute the diagnostic criteria, but it's almost impossible to extrapolate from that information what it means to have AS. For that reason we devote this chapter to what Asperger Syndrome is from a clinical diagnostic viewpoint and chapter 2 to how it manifests in terms of symptoms and behaviors.

Asperger Syndrome was named for Dr. Hans Asperger, a Viennese pediatrician whose paper describing the disorder, "'Autistic Psychopathy' in Childhood," was published in 1944 in German. It did not become widely known until Dr. Uta Frith translated the paper into English in 1991. In the most basic terms, Asperger Syndrome is a neurological disorder characterized by what psychiatrist Dr. Lorna Wing terms a "triad of impairments affecting: social interaction, communication, and imagination, accompanied by a narrow, rigid, repetitive pattern of activities."[1] Asperger Syndrome shares these qualities with several disorders that are, like AS, classified as *pervasive developmental disorders* (PDDs). Although we have yet to learn the cause of Asperger Syndrome or other pervasive developmental disorders, several of them—including AS—are often grouped together under the now common but unofficial term *autism spectrum disorders,* or ASDs.

— ◆ ◆ ◆ —

Pervasive Developmental Disorders

Asperger Syndrome is listed in the *DSM-IV-TR* as one of five pervasive developmental disorders. Technically, all of the disorders included here are PDDs, but for the purposes of this book, when we refer to "autism spectrum disorders" we are specifically excluding Rett's disorder and childhood disintegrative disorder. The five pervasive developmental disorders are:

Asperger Disorder (see text)

Autistic Disorder

This is what may be best viewed as the classic Kanner's autism. Using the *DSM-IV-TR* criteria, an individual must meet six of twelve criteria to be diagnosed with autism: two in the area of social development, two in communication, and two in the area of atypical interests. Autistic disorder is characterized by severe deficits and abnormalities in verbal and nonverbal communication and social interaction. Children with autistic disorder typically exhibit perseverative, stereotyped, and repetitous behaviors. While some may have average IQs, a substantial percentage have lower IQs. In addition, these children may have unusual responses to sensory stimuli, seeming lack of interest in other people, abnormally intense insistence on routine and sameness, and unusual attraction to specific objects or parts of objects. Autistic disorder can range from mild, so-called high-functioning, autism (HFA) to severe. No two persons have the same profile in terms of symptoms, onset, or prognosis.

Pervasive Developmental Disorder–Not Otherwise Specified (PDD-NOS)

PDD-NOS has been described as the subthreshold—or "close but no cigar"—diagnosis and is often referred to as "atypical autism."[2] This diagnosis is given when an individual does not meet the diagnostic criteria for another PDD, or if the symptoms are felt to be less severe than autistic disorder. Although it is often stated that the PDD-NOS diagnosis is given to children who present with symptoms after thirty months of age, younger children do receive this diagnosis. A child with a language delay may be given a diagnosis of PDD-NOS rather than Asperger Syndrome. This does not mean that a child with PDD-NOS is any more or less impaired than a child with AS or autism, but rather that his or her behaviors don't fit neatly into current diagnostic criteria.

Rett's Disorder
Rett's is believed to be genetic in origin and shares many features with autism and PDD-NOS. Rett's affects girls almost exclusively and is considered to be a rare disorder with a probable genetic basis. Children with Rett's start out with normal development and lose skills over time.

Childhood Disintegrative Disorder (CDD)
Children with CDD develop normally and then at some point in the early years begin to show autistic symptoms. While children with autism and PDD-NOS may have several words before they lose language, children with CDD are often speaking in complete sentences when they begin to lose their language.

Asperger Syndrome differs from other pervasive developmental disorders in that those children who have it usually hit major developmental milestones on time or even early. In most cases, a child with AS appears to be developing normally in terms of expressive speech, motor development (sitting, crawling, standing, walking), and may be "on schedule" for basic self-help skills, toilet training, self-feeding, and manipulating common objects. Among the first things parents and professionals may notice is that the child's interests and styles of social interaction are obviously different from those of most of his peers. For example, even the most talkative child will usually be deficient in the use of nonverbal language, particularly pointing; have little, no, or an unusual style of eye contact; and rarely if ever show an interest in what others around him—particularly peers—are doing or saying. It's usually not until a child reaches preschool or early school age that the characteristics and deficits that define AS become blatantly apparent. Our OASIS Survey on Diagnosis found that 52 percent of our respondents' children received their AS diagnosis between the ages of four and eight years of age. Another 11 percent were diagnosed at age four, and 21 percent between the ages of ten and twelve.

No one is certain how common AS may be. Most authorities place the incidence of AS somewhere around 1 in 250 to 1 in 500 persons. We do know that the rate of diagnosis for autism, Asperger Syndrome, and PDD-NOS has increased dramatically over the past decade. A landmark 1989 study[3] placed the prevalence of AS between 10 and 26 children per 10,000. Just four years later, the same researcher revised that 1989 estimate upward, to 71 children per 10,000 births—an increase of about 180 percent. Because, statistically, rates of autism spectrum disorders are up across the boards, we assume that AS is more common, or more commonly diagnosed, than it was before 2001. (For more on statistics, see page 18.)

We know that AS is much more common among boys than girls. Four out of every five persons diagnosed with AS are male. However, as awareness about AS grows and more children are diagnosed, an increasing number of women and girls are being identified as having AS.

• • •

Women and Girls with Asperger Syndrome

As difficult as Asperger Syndrome can be to diagnose in males, it seems that it is even more challenging to detect in women and girls. It is interesting to note that in children with nonverbal learning disability (or disorder; NLD), a learning profile that fits many children with Asperger Syndrome, females are diagnosed at the same rate as males (1:1 ratio).[4] It's been suggested that one of the reasons for the lower AS diagnosis rate in females is that girls are labeled as NLD while boys are diagnosed with AS.

Girls and women with AS may present with different symptoms than boys and men, but their problems with core social deficits, theory of mind, and the resulting social confusion are usually essentially the same. In some ways, these differences may seem even more striking, since our culture expects girls and women to be more understanding of and intuitive about the thoughts and desires of others.

Regardless of the official figures for AS in girls, we have seen a definite increase in the number of parents of girls who visit the OASIS Web site and forums.

There is a glaring lack of research on and resources for women with AS. Interestingly, however, women with Asperger Syndrome (among them Liane Holliday Willey and Dawn Prince-Hughes) have written some of the most illuminating and compelling autobiographical accounts of their lives. One possible reason for the paucity of research may well be cultural. Girls and women are simply permitted a wider range of "acceptable" behaviors than are boys. For example, a little boy who is too uncoordinated to play sports and who falls apart at the first sign of competition may be viewed quite differently from a little girl who does the same. In other environments, behaviors that are perceived as negative in a boy may well be perceived as positive in a girl. One parent tells of parent-teacher conferences in which a list of behaviors her son was exhibiting in school were viewed as negative—he spends too much time on the computer, refuses to "go with the flow," and isn't interested in the same things as other boys in the class—while those same behaviors were perceived as positive for a little girl in the same group. She did not care for frilly dolls like most of the other girls, she always had an original way of doing things, and unlike the other girls in the class, they had to drag her away from the computer.

It may well be that girls with such behaviors are receiving diagnoses other than AS. The majority of women with AS who participated in the OASIS survey stated that they had received a diagnosis of obsessive-compulsive disorder (OCD), depression, or an anxiety disorder prior to discovery of their AS diagnosis. Of course, many were diagnosed before AS became as widely known. However, it raises the question of why they did not receive the more typical misdiagnoses boys receive, such as ADHD.

The following may be reasons that AS manifests differently in girls:

- Girls in general tend to be less aggressive, and if they are not a behavioral problem in school, it is less likely that they will be referred for an evaluation. However, it is important to note that many parents who responded to the OASIS survey did indicate that their daughters also had problems with tantrums and outbursts.

- Certain behaviors that are viewed as negative in boys—being passive, unathletic, submissive, noncompetitive—may be interpreted as less troubling in girls.
- Female peer groups, at least at a young age, may be more supportive of differences than male groups. Liane Holliday Willey, an adult with AS, often comments that it was other girls who offered her guidance as to proper behavior. Several parents mentioned that their daughters were "mothered" by other girls in class who, as one mother wrote, "take care of her and make sure that she does the right thing." This type of peer nurturing may be less likely to occur among boys.
- Special interests may seem more gender appropriate. For example, though there were a few girls who collected things such as G.I. Joe dolls and showed an intense interest in *Star Trek* and Pokémon, the majority of the girls were interested in dolls, animals, drawing, music, singing, dancing, and other "typical" girl interests.
- Daydreaming, lacking common sense, and other behaviors that suggest one is not always "with it" are not viewed as negatively in girls as they are in boys. In fact, the "ditzy" girl has long been a mainstay of popular media, and girls are sometimes reluctant to appear "too smart."

This is not to say that girls with Asperger Syndrome have things any easier than boys with AS. Parents participating in the OASIS survey for parents, and women with AS who answered questions in the survey for women with AS, reported difficulties in all of the same areas as males with AS. Among these are lack of friendships and inability to make friends, problems with gaze modulation, lack of organization, tantrums and rage, and extreme naiveté. At the same time, parents indicated the following about their daughters' AS characteristics: "more subtle," "placid," "more rule-oriented," "quiet in class," "more interested in pleasing people," "have better coping/masking skills," "very affectionate," and "more flexible than boys with AS." They also mentioned that their daughters were depressed and more aware of their differences.

An area of great concern to parents of girls with AS involves sexuality. Although girls with AS physically mature at the same rate as typical young women, their social naiveté often puts them at great risk for sexual predators. Unfortunately, it is not rare to hear from parents of girls with AS who describe instances in which their daughters have found themselves in compromising situations without truly understanding how they got there. Women with AS have described similar incidents. Because girls with AS lack the ability to read body language and have difficulty determining another person's true motives, girls and women with AS are at greater risk for date rape, sexual assault, or being taken advantage of.

Another area of concern for parents of daughters with AS has to do with personal hygiene. Neatness, good grooming, and fashion sense are generally considered more important for girls than for boys. As one woman with AS posted in the OASIS survey, "Society seems more tolerant of boys with body odor, unkempt hair, poorly groomed nails, etc." Hormonal changes at the onset of puberty are another frequent topic of discussion. Both parents of girls and women with AS mentioned difficulties with premenstrual syndrome (PMS).

When we asked AS women what they would like people to know about AS, they said:

> "We are loners and we may come across as being downright rude to other people. We do not mean to hurt anybody's feelings. However, we can do a good job if just left alone. Please do not put us in teams, but let us choose our work partners. We can be and often are great assets to the company and institution."

> "We do work, we do get married, and we do have children."

> "Most people see us as just shy and scatterbrained."

Asperger Syndrome and other pervasive developmental disorders are neurological disorders. A person with AS has no more control over how he or she views the world and interprets what is seen, heard, felt, or understood than a person who has suffered a stroke or developed Alzheimer's disease. Asperger Syndrome is the result of anomalies in the physical brain, not emotional or behavioral problems, although those certainly can *result* from it. Although effective interventions can help people with AS learn to respond more appropriately, there is no way to change what the world "means" for them. When we speak of "treatment" and "intervention," we are referring to methods of addressing issues, not effecting a "cure." There is no known cure for any autism spectrum disorder. Barring a miraculous scientific breakthrough, your child probably will always be a person with AS.

Although research is continuing and scientists have discovered genetic anomalies that they believe are related to autism, we have yet to discover the precise cause of AS, a biological or physiological "marker" or distinct, telltale "sign." Evidence suggests that the genetic contribution to autism will more than likely be shown to result from the interactions among several genes, perhaps even twenty or more. There is no "one thing" a person with AS may have that is exclusive to AS. Asperger Syndrome is identified and defined by the pattern of its presentation—the symptoms, behaviors, strengths, and deficits—not by its "cause."

• • •

The Genetics of AS and Autism

Numerous studies have established a genetic component in the development of autism. Studies of monozygotic (identical) twins have shown that autism occurs in both twins in 64 percent of cases. Among dizygotic (fraternal) twins, autism occurs in both at a rate of about 10 percent. A sibling of a child with autism is fifty times more likely to have autism than a sibling without autism in the family.

From the first papers published on autism and Asperger Syndrome, by Dr. Leo Kanner and Dr. Hans Asperger respectively, authors have noted the frequency with which parents—usually fathers—present with traits and behaviors similar to those of their AS children, although the parents' symptoms are usually milder. Today these family members would be considered to fall under the broader autistic phenotype, or BAP. Studies have established that in cases where one identical twin has autism but the other twin does not, 90 to 95 percent of the seemingly unaffected twins will have language or social disturbances, as will 30 to 40 percent of fraternal twins. Nonautistic siblings also have a much higher rate of language and social disturbances.

These findings suggest two possibilities: the involvement of more than one gene (which is the case in most genetically transmitted diseases) and the influence of other, as yet unknown, environmental factors on the development of autism. If autism arose out of a single genetic defect, 100 percent of monozygotic twins would be expected to have autism.

Studies of families of persons with autism indicate a higher than average prevalence of autism and autism-related disorders among first-degree relatives (parents, siblings). Of 99 families surveyed in one Yale study, nearly half—46 percent—reported a family history of AS or a related disorder (19 percent fathers, 4 percent mothers). In addition, 6 percent of fathers and 2 percent of mothers had language disorders.[5] Although one could argue that early researchers were wrong to view unusual parental behaviors as the cause of autism, there is no denying that in many families such behaviors do exist. In a study that compared the families of children with autism to the families of children with Down's syndrome, the parents of persons with autism were more likely to have "aloof, rigid, hypersensitive, and anxious personality traits and of speech and pragmatic language deficits. They also had more limited friendships."[6] Other studies have found higher rates for other disorders, several of which are frequently seen in persons with AS. First-degree relatives have higher than normal rates of social phobia, simple phobia, and major depression.[7]

ASPERGER SYNDROME IN RELATION TO PERVASIVE DEVELOPMENTAL DISORDERS AND AUTISM SPECTRUM DISORDERS

Throughout this book and elsewhere, you will encounter the terms *pervasive developmental disorder* (PDD) and *autism* (or autistic) *spectrum disorder* (ASD). Although often used interchangeably, they are not the same. Although these points may seem academic, parents, educators, and other professionals often draw premature erroneous conclusions about the nature of AS and the needs of people who have it based on common misunderstandings about these terms and the concepts behind them.

The term *pervasive developmental disorder,* or *PDD,* is the official category under which the Asperger Syndrome diagnosis is classified in the *Diagnostic and Statistical Manual of Mental Disorders, Fourth Edition— Text Revision (DSM-IV-TR),* the gold-standard reference on psychiatric and neurological disorders. There are five PDDs (see box on page 10), three of which—AS, autistic disorder, and pervasive developmental disorder–not otherwise specified (PDD-NOS)—are often thought of as being part of the autism spectrum and are commonly grouped together as ASDs. However, there are also those who believe that the term *ASD* applies only to so-called high-functioning forms of autism. The two other PDDs—Rett's disorder and childhood disintegrative disorder—are not always referred to as ASDs, even though persons with those diagnoses may have autistic behaviors.[8]

When we consider autistic disorder, AS, and PDD-NOS, the idea of an autism spectrum that links them seems logical. Not only do these three disorders share Dr. Lorna Wing's triad of impairments, but the nearly infinite variations in the presence of symptoms and behaviors and their severity also seem to span a wide range. For example, someone with AS may have a very high IQ and be at or above grade level in terms of academics yet have perseverations (repetitive behaviors) or feel compelled to engage in behaviors such as rocking that are more commonly seen in children with autistic disorder. The differences that distinguish one PDD from another involve such factors as age at onset of symptoms, degree or severity of symptoms, combination of symptoms, and the presence of other mitigating traits, skills, or characteristics.

— ● ● ● —

The Statistics

How Many People in the United States have Asperger Syndrome?

We really don't know. No one has counted heads yet, and even if there were such a count, there are certainly a significant number of people who are mis-, under-, or undiagnosed. The Autism Society of America, the oldest autism organization in the United States, claims that there are currently 1 million to 1.5 million Americans with autism out of a national population of 293 million. Interestingly, current figures for autism spectrum disorders in the United Kingdom, with a population of about 60 million—only 20 percent of that of the United States—are about 535,000. In the United Kingdom, 211,700 persons have Asperger Syndrome. If the same rates of prevalence held for the United States based on current census figures, we might expect to find more than 1 million persons with Asperger Syndrome or high-functioning autism.[9]

Are the Rates of AS and Other ASDs Rising?

Yes. In the past fourteen years there has been a rampant increase in the number of reported cases of autism spectrum disorders, including Asperger Syndrome. An analysis of prevalence studies conducted between 1966 and 1984 found autism at a rate of .4 cases per 1,000. Between 1986 and 1997, the rate more than doubled, to 1 per 1,000. The recent study of a suspected cluster in Brick, New Jersey, found 4 per 1,000, or 1 in 250.[10] On January 1, 2003, the *Journal of the American Medical Association* published the results of a Centers for Disease Control study of 987 children in Atlanta, Georgia, that demonstrated that the figures from Brick, New Jersey, were not "unusually high" but most likely reflect the prevalence of autism spectrum disorders today. As the largest U.S. prevalence study to date, the CDC study found the prevalence of autism was 3.4 per 1,000, with a male-to-female ratio of 4 to 1. The study's authors write, "This overall rate is ten times higher than rates from three other U.S. studies . . . in the 1980s and 1990s." The Atlanta study also confirmed what other researchers had found among other population samples: More than two-thirds of those diagnosed with autistic disorder were cognitively impaired and 8 percent had epilepsy.[11] Today autism spectrum disorders affect anywhere between 1 in 166 and 1 in 250 children.[12] This makes ASDs more common than childhood cancer, Down's syndrome, muscular dystrophy, or cerebral palsy. (Just five years ago, in our first edition, the most current figures placed the prevalence at between 1 in 250 and 1 in 500.)

The U.S. Department of Education has also noted a dramatic rise in the number of students classified as having autism under the Individuals with Disabilities Education Act (IDEA): from 15,580 (ages six to twenty-two) in 1992 to 137,708 (ages three to twenty-two) in 2002. That is an increase of 662 percent.[13] While the annual incidence of autism under IDEA has increased anywhere from 18 percent to 28 percent during those years (average 22.5 percent), the annual growth for all other IDEA classifications showed significantly smaller increases—an average of just 2.8 percent.[14]

What Accounts for This Rise?

Are the statistics rising because of an actual increase in autism in general or is it because more children are being identified? While some of the rise may be the result of better diagnosis, one finding from the Atlanta study questions that. In his accompanying editorial, Dr. Eric Frombonne noted that 18 percent of the children that study identified as having an ASD were not previously suspected of having such a problem or diagnosed. If the previously unidentified children are representative, it suggests that nearly one in five children with an ASD are still not being accurately diagnosed. Further, there may also be what Frombonne terms "diagnostic substitution" at work; in other words, a child who is today diagnosed with autistic disorder or PDD-NOS might have received the diagnosis of mental retardation years ago.[15]

What Could Be Causing This Increase in Autism?

Theories abound, but no one really knows. Scientific evidence points to a basic defect in fetal development of the neural tube, the primitive structure from which the brain evolves, occurring between day 20 and day 24 of gestation. Clearly, there is a genetic component to autism, but if genetics were the sole factor in determining autism, the rates of autism would be expected to be near-constant (or even decreasing, since many persons with autism would be presumed not to have children). Whether the defect that gives rise to autism is purely genetic, the result of environmental insult, or a combination of the two is a question science has yet to answer.

AS is more likely to occur in families where other members have AS or other forms of autism. There is growing recognition that parents and other relatives of persons with AS, autism, or PDD-NOS may show similar but milder forms of certain traits. There is also the fact that with timely and intensive intervention, children diagnosed with one form of ASD may, years later, present with symptoms that suggest another one. Current research has yielded compelling if early evidence that families containing a member with AS are more likely to also include members who have AS, AS-type traits, or other forms of ASDs, as well as learning disabilities and a history of clinical depression. This suggests that there may be a common genetic factor in these disorders.

In more practical terms, many states and school districts consider Asperger Syndrome a medical diagnosis that comes under the umbrella classification of autism, which may be the classification your child receives for special education services. Finally, if your child receives a diagnosis, the universal diagnostic code number used for insurance purposes for Asperger Syndrome (299.80) is also the code for PDD-NOS and Rett's disorder.

As of this writing, the five pervasive developmental disorders share a classification based on their common symptoms. However, some experts question whether they are indeed as closely related as they appear. Although the autism spectrum is indeed a handy concept, neither it nor the PDD category itself is based on overwhelming scientific evidence that these disorders share a common cause (etiology), course, response to treatment, or outcome. As research into all forms of autism continues, we may discover aspects of etiology or prognosis that result in new classifications or subclassifications of the three existing ASDs.

Some experts argue that the differences between AS and the other two ASDs outweigh the similarities, in both degree and kind. Others focus on and choose to identify their child's issues in terms of a combination of symptoms and syndromes that are commonly seen among people with AS but "is not" AS. It's possible for a person to have a range of issues common to AS and not have AS itself.

Some children with AS have no symptoms commonly associated with autistic disorder; others do. While only 10 percent of our OASIS survey respondents indicated that they view AS as a condition distinct from autism or PDDs, 56 percent said they did not consider their child with AS "autistic." Even so, there may arise situations in which using the term *autism* is recommended; for example, in dealing with doctors and other medical professionals and law enforcement personnel who may be unfamiliar with AS. For better or worse, *autism* is a highly charged term that communicates that the person's condition is serious and that his or her ability to communicate effectively is severely compromised.

— • • • —

Common AS Behaviors That Are More Likely to Be Considered "Autistic"

Echolalia

Echolalia is a particular speech pattern in which the individual repeats what he or she has heard. Officially, there are two types of echolalia:

- **Immediate echolalia:** This is when the individual immediately echoes back words. It has been suggested that because a child with AS has poor language comprehension, he or she repeats what has just been said to buy more time to understand the question and formulate a response. For example, when one boy was asked, "Do you want dinner?" after a relatively long pause, his response was "Do I want dinner?" And after another pause, he said, "Yes. What are we having?" In this case, he used his echolalia as a holder to give him time to process the question and provide the appropriate answer. Another child who is asked the very same question might echo "Do you want dinner?" in this case reversing the pronoun. However, even with pronoun reversal, it should be assumed that the child is still trying to understand the question since "it ends up with language coming out pretty much as it went in."[16]
- **Delayed echolalia:** There are two main types of delayed echolalia: functional and nonfunctional. In *functional* echolalia, children will take a word or phrase and overgeneralize its meaning. For example, a child might use a phrase he has learned from a video or favorite movie and apply it to a real-life situation. Rather than say "I bumped my head," a devotee of *Thomas the*

Tank Engine might say "James ran off the track." In *nonfunctional* echolalia, a child may repeat entire movies, television programs, commercials, or radio programs he has memorized. While some of us might marvel at a child's ability to repeat lengthy scenes from movies or passages of text, it should not be regarded as a "talent" so much as evidence of a problem in language processing sometimes called "chunking." Even when parents and others can "translate" the words into the child's meaning, as in the "James ran off the track" example, it is still highly irregular and warrants intervention.

• **Stress echolalia:** We and some other parents have noticed a third type of echolalia that occurs when a child is under extreme stress or feels cornered. This type of echolalia involves the child repeating the last few words spoken to him, but in an intense, rushed manner that often involves echoing the word or phrase anywhere from two to more than a dozen times. Patty recalls that, before he was diagnosed, Justin would become echolalic whenever she reprimanded him strongly. If she said "Pick up your toys right now," he might become very upset and repeat "toysrightnow, toysrightnow, toysrightnow" as if it were one word.

• **Pallilalia:** This is the noncontexual, inappropriate, or meaningless repetition of a word, syllable, or phrase.

Perseveration

Individuals with Asperger Syndrome who show repetitive behaviors and interests are sometimes described as exhibiting *perseveration*. For example, the child might play with the same toy, using the exact same motions in the same sequence (for instance, crashing a toy car into a wooden block or starting a jigsaw puzzle and being unable without major tantrums to interrupt work on it until it is complete). They exhibit a single-mindedness and concentration that can range from impressive to frightening depending on the situation. In the case of perseveration of thoughts, a child might get "stuck" on a certain event or situation and be unable to let go of it. He may perseverate on a specific fear or on an event that happened long ago. Or a child who wishes to engage in his special interest may not be able to let go of it. For example, a child who is waiting for the latest Harry Potter movie to arrive in theaters may talk and talk and talk about it and be unable to change his focus to something else.

Not surprisingly, many of these children are diagnosed with obsessive tendencies. Some perseverations can be diminished or extinguished through behavior modification techniques, including applied behavior analysis (ABA). (See page 175.)

Unusual Eye Contact or Gaze Avoidance

Many individuals with Asperger Syndrome exhibit gaze avoidance and have difficulty making "normal" eye contact. Although this behavior can be disconcerting to a listener because it seems as if the person with AS is not listening, many individuals with AS have described the process of making eye contact as painful, uncomfortable, and even impossible. Often when individuals with AS do make eye contact, they tend either to look too little or stare too intently. In addition to the sensory overload that occurs with direct eye contact (which, if we think about it, even neurotypicals can have trouble with; consider for a moment the staring contest), it also could be troubling to children with AS because they have difficulty doing two things at once and find "looking" and "listening" simultaneously nearly impossible. This leads one to consider how important it may be to teach such children to "look at me" in every social situation.

Certainly, the child who is not looking cannot learn to imitate the actions of another or follow nonverbal cues or communication. However, many teachers have commented that children with AS seem not to be listening because they don't look directly at them, but later when they ask such children a question they discover that the children were indeed paying attention and did learn the material. Other individuals with AS make appropriate eye contact when talking but look away when listening or trying to process an answer. Whether or not a child with Asperger Syndrome should be forced to make eye contact is a subject of great debate. In terms of social success, learning to make appropriate eye contact is important, but many believe a child should not be expected to make contact when it is so stressful. One mother suggested a compromise. She told her son to look at the cheek or chin of the person rather than directly into his or her eyes, which he found less threatening.

Stereotypies

Stereotypies are repetitive motor movements such as hand flapping, finger flicking, walking on tiptoe, rocking, spinning, twirling, chewing, pulling, and picking. You may hear them referred to as "stims" (self-stimulating behavior), but that term may be misleading, for several reasons. One is that we have no way of knowing if self-stimulation is the cause or the effect of the behavior. In some cases, obsessive-compulsive disorder or a tic disorder may be the cause of the behavior. Some individuals with such disorders will tell you that engaging in these types of movements is not so much stimulating and enjoyable as it is a necessary "release," much like a sneeze.

Most of us exhibit some type of repetitive behavior: flexing our toes when we cross our legs, examining our fingernails, biting our nails, popping our chewing gum, smoking a cigarette, or needlessly clearing our throats before we speak. In children with AS, however, these behaviors are different. They tend to be less socially acceptable and more intense, in both their execution and duration. Sometimes while engaging in them a child seems to be totally out of reach. Parents of children with AS have noticed that their child's stereotypies seem to increase when their child is under stress. Whether they should intervene to stop a child's stereotypies through behavior modification, nagging, punishing, or somehow physically preventing is not always clear. It has been suggested that the stereotypies release a child's stress and that if one is eliminated another will appear in its place. One goal of behavior modification is to recognize that the compulsion to engage in the behavior may never go away and so try to change its expression or topography; for instance, to substitute running one's hand through one's hair instead of pulling the hair out. Another approach is to give the child something to manipulate or squeeze unobtrusively whenever the urge strikes. Small Koosh balls in a pocket, strips of Velcro placed under a desk, and other sensory-rich objects can be used.

More often than not, outside the privacy of home, stereotypical behaviors appear odd and are socially stigmatizing. Some families have used behavior modification to extinguish or change their child's behavior. This is always recommended when the behavior is socially inappropriate (touching one's genitals, masturbating, nose picking, screaming), socially risky (pinching, smelling, hugging, kissing, and touching strangers), or potentially harmful to the person herself (hair pulling, skin picking, self-biting, lip chewing) or others (hitting, biting, pinching, choking), or when it interferes with learning.

We are not implying that one view is more correct or accurate than another, only that you are more likely to hear professionals describe AS in terms of autism, pervasive developmental disorder, and the autism spectrum. As of this writing, however, most professionals subscribe to the concept that AS is a type of PDD or ASD. Further, those who have worked closely with individuals across the spectrum will tell you that the differences in behaviors and symptoms across the disorders is more in degree than in kind.

ASPERGER SYNDROME "ON THE SPECTRUM"

You may hear of AS described as a "high-functioning" form of autism. While that is an easily understood description, we agree with Dr. Ivar Lovaas and find the terms *high functioning* and *low functioning* discriminatory. This is not simply a matter of semantics or a desire to be politically correct. The fact is, individuals with ASDs each have within themselves a spectrum of abilities and challenges. We have seen young children with serious deficits in language and speech who are more independent in self-care than some older adolescents with AS who have IQs over 130. The term *high functioning* is often applied to AS because persons with this diagnosis typically have a normal or above-normal IQ and many, though not all, exhibit exceptional skill or talent in a particular area, often their area of special interest. (This should not be confused with the autistic savant phenomenon, depicted in the film *Rain Man,* where a person with autism demonstrates incredible feats of calculation or memory, or a creative talent.)[17]

Another distinguishing feature of Asperger Syndrome, as defined by the *DSM-IV-TR* and as described in much of the medical literature, is the absence of a "clinically significant delay in language." In other words, young children with AS have early language development that ranges from normal to precocious. This is in contrast to children with autistic disorder or PDD-NOS, who may completely fail to acquire language or who acquire a number of words and communicative behaviors that seem to fade or disappear sometime around the second birthday. This is yet another example of how misleading the current diagnostic criteria can be. For while early language development appears to be normal in children with AS, there is growing evidence that the deeper language deficits are always present. Further, some children with early language delay are later diagnosed with AS.

A MILD FORM OF AUTISM?

Some consider Asperger Syndrome a "mild form" of autism or, to use AS expert Uta Frith's description, "a dash of autism." Certainly the prognosis for a child with a normal IQ, speech (albeit abnormal), and a desire for social relationships is somewhat more optimistic than that for a child with a lower IQ who lacks speech and a desire to relate to others. It is important to remember that Asperger Syndrome is a serious, lifelong disability that requires individualized expert intervention and should be treated as such.

We have heard from many parents who have been told by doctors or other professionals that "Asperger Syndrome just means your child has a few little 'autisticlike' behaviors but isn't really autistic," or "Asperger Syndrome isn't as serious [or difficult or lasting] as some other pervasive developmental disorders." You may have heard Asperger Syndrome described as mild autism, but as one mother aptly put it, "My son doesn't have mild anything." If a professional attempts to downplay the seriousness of Asperger Syndrome or refuses to give your child a diagnosis because he or she feels that your child may "grow out of it," consider consulting another professional.

Though the assumption might be that a child who is highly verbal and more empathic might do better than a child who is less verbal and struggles socially, we simply do not know how things will turn out. However, we do know that early intervention has made an incredible difference for many children. For example, today there are children who appear at age eight or older to have AS but who at age three were nonverbal, socially withdrawn, and tested with extremely low IQs. Through early intensive intervention, ideally before elementary school, these children were not only sufficiently verbal and socially skilled to join mainstream classrooms but showed average to above-average IQs on retest. At the other extreme are children with highly developed language and high IQs who are struggling tremendously. And somewhere in the big middle are those who require supports and services, who manage to make great strides, but for whom there will always remain challenges and limitations.

We also have noticed a troubling trend. We've heard from countless parents and teachers who describe children with AS excelling academically only to plateau or plummet somewhere between the late elementary and middle school grades. Suddenly schoolwork requires more independence, organization, social reasoning, and abstract and conceptual thinking. We explore this issue later in chapter 11.

Prognosis for any of our children depends less on the actual diagnosis than on the support, intervention, and care they receive. Even the most able individual with Asperger Syndrome may always require some form of assistance. The message is clear: Any child with AS or other PDD needs timely, early, intensive intervention, regardless of what strengths he or she appears to possess.

ASPERGER SYNDROME: THE OFFICIAL VERSIONS

Today, in the United States and Canada, a person will be diagnosed with Asperger Syndrome if he or she meets the diagnostic criteria as published in the *DSM-IV-TR*.

— • • • —

DSM-IV-TR Diagnostic Criteria for Asperger's Disorder, 299.80

A. Qualitative impairment in social interaction, as manifested by at least two of the following:
1. marked impairment in the use of multiple nonverbal behaviors, such as eye-to-eye gaze, facial expression, body postures, and gestures to regulate social interaction

   2. failure to develop peer relationships appropriate to developmental level

   3. a lack of spontaneous seeking to share enjoyment, interests, or achievements with other people (e.g., by a lack of showing, bringing, or pointing out objects of interest to other people)

   4. lack of social or emotional reciprocity

B. Restricted repetitive and stereotyped patterns of behavior, interests, and activities, as manifested by at least one of the following:

   1. encompassing preoccupation with one or more stereotyped and restricted patterns of interest that is abnormal in intensity or focus

   2. apparently inflexible adherence to specific, nonfunctional routines or rituals

   3. stereotyped and repetitive motor mannerisms (e.g., hand or finger flapping or twisting, or complex whole-body movements)

   4. persistent preoccupation with parts of objects

C. The disturbance causes clinically significant impairment in social, occupational, or other important areas of functioning.

D. There is no clinically significant general delay in language (e.g., single words used by age two years, communicative phrases used by age three years).

E. There is no clinically significant delay in cognitive development or in the development of age-appropriate self-help skills, adaptive behavior (other than social interaction), and curiosity about the environment in childhood.

F. Criteria are not met for another specific Pervasive Developmental Disorder or Schizophrenia.

Reprinted with permission from the *Diagnostic Manual of Mental Disorders, Fourth Edition, Text Revision*, Washington, D.C.: American Psychiatric Association, 2000.

It is interesting to study other diagnostic criteria and guidelines, which differ in small but important ways from these. The World Health Organization publishes *The International Classification of Diseases*. In its tenth edition, published in 1993, it included Asperger Syndrome for the first time.

For some, the *DSM-IV-TR* diagnostic criteria raise more questions than they answer. Although it may be very clear to you that there is something different, unusual, or abnormal in your child's behavior or the way in which he relates to others, it's not always easy to match the diagnostic criteria to real-life behaviors. For example, what exactly is meant by terms such as *qualitative, significant, appropriate, spontaneous, nonfunctional, persistent,* and *abnormal?* We generally consider it "normal" to cringe at the sound of fingernails on a blackboard. How "abnormal" is it to have the same response to the sound of someone chewing gum? Where do you draw the line between inherent shyness and inability to make appropriate social contact? When is absentminded hair twirling a common habit and when does it become a stereotypical behavior? At what point does a hobby or fascination with the latest fad become a "special interest" bordering on obsession? The *DSM-IV-TR*'s accompanying text can help to clarify some of these questions for clinicians and parents alike.

In 1995, Dr. Tony Attwood co-authored a rating scale to be used by parents and teachers to help identify primary school–age children who might have the disorder. Rather than list diagnostic criteria, it instead poses easy-to-understand questions, which parents, teachers, and others who know the child answer using the scale from zero to six. Zero would indicate the type of behavior typical of most children of the same age. Six indicates behavior that occurs frequently. You might also consider using the Australian Scale (and perhaps having several people who know your child well complete copies, too) if you are stuck dealing with a doctor, educator, or other professional who has had little or no experience with AS or who balks at its validity.

According to Dr. Attwood, "If the answer is yes to the majority of the questions in the scale, and the rating was between two and six (i.e., conspicuously above the normal range), it does not automatically imply the child has Asperger Syndrome. However, it is a possibility, and a referral for a diagnostic assessment is warranted."

— • • • —

The Australian Scale for Asperger Syndrome

1. Does the child lack an understanding of how to play with other children? For example, is he or she unaware of the unwritten rules of social play?

0 1 2 3 4 5 6
rarely   frequently

2. When free to play with other children, such as school lunchtime, does the child avoid social contact with them? For example, he or she finds a secluded place to sit or goes to the library.

0 1 2 3 4 5 6
rarely   frequently

3. Does he or she seem unaware of social conventions or code of conduct and make inappropriate actions and comments? For example, when making a personal comment to someone, the child seems unaware how the comment could offend.

0 1 2 3 4 5 6
rarely   frequently

4. Does the child lack empathy, i.e., the intuitive understanding of another person's feelings? For example, does he or she not realize an apology would help the other person feel better?

0 1 2 3 4 5 6
rarely   frequently

5. Does the child seem to expect other people to know his or her thoughts, experiences, and opinions? For example, does he or she not realize you could not know about something because you were not with the child at the time?

0 1 2 3 4 5 6
rarely   frequently

6. Does the child need an excessive amount of reassurance, especially if things are changed or go wrong?

0 1 2 3 4 5 6
rarely   frequently

7. Does the child lack subtlety in his or her expression of emotion? For example, the child shows distress or affection out of proportion to the situation.

0 1 2 3 4 5 6
rarely   frequently

8. Does the child lack precision in expression of emotion? For example, he or she doesn't understand the levels of emotional expression appropriate for different people.

0 1 2 3 4 5 6
rarely   frequently

9. Is the child not interested in participating in competitive sports, games, and activities?

0 1 2 3 4 5 6
rarely   frequently

10. Is the child indifferent to peer pressure? For example, does he or she not follow the latest craze in toys or clothes?

0 1 2 3 4 5 6
rarely   frequently

11. Does the child take in literal interpretation of comments? For example, he or she is confused by phrases such as "pull your socks up," "looks can kill," or "hop on the scales."

0 1 2 3 4 5 6
rarely   frequently

12. Does the child have an unusual tone of voice? For example, the child seems to have a foreign accent or monotone that lacks emphasis on key words.

0 1 2 3 4 5 6
rarely   frequently

13. When talking to the child, does he or she appear uninterested in your side of the conversation? For example, does he or she not ask about or comment on your thoughts or opinions on the topic?

0 1 2 3 4 5 6
rarely   frequently

14. When in conversation, does the child tend to use less eye contact than you would expect?

0 1 2 3 4 5 6
rarely   frequently

15. Is the child's speech overprecise or pedantic? For example, he or she talks in a formal way or like a walking dictionary.

0 1 2 3 4 5 6
rarely   frequently

16. Does the child have problems repairing a conversation? For example, when the child is confused, he or she does not ask for clarification but simply switches to a familiar topic or takes ages to think of a reply.

0 1 2 3 4 5 6
rarely   frequently

Cognitive Skills

17. Does the child read books primarily for information, not seeming to be interested

0 1 2 3 4 5 6
rarely   frequently

in fictional works? For example, he or she is an avid reader of encyclopedias and science books but not keen on adventure stories.

18. Does the child have an exceptional long-term memory for events and facts? For example, he or she remembers the neighbor's car registration of several years ago, or clearly recalls scenes that happened many years ago.

0 1 2 3 4 5 6
rarely   frequently

19. Does the child lack social imaginative play? For example, other children are not included in the child's imaginary games or the child is confused by the pretend games of other children.

0 1 2 3 4 5 6
rarely   frequently

20. Is the child fascinated by a particular topic and an avid collector of information or statistics on that interest? For example, the child becomes a walking encyclopedia of knowledge on vehicles, maps, or [sports] league tables.

0 1 2 3 4 5 6
rarely   frequently

21. Does the child become unduly upset by changes in routine or expectation? For example, he or she is distressed by going to school by a different route.

0 1 2 3 4 5 6
rarely   frequently

22. Does the child develop elaborate routines or rituals that must be completed? For example, he or she lines up toys before going to bed.

0 1 2 3 4 5 6
rarely   frequently

Movement Skills

23. Does the child have poor motor coordination? For example, he or she is not skilled at catching a ball.

0 1 2 3 4 5 6
rarely   frequently

24. Does the child have an odd gait when running?

0 1 2 3 4 5 6
rarely   frequently

Other Characteristics

For this section, indicate whether the child has shown any of the following characteristics:

a. Unusual fear or distress due to:
- ordinary sounds—e.g., electrical appliances ☐
- light touch on skin or scalp ☐
- wearing particular items of clothing ☐
- unexpected noises ☐
- seeing certain objects ☐
- noisy, crowded places—e.g., supermarkets ☐

b. Tendency to flap or rock when excited or distressed ☐

c. Lack of sensitivity to low levels of pain ☐

d. Late in acquiring speech ☐

e. Unusual facial grimaces or tics ☐

Reprinted (with minor editing) with permission from Dr. Anthony Attwood. This scale appears in Dr. Attwood's *Asperger's Syndrome: A Guide for Parents and Professionals* (London and Philadelphia: Jessica Kingsley Publishers, 1998), pp. 17–19.

In addition, there are two relatively new AS-specific assessments, both of which are designed to be used by teachers and parents as well as doctors and other professionals: the GADS (Gilliam Asperger's Disorder Scale) and the ASDS (Asperger Syndrome Diagnostic Scale). In addition, the widely used Vineland Adaptive Behavior Scales can also be used to help diagnose AS.

˙SEEING THE WORLD DIFFERENTLY

To begin to understand what it's like to have AS, we need to consider what it means to not have AS. We pride ourselves on our individuality. Our society celebrates the individual who does what he thinks is right, who goes his own way. In truth, however, one sign of being neurologically typical, or "neurotypical," is that we behave, think, and act in ways that are similar enough that, in most social situations, we have a fairly accurate idea of what to expect from others; we have a fairly accurate idea of what others expect from us; and we have the ability to say and do things that will meet those expectations. One big advantage that a neurotypical person has over someone with a social disability like AS is that he moves through the world and relates to others with the understanding that others do have expectations of his behavior and a general idea of what those are.

In fact, we're so good at this that we often meet the expectations of others even when we really don't want to. If you think that makes most of us sound less like independent-thinking individuals and more like sheep, you may find common ground with some people with AS. Some individuals with AS and other PDDs don't understand why most people feel it's important to make small talk, dress in the current style, feign interest in people or topics they could not care less about, or tell white lies. If your friend asks, "Do you like my new hair color?" someone with AS might reason that the friend really wants to know the truth. However, without even thinking, most of us "instinctively" know that our friend only wants—and only expects—to be told how flattering this particular Bozo-ish shade of red is on her. So we do the socially appropriate thing: we tell a white lie, which is not truthful and yet not "wrong." This degree of moral ambiguity and rule-bending that we accept as part of normal social interaction is unthinkable and can be quite confusing to a person with AS.

How did we learn when and how to tell this kind of lie? Moreover, how did we learn that it was not only okay to do but also the best thing to do? How did we learn to lie to our friend in this situation but not in another? If pressed, we can each offer a careful, blow-by-blow account of how we came to that decision, but that's just Monday morning quarterbacking. In the moment, we did not even think about how we would respond. In less than a millisecond, we knew to say "You look great." And our friend, who herself may have been thinking, *I know this color was a mistake,* replied "Thank you."

What accounts for this amazing ability? It provides the software that shapes the content and style of our conversation to fit perfectly the expectations of the person to whom we are speaking. It automatically adjusts our body posture, gestures, volume and tone of voice, word choice, and physical proximity. It alerts us to when we are being lied to, misled, pressured, or embarrassed. It regulates how much we ask of someone else in conversation and how much we reveal. Even more incredibly, it allows us to glean accurate information about things that weren't even specifically addressed in conversation, things that we'd have no other way of knowing. It allows us to have some knowledge of what other people are thinking; to predict in general terms and with pretty amazing accuracy what they will say and what they will do. It gives rise to having "funny feelings," "suspicions," "hunches," and "second thoughts" about a person or a situation. It convinces us to take an action that in the moment seems irrational but is "right": avoiding a particular stranger on the street, for instance, or surprising a potential love interest with a meaningful look or a kiss.

All of this is possible because most people possess "theory of mind," which is essentially the innate capacity to understand that other people can have desires, ideas, and feelings different from our own. In addition, most of us also have an innate ability to "read" nonverbal social cues, to naturally pay attention to what most of us consider the relevant information from our surroundings, and to instantly process all of that with little or no conscious thought. In contrast, people with AS lack or have an incomplete understanding of theory of mind. They do not know, automatically and instantly, what to expect or what is expected of them in social situations. Intelligence and disposition have nothing to do with our ability to read the minds of others. Despite a high IQ and a loving, generous disposition, a person with AS may still find himself saying or doing the "wrong" thing or, even worse, not being able to defend himself against being deliberately misled by others or from being misunderstood. For now, however, it is important to understand that mindblindness is common to some degree in all ASDs. It lies at the heart of the disability AS entails and is often at the root of the behavioral challenges and social difficulties people with AS face.

Throughout the rest of the book, we will look at the many facets of AS in more depth and explore how understanding AS can help you to understand and support your child.

Chapter 2

WHAT ASPERGER SYNDROME LOOKS LIKE

AS SYMPTOMS

BEYOND the basic "triad" of social disabilities typical of all pervasive developmental disorders, AS has its own "second-tier" core of common symptoms. In every instance, there can be wide variability in the range and severity of symptoms. The following are the most common AS behaviors. As you read, it is important to remember that every person with AS is different. Even when considering a trait as commonly shared as the special interest, you will find among individuals with AS wide variations in terms of intensity. Two persons with AS may give you very different descriptions of what it means to have AS.

Preoccupation with a Special Interest

Many persons with Asperger Syndrome are often identifiable by their all-consuming interest in one or more particular topics. In our OASIS survey of parents, 100 percent indicated that their child had one or more special interests, as did 99 percent of adults and teenagers with AS. The top five most prevalent special interests were peer-appropriate fads or interests (e.g., Pokémon); video or computer games; works of art, movies, fictional books, or television programs; and computers. Among adults with AS, the most common special interests were specific concepts or ideas; computers; and works of art, fictional books, movies, or television programs. Sometimes the object of fascination is something peers and even adults can relate to—dinosaurs, trains, cars, Pokémon, or other trends; *Thomas the Tank Engine, Star Trek, Star Wars, Lord of the Rings,* or other popular fictional works; a celebrity or historical figure, a historical object or event such as the voyage of the *Titanic*; subjects such as math or astronomy; technology such as computers or video games; or sports.

More noticeable are the special interests that concern objects, persons, events, or abstract concepts that, by neurotypical standards, range from peculiar to downright bizarre. Children with AS have been known to be obsessed by such things as bleach bottles, alarms and alarm systems, street lamps, lawn mowers, junipers, organs and organ music, road signs, maps, clocks, time, directions (north, south, east, west), the British royal family, telephone books, issues of *TV Guide,* sports announcing, game shows, and insects.

A person with AS might collect items related to the special interest and, as he or she grows older, collect information as well. So, for example, a child at three might collect *Thomas the Tank Engine* toy trains and play with them exclusively. Once he starts reading, he might read about trains exclusively, or collect local train schedules and maps, and then feel compelled to talk about what he has learned. "Walking encyclopedia" is often an accurate description of the amount and depth of information children with AS accumulate. However, not everyone follows the same pattern. Some persons with AS maintain a constant level of involvement: for instance, playing with Batman figures but not necessarily learning and talking about the evolution of the character from its inception.

Although much is written about a child's single special interest, most persons with AS have more than one at a time. In our OASIS survey, only 18 percent of children and 10 percent of adults had just one interest. The majority had two (34 percent for children; 29 percent for adults), three (32 percent for children; 26 percent for adults), or four (10 percent for children; 13 percent for adults). Interestingly, the number of interests appeared to increase as some grew older. Fifteen percent of adults indicated that they had six or more interests. Both parents and adults with AS indicated that the first special interest emerged very early: at age two to three (66 percent of children; 25 percent of adults), or four to five (12 percent of children; 29 percent of adults). Eighteen percent of parents indicated that their child's special interest was apparent at the age of one. Thirty-five percent of adults said their first special interests began when they were between six and eleven.

• • •

What Role Does the Special Interest Play in the Lives of Persons with AS?

Respondents were asked to check all categories that applied.

Role of the Special Interest	Children	Adults
Interest	80%	64%
Fun	73%	46%
Security, comfort	65%	32%
Relaxation	62%	38%
Stress reduction	55%	38%
Facilitation of social interaction	54%	39%
Avoidance of social interaction	39%	21%
Development of a special talent or skill	32%	36%

The line between a person sharing an interest in a hobby or profession and an AS-style special interest is usually immediately clear upon hearing a person with AS talk. Not surprisingly, the number one way kids with AS pursue their special interest is by talking about it (77 percent). In contrast, adults with AS are more likely to read about their special interest than to talk about it. A special interest "exchange" is noticeably one-sided, run-on, and more a monologue than a conversation. Persons with AS are often unaware of the repertoire of nonverbal and verbal cues listeners may use to stop or redirect the conversation, so they may not notice that the person to whom they're speaking is changing the subject, breaking eye contact, affecting an uninterested look, turning away, or even walking away. Unfortunately, this can leave the impression that a person with AS is, to put it nicely, overbearing, self-centered, or rude. This can erect barriers to social interaction instead of building bridges, as sharing a hobby often does.

Also, immersion in the special interest may come at the expense of other, more socially appropriate activities. The play date that collapses under the weight of a child's insistence that his friend play only "name that freight car" or listen to him recite, by name, the most significant dinosaur finds and the museums in which they are now housed, is a social setback from which it may be difficult to recover.

— ● ● ● —

How Parents Cope with Special Interests

Or, meet the other moms who have eight more Pikachus—or Sponge-Bobs or Harry Potters or One Rings—hidden in the closet. We asked: Because of the special interest and the individual's behavior or expected behavior related to it (e.g., difficulty shifting focus, tantrums, getting upset), have you or others close to the individual ever . . .

made a special trip to replace or purchase an item related to the special interest?	76%
deliberately avoided a particular place or event out of concern that it would spark and/or reinforce the special interest (e.g., avoiding the store that displays Pokémon cards at the checkout)?	48%
been late for an appointment or other scheduled event, including work or school, for reasons related to the special interest?	42%
driven out of your way to accommodate the interest (e.g., taken a certain route that goes alongside railroad tracks)?	41%
made special plans for vacations and holidays to accommodate the special interest?	35%

made repeated trips to places or events that most people would be satisfied to see or to experience once or twice in a lifetime?	27%
left a social gathering because the individual's special interest was dominating the event and attempts at redirection did not work?	20%

Special interests can range from mildly annoying to intolerable. Fifty-seven percent of parents said that they had tried to control or curtail their child's special interest, usually by restricting access to it or placing limits on the circumstances and the length of time it could be discussed. Over a third of the parents told us that they had reduced the degree to which they would accommodate the special interest, and 21 percent refused to participate in activities related to the special interest. One positive aspect of a special interest is its power as a motivator or reinforcer. Making access to the special interest contingent on clearly specified behavior can be very effective. Special interests can also be used more informally as a reward for appropriate behavior—for example, an interest-related gift for the child who completes an assigned task.

It's important to bear in mind that special interests do serve a function. Persons with AS truly enjoy their special interest. In a world that can be wildly unpredictable, the special interest is an oasis of predictability, calm, and control. The special interest can provide a sense of accomplishment, mastery, and happiness. When asked to describe the individual's level of involvement with a special interest in times of stress, 43 percent of parents and 30 percent of adults with AS said that it "increases significantly"; 33 percent of parents and 30 percent of adults with AS said that it "increases a little."

Often those special interests can build bridges to interaction and enjoyment with others who share similar interests. By joining a club that focuses on a particular interest, the individual may have a real opportunity to interact with others. For 28 percent of children and 25 percent of adults with AS, the special interest became a common ground for friendship. Similar percentages said that the special interest was the common ground for inclusion in an informal peer group or organization. Meetings of Magic the Gathering enthusiasts or model railroad hobbyist clubs are just two examples of such social opportunities.

Some educators recommend using a special interest to help develop skills. For example, one of Barb's son's teachers used his love of mathematics to foster an interest in expository writing. She assigned him books on mathematical topics, and child and teacher discussed these subjects in a journal they passed back and forth. If you and your child's teacher give it some thought, you may find many ways to base lessons on a wide range of topics on a special interest. Justin's interest in WWII aircraft has yielded knowledge of geography, science, and history.

Odd though it sounds, a restricted special interest can broaden a child's world. Nearly half of our parents said that they sometimes use the special interest to encourage their child to try new things; 22 percent said they used it that way often. It can also be a way to spend special time with your AS child. Carol, whose son's special interest is the history of technology related to car engines, said, "I take pleasure in the pleasure George derives from his special interest. I regularly set aside time that's just for him and me, a 'free zone' where he knows he can talk to me about this and know that I will give him my full attention, ask him questions, and not rush him because I'm preoccupied with dinner or driving him someplace. I find this time very special and fulfilling for both of us."

Persons with AS can sometimes channel their special interest into a satisfying career. This is especially true if the interest can be applied to a profession that makes few social demands (i.e., it allows independent as opposed to team work and limited interaction with the public) and attracts people with similar traits or a generous tolerance for social differences. The "new frontier" of computer- and Internet-related jobs has proved a boon for persons with AS.

Noticeably Stiff, Pedantic, One-Sided Conversational Style

This is most clearly noticeable when a person with AS is talking about a special interest. Listeners may get the impression that they are being lectured *at* rather than spoken *to* by someone more intent on showing off his knowledge in the minutest detail than in participating in a reciprocal conversation. A child with AS may have an impressive, adultlike vocabulary, often adopting an overly formal, almost old-fashioned manner of speaking. No one has yet determined why this is so. One possibility is that among the many social behaviors children with AS do not master is that of imitating and "acting like" others their own age. AS seems to limit the degree to which a child can absorb and model the age-appropriate behavior of peers.

Problems in the Social Use of Language

The difficulty persons with AS have in the social use of language can range from subtle to striking. Even though your child may be sophisticated in her expressive use of language (what she says), most persons with AS have "hidden" yet deep and pervasive deficits in their understanding of what is communicated to them, through the use of words (semantics and pragmatics) and the flow of nonverbal information we transmit constantly through tone, rhythm, inflection of voice; body language; facial expression; and gaze modulation. Even children with apparently good expressive language skills may reveal surprising limitations when in the grip of strong emotions, such as anger and frustration. These deficits give rise to such common AS-related behaviors as overly literal interpretation of metaphors and images and its "mirror" deficit, incomplete understanding of oral communication that is insufficiently explicit. As a result, your child might become alarmed at such common Momisms as "I've talked until I'm blue in the face" (to which Patty's son pointed out, "Mom, your face isn't really getting blue") or "I'm losing my patience" (which your child may offer to help you find).

Language can prove troubling for children with AS in other ways as well. One adult who describes herself as having some AS traits recalls being totally confused as a child when she learned there was no lake on Lake Drive or no one named Ed at Ed's Restaurant. "I took language not only literally but very visually. After I learned to read and could make out the word *color* within the word *Colorado*, I fully expected the Colorado River to be colored blue, pink, yellow, and other 'nonriver' shades."

Parents of children with AS also notice that the parts of messages they assume will be understood often are not. For example, for most children, "Get ready for school" is interpreted as "Go upstairs, brush your teeth, wash your face, put on clean underwear, pants, a shirt, shoes, and socks, gather your book bag. . . ." That is not necessarily the case for a person with AS. Behaviors that we may attribute to laziness, lack of organization, or lack of skill may in fact be caused by an individual's inability to fully process language, to keep front and center in her mind what she is supposed to do, in what order.

Persons with AS also have deficits in other areas key to carrying out such a seemingly simple instruction—problems with fine and gross motor skills, planning, organization, and conception of time, to name a few. Most parents can recount dozens of examples when the information inside the message did not seem to reach its destination. For some children with AS, the process of getting ready for school must be broken down into short, clear, sequential oral instructions or visual reminders, often with a lot of prompting and supervision, regardless of how bright the child or how many times (even hundreds of times) you two have been through the same routine. Looking back, parents with AS—and our kids—recall many instances of flaring tempers and tears over such situations that were wrongly miscast as bad behavior. As we explain later in chapter 9, there are time-tested methods that teach skills and independence parents can use to avoid the cycle of dependence and learned helplessness that too many families fall into.

Inability to Correctly Interpret or Express Nonverbal Communication

We rarely give it much conscious thought, but most of us instinctively know that it's not what you say but the way you say it that fully communicates what you mean. Because persons with AS lack the ability to interpret and use nonverbal forms of social communication, they often appear socially naive and inept. Part of this is due to the challenges of coping with spoken language, as outlined above. Another part has to do with an inability to understand nonverbal language. Some experts estimate that up to 90 percent of communication is nonverbal. It's easy to understand why someone who devotes the bulk of his attention only to that verbal 10 percent can miss or misinterpret the full message.

Some individuals with AS have a great deal of difficulty listening and looking at the same time. They may understand the "words" but miss the context because they are unable to concentrate on the non-verbal actions and subtle cues being offered. Thanks to brain imaging technologies, we know that the brains of some people with AS are structurally and/or functionally different. This may explain why AS forces attention on things most people ignore while it causes people with AS to ignore or simply not "register" information most individuals seem "programmed" and compelled to observe and act upon. At the same time, it seems clear that even individuals with AS who do attend to the verbal and nonverbal language of others do not necessarily interpret what they perceive correctly or with the degree of fluency or subtlety necessary.

In a revealing study, Dr. Fred R. Volkmar and Dr. Ami Klin and their colleagues at the Yale Child Study Center were able to track the eye movements of persons with and without AS or high-functioning autism (HFA) and compare them. They showed the subjects a video-tape of the emotionally charged film *Who's Afraid of Virginia Woolf,* starring Elizabeth Taylor and Richard Burton. Interestingly, most of the "action" during this evening in the life of a poisonous marriage is in the actors' words. The researchers discovered that the neuro-typical viewers watched everything on the screen but paid particular attention to the faces of the actors, particularly the eyes. Persons with AS or HFA, however, focused on the mouths of the actor speaking, in contrast to the neurotypical controls, who focused on the whole faces of both the actor speaking and those being spoken to.

Since we learn to use appropriate facial expression, body language, and gestures through observation and imitation, it's not surprising that persons with AS, who are limited in their ability to notice these in others, would be at a disadvantage in developing their own. There is also the possibility that deficits in this area may also be related to problems with motor skills.

Lack of Empathy Regarding Feelings of Others

The term *empathy* crops up a lot in ASD-related discussions. Most people assume that it means only the ability to understand and relate to the feelings of others. But there's more to empathy than that. For example, persons with AS also lack "empathic response," the inherent desire to share attention with others, as when a child points out an object of interest to another person, or when he expresses interest in something that interests someone else.

The idea that children with AS seem to have no feelings for others or no ability to sympathize is mentioned prominently in the literature. It fuels oversimplified popular media depictions of persons with AS as being "emotionless," "disconnected," or "like robots." This is an impression with which many parents and people who work closely with our children would beg to differ. Persons with AS are not cold, mean, or uncaring. Their apparently limited empathy is one aspect of their problems with theory of mind (TOM), as we discussed earlier. Because of this "mind-blindness," a child with AS may literally not understand why you would be angry that he tracked mud across the kitchen floor you just mopped, why a sibling gets angry when he grabs her toy, or why his friend does not wish to share her snack (after all, you may hear, "I told her that I wanted it").

Educators and others who know just a little about AS often express surprise at how "nice" and "kind" our children can be. In fact, we have heard from many parents who were told, "Your child is too affectionate" or "too caring," or "too emotionally connected" to have a PDD. Children with AS can be very affectionate and loving. While they may have difficulty reading people at school or in other social situations, they can be surprisingly perceptive about the emotional states of parents, grandparents, siblings, friends, and beloved teachers, baby-sitters, and others. Parents of children with AS have speculated and many adults with AS have expressed that it is not that they don't "feel" at all, but rather that they feel too much. Often these feelings are overwhelming and confusing. It is not always that children with AS lack emotion, but rather that they lack the ability to express it appropriately.

Negativistic Worldview

For reasons that have yet to be fully explained, many children with AS seem to see the glass of life as perpetually half empty and, depending on their mood that moment, dingy and cracked as well. Often their emotional responses are much more or much less intense than one might expect. For example, a child may cry hysterically over something that would seem to most people not worth the tears, and later show no emotional response to something others view as sad. One mother recalls having her AS son comment out loud at a family funeral, "Part of me wants to laugh and part of me wants to cry." He was clearly feeling something (in this case sadness); he just wasn't sure how to express it. Or perhaps a child simply may not share in another's enthusiasm and lacks the social skills to fake it. After Justin had chosen new curtains and a matching bedspread for his room, Patty recalls saying brightly, "Wow, your room really looks great! Don't you think so?" Justin calmly replied, "Mom, I'm sorry, but is it okay if I just don't get as excited about these things as you do?"

Some of these children complain, whine, protest, and argue more than most other children and often more than a given situation warrants. Many of them also have prodigious memories, but parents often remark on how vivid and persistent bad memories are, while happy moments seem somehow out of reach. It's as if the child's emotional response to a difficult time or situation literally overwhelms whatever pleasant experiences she may have had. Parents of children who have AS and some degree of obsessive behavior know well the seemingly constant "replaying" of the unhappy moment and the memory of it that can persist for years. Add to this the fact that some children with AS simply do not express happiness or pleasure with quite the same verve and enthusiasm you expect, and you may get the impression that they are apathetic or uncaring.

Of course, most children with AS are neither apathetic nor uncaring. It's important to put these comments in the context of the child's daily life, which, for many of them, is stressful. One child expressed the sentiment that a "good day" was a day when nothing went terribly wrong. Honestly, how many days like those do some of our children have? Probably not many. We know that children with AS are at much higher risk for depression. We also know that these are children who because of their inflexibility, literal-mindedness, and trouble dealing with the unexpected probably do perceive that more "bad things" happen to them.

Difficulty Relating Socially with Others, Particularly Same-Age Peers

Though it is becoming increasingly apparent that children with AS probably showed some telltale, atypical social behaviors years before they were diagnosed, the extent of their social disability is rarely obvious until preschool or kindergarten, when they are faced with the increased social demands of a peer group. Before then, most play dates likely consisted of two or more children engaged in parallel play; that is, playing "near" but not "with" one another. As children get older, they typically learn and naturally seek out cooperative play with others. Children with AS, however, tend not to, or when they do play with other children, the play is one-sided and lacks the social give-and-take of a typical peer relationship.

Their difficulty interacting with peers is the culmination of all the important symptoms mentioned thus far. It's not so much that they are lost in their own worlds in the same way that a child with a different type of PDD might be. Rather, it's that they seem not to know how to enter a conversation or a social situation. Several factors probably come into play here, among them their impoverished ability to observe and adopt socially appropriate behavior, their one-sided conversational style, and their unusual manner of speaking. Their special interest may preclude their being interested in or willing to tolerate play that involves anything else.

Unlike typical children in a play situation, children with AS seem unable to "go with the flow" or tolerate the frequent shifts in focus and activity that free play involves. A child with AS may become upset when another child will not play what he wants to play for as long as he wants to play it. Alternately, children with AS may drift off and not pay attention to the other children. Unfortunately, what constitutes fun for some of our children is not enjoyable to their peers and what constitutes fun for other children is not always enjoyable for ours. While many children with AS do well one-on-one with peers, most typical children by the time they reach school age are able to interact with more than one playmate at a time and are capable of playing at an activity they may be ambivalent about for the sake of playing. Sustaining attention with more than one child can be difficult and stressful for a child with AS, and feigning interest for the sake of social interaction may be near impossible.

Children with AS are often hampered in developing peer relationships by the fact that they have two built-in "outs." One, they often have no trouble playing by themselves and may actually prefer to do so. Two, they usually find it much easier to talk with and be tolerated or even accepted by sensitive older children, teenagers, and adults. Our children feel more socially at ease around people who can carry the conversation, socially speaking. Despite our children's deficits in terms of social observation and theory of mind, they do sense clearly, even painfully, when they are not being accepted.

When your child seems happiest playing alone or engages in productive, rewarding activities on his own (at the computer, for instance), it can be hard to fully appreciate what he is "missing." We have noticed that parents of children who are highly skilled in some independent endeavor or who are academically exceptional may be less likely to see the value of developing peer social skills. It is important to remember that no matter what talent or skill your child has, no matter how little he may seem to miss being around other children, learning to be among peers is a critical skill. Why? Our social experiences throughout childhood teach us much about others and ourselves. Like all children, ours need opportunities—structured, brief, few, and supervised though they may be—to know others, to tolerate someone else who makes a different choice or has a different thought, to experience what makes other people valuable, enjoyable, and worth spending time with.

BEYOND THE CORE: THE "OTHER" TELLTALE SIGNS OF AS

Complicating the already busy picture for most individuals with AS is the common presence of a legion of other deficits, disabilities, and syndromes. Not all of these are recognized in various diagnostic criteria, but most are known to those familiar with AS. The fact that not all are included under official diagnostic criteria doesn't mean they are less prevalent, less important, or have less impact on the person with AS. These other issues can be problematic in and of themselves even in someone not challenged by AS. However, when you mix the core social skills deficits of AS, sensitivity to noise, and a birthday party, you have the grist for the "party from hell" story every parent seems to have.

Having AS compromises the ability to cope or create compensatory strategies for dealing with something like tactile sensitivity, anxiety, or motor clumsiness. For example, one problem people with AS often have is an inability to know that other people might know something they themselves do not. A neurotypical child who experiences extreme distress over a clothing tag touching the back of her neck has the theory of mind to ask someone else to cut it out for her. A child with AS might simply fall into a tantrum, the cause of which appears inexplicable to those who do not understand how the disorder manifests in that particular child. Or a neurologically typical but physically awkward person might compensate by learning to anticipate the movement of strangers in a crowd, a feat that involves a level of theory of mind, physical grace, and the ability to attend to numerous stimuli simultaneously—three skills that many with AS simply do not have or cannot exercise comfortably without tremendous effort.

Unfortunately, professionals who specialize in only one area (for example, speech therapists, audiologists, educational counselors, occupational therapists, and so on) may "diagnose" the person with AS not as having AS but as having one or several of the disorders, syndromes, or disabilities that commonly are seen with it, such as central auditory processing disorder or sensory integration disorder. Worse, they may attempt to explain every aspect of a child's PDD symptoms as stemming from one particular "cause." We hear from many parents whose children have collected a "charm bracelet" of related diagnoses before the core disorder—AS—was identified. Sadly, we also hear, "But he doesn't have a serious problem, he has gravitational insecurity [or tactile defensiveness or noise sensitivity or whatever]." Again, AS is a pervasive developmental disorder and is so considered because its effects are systemwide. No one with AS has "just one" symptom or behavior, though there may be persons with and without other disorders who do. The presence of any of the following does not rule out AS; indeed, the presence of several together suggests that further evaluation for AS or another disorder may be warranted.

Emotional Lability and General Anxiety

An individual with AS lives under stress. He may become easily and quickly upset over something that would not bother most people. Common behaviors range from general grumpiness and low-key whining to violent tantruming that may involve physical aggression directed toward oneself or others. One hallmark of the AS tantrum is its seemingly instant onset and its supersonic trajectory from calm to complete meltdown in a matter of minutes, if not seconds.

To those unfamiliar with AS, these tantrums seem to come from out of the blue. However, there is usually a trigger, or antecedent, but it may not be immediately obvious. Children may be at a loss to identify, articulate, or explain what prompts the outburst. Parents find themselves playing detective to discover the culprit, then acting like Secret Service agents, casing out every situation for potential triggers. Tantrum antecedents range from extreme confusion and stress because of theory of mind and socialization problems; avoidance of touch or tactile stimulation; sensitivity to certain sounds, smells, tastes, textures, or light; or what many parents recognize as simply mental fatigue from the stress of coping. One result of this is that our children sometimes strike others as emotionally immature, manipulative, and spoiled, and we parents as overprotective or indulgent. In fact, all we're doing is protecting our kids from a world that can be too loud, too busy, too quick, or too confusing.

People with AS can be extraordinarily sensitive to what they consider "criticism," which may in fact be only a request, suggestion, or mild reprimand. A child with AS may become very angry or very sad because an adult has reminded him to remove his hat inside or because there are no lemon lollipops at the doctor's office. In uncomfortable or new situations, a child's stress can prompt negative or inappropriate responses. For example, an AS child who witnesses another child being hurt might laugh. This could be interpreted as lacking empathy, but it is more likely that the child is nervous or doesn't know what the appropriate response should be.

Sensory Integration Problems

A person with AS may react strongly to touch, smell, sound, tastes, and visual stimulation. He or she may be overwhelmed to the point of feeling panic or nausea by the sensation of sitting in a doctor's exam room without clothing, the antiseptic smells, the taste of the tongue depressor, the feel of the paper on the examination table. In school, the touch of chalk, the texture and scent of a new textbook, and the sharp crackle of the PA system may be literally unbearable. At the shopping mall, the "white noise" of a large space, the scent of several perfumes, or the bright reflection of halogen lighting on chrome and glass counters can set off panic or tantruming.

Auditory Integration Problems

Many people with AS also have a central auditory processing disorder (CAPD), of which there are several forms. Behaviors typical of CAPD include the inability to follow oral directions that involve two or more steps (e.g., "When you finish breakfast, bring your dishes into the kitchen, rinse them, stack them in the sink, then use the dishcloth to wipe the table"), difficulty attending to conversation or other aural input in the presence of competing sounds or distractions, and repeatedly asking others to repeat themselves. For those who also have auditory sensitivity (also part of CAPD), the sounds of a child crying in the next room can be overwhelming; the pitch of a telephone's ring or a beeper may be physically painful. While some are sensitive to sound at high volumes, many are made uncomfortable by certain sounds and pitches, regardless of volume. A child might cringe at the sound of a distant leaf blower and yet enjoy banging loudly on a drum. Some parents have noticed that sometimes the ability to control the noise makes it tolerable. These same children may also have difficulty regulating their own voices. They may not realize they are speaking too loudly and some find it impossible to whisper.

• • •

Hearing and Noise

Anxiety, depression, tantruming, avoidance behavior, crying, screaming, running, and totally shutting down to the point of putting oneself to sleep are some of the ways a person with AS or other PDD may react to sound. For those of us whose brains process sound normally, it can be difficult to imagine the sheer panic a child might experience at something like the sound of a car starting or water running down the bathtub drain. Most of us simply assume that only loud, sudden noises might be distressing. However, persons with AS who have central auditory processing problems may be as unnerved by what most of us consider the near-silent hum of fluorescent lights as we would be by a loud car alarm. A surprising number of children in our survey were very troubled by the sound of other people chewing food, for example.

When we asked parents about their children's patterns of sound sensitivity, we found that while only 23 percent were always sensitive to noise in general, 43 percent were sensitive only when tired or "overloaded." Forty-eight percent were always sensitive to particular sounds, regardless of their emotional state. Central auditory processing difficulties also seem to play a role in expressive communication. Sixty-eight percent of our parents indicated that their child had trouble modulating his or her own voice (e.g., didn't really know how to whisper or was unaware when talking too loudly). Interestingly, 32 percent said that their child "often says that people are 'yelling' at him/her when most people would feel that a normal voice volume was being used."

As for the types of noise the children found most troubling, the results will probably be surprising to someone who does not know a child with AS. When we asked parents which of forty-four sounds provoked "extreme discomfort, panic, fear, [the child] would try to avoid at any cost," these were the top five responses:

Noise at a fairly crowded sports event or similar event where many people are screaming	35%
Sudden loud noises	34%
Sirens and alarms	34%
High-pitched whistles	33%
Sound of fireworks	28%

Among other frequently mentioned sounds or environments were a baby or young child crying, 25 percent; a school cafeteria, 24 percent; school assembly, 21 percent; balloon popping, 19 percent; and loud music, 17 percent.

Over 40 percent of our respondents said that their children experienced "moderate discomfort; would prefer to avoid but can tolerate" the following sounds: sudden loud noises; sirens and alarms; school bells; car alarms; loud music; movie theaters; a school assembly; a school cafeteria; high-pitched whistles; a balloon popping; a typical, fairly crowded restaurant; a baby or young child crying; a gymnasium; and a fairly crowded sports event or similar event where many people are screaming.

When asked to describe how often a child behaved in the following ways, parents' answers ranged from "about half the time" to "all of the time or almost all of the time."

Will cover ears with own hands 71%

Will become agitated 69%

Will go to places where sound may be a problem, but is
    visibly agitated, tense, or nervous 62%

Will become angry 62%

Will go to places where sound may be a problem, but
    does so reluctantly 53%

Will become irrational 51%

Refuses to go places where problem sounds occur or
    may occur 43%

Will shut down emotionally 40%

In addition, parents indicated that their children had difficulty understanding what was said in the classroom (68 percent). Parents also noted other unusual responses to sound. Sixty-four percent said that at least half the time, their child becomes easily distracted by noises that most people would not notice, and over 52 percent indicated that their child seems to respond to questions at a noticeably slower rate than would be expected. Eighty-nine percent of our parents said they had "avoided situations in which the child could easily become overloaded."

Other hearing-related behaviors noted to occur more than 75 percent of the time were difficulties with following all but the simplest oral directions and understanding oral statements made in a moderately crowded or noisy place. About 50 percent of parents said their children had significant difficulty attending to simple oral statements made in the presence of everyday background noise, such as a television or radio playing.

Motor Clumsiness

The majority of those with AS struggle with some degree of fine- and gross-motor skills deficits. They have trouble tossing and catching a ball, dressing and undressing, tying shoes, holding a fork properly, balancing, hopping, or following directions related to physical movements (e.g., "Raise your right hand over your head," "Hop up and down on your left foot"). Many individuals have an unusual gait and problems with spatial judgment; they literally may not know where their bodies are in space. This may account for their unusually high rate of spills, trips, and bumps into things. Many are also dysgraphic and have a great deal of difficulty with handwriting, some to the point that holding a pencil is literally painful.

Atypical Responses to Stimuli

Some individuals with AS seem to experience sensory stimuli differently. They may have difficulty describing the degree and type of pain they experience, and/or their responses may seem out of proportion or inappropriate, over- or underreactive. The same person who has no problem getting an injection may scream when you place a stethoscope to his skin; a child who eschews being touched lightly might enjoy jumping off the couch repeatedly and coming down hard on his knees. This probably results from some form of sensory integration dysfunction. (See page 206.)

Unitasking

Paying attention to more than one thing at a time can be challenging for a person with AS. They may struggle to maintain eye contact while talking or listening, to follow a series of directions as they are being given, or to listen and write notes in class simultaneously. As mentioned earlier, a child with AS may appear not to be paying attention and yet can recall everything that was said. This seems to suggest that some people with AS can watch the teacher *or* listen to the teacher but cannot do both at the same time easily. It also may explain why so many have difficulty with team sports. Not only do they have to pay attention to what they are doing but they have to heed what their teammates are doing. This same "unimodal" approach might explain why individuals with AS find social interaction so difficult.

Problems with Organization

Asperger Syndrome compromises executive function (EF), or the brain's ability to plan and carry out the steps to complete the task or behavior at hand. Executive function also controls inhibitions (e.g., the ability to think before you act) and makes it possible for a person to generalize or apply knowledge gained in situation A to situation Z, regardless of how different the two are. People whose executive functioning is impaired (a recent study found that 90 percent of persons with AS tested below average in EF tests) are not adept at responding to situations or tasks in an organized, efficient way. This may be evident in a student who sits at his desk to do his homework but literally does not know where to begin. He may need prompting to gather the necessary supplies and books. Children with EF problems may exhibit so-called learned helplessness. Children with AS often seem behind their peers in doing simple things for themselves independently, such as getting their own breakfast, following a morning routine without prompting, or arriving at school with everything they need in their backpack.

Other Typical AS Behaviors

People with AS have difficulty with transitions (e.g., moving from classroom to classroom in the upper grades), surprises, changes in schedule and routine, unfamiliar environments, and novel situations. They may be challenged, even baffled, by certain abstract concepts, such as those relating to time and future events or, from our earlier example, the "white lie." Confusion about time and sequence is often a stressor. A child with AS who is told that he may watch television or ride his bicycle before bedtime may finish his television program, then be surprised and upset when told it is time for bed. For most children, the fact that making a choice means getting to do only one thing and not the other is communicated clearly by the word *or.* Someone with AS may not glean that doing one thing automatically eliminates the possibility of doing the other one, too. That information needs to be presented explicitly.

Because AS makes it difficult to generalize information from one setting or situation to another, you may notice your child asking questions to which you would expect he would know the answer. One parent told us of her son's anxiety over where they would buy the Halloween pumpkin. She did not realize that because the store where they bought the pumpkin the year before had closed, her son did not know (because no one had explicitly told him) that other stores could also be expected to have pumpkins. The inability to generalize is responsible for much of the low-level "background" stress people with AS seem to experience. Imagine for a moment believing that nothing you know about going to your bank's local branch, for example, would apply in another branch office. Multiply this by the dozens of situations children with AS confront each day and you get some idea of the uncertainty and anxiety they may experience.

THE "MASK" OF AS: WHEN SYMPTOMS LOOK LIKE STRENGTHS

Once you suspect that there may be a problem, it's easy to fall into the trap of seeing everything in terms of that problem. Yes, especially after your child is newly diagnosed, it seems that Asperger Syndrome "explains" just about everything. However, never forget that there will also be things about your child that owe more to her being who she is than to her being a person with AS.

Particularly during the sensitive period between recognizing a problem and learning to cope, don't lose sight of your child's areas of strength, and try to put them in context. Children with AS often have impressive skills and characteristics: They may be academically precocious, uninterested in the fads that other children drive their parents crazy over, capable of amazing feats of memory and concentration, more emotionally attached to you than their peers are to their parents, and even be considered your adult friends' favorite child to talk to because they seem "so grown up." Best of all, yours is probably simply a great kid. These are wonderful characteristics that, if channeled properly, can be used to your child's advantage. There is something statistically unusual but certainly nothing wrong with reading at age two, being ambivalent about the latest cartoon craze, knowing the bird (and flower and tree and motto and per capita income ranking) of all fifty states, and being comfortable talking to adults.

The potential problems lie not in these behaviors themselves but in the reasons why a child engages in them to the degree that they do. Some parents of children with AS recall feeling blessed to have avoided the terrible twos. Looking back, before they suspected a problem, they recall a toddler who never screamed for a particular brand of cereal and never got into things as much as other kids did. One mother remarked, "If I had left him to crawl around in a room full of cleaning products and poisons, he would never even have touched them," and she is probably not exaggerating. What these descriptions of "good" babies overlook is that a toddler who screams for Cocoa Puffs is engaged in the crucial testing of his communication and theory of mind "systems." The child who could be "trusted" in a room full of hazards can "be good" because either AS itself or the neurological anomaly that results in AS seems to short-circuit the natural impulse to explore and experiment with the environment.

It is only natural and right to count our child's outstanding characteristics as pluses. Doing this with AS, however, can be misleading. We speak from our own personal experience here, and between us we have spoken to or corresponded with hundreds of parents on the brink of diagnosis. Regardless of how extreme a child's behavior, no matter how certain a parent may be that, yes, something is definitely amiss, there is an almost reflexive drive to "balance the books," so to speak. Sometimes that involves citing true skills, such as an advanced understanding of mathematics or a natural mechanical ability. Other times, however, parents are unknowingly describing AS traits that sometimes manifest in what at first glance appears to be acceptable, exceptional, or desirable behaviors. The child who does not "go with the crowd," the child who never demands to go outside to play, the child who spins wildly imaginative tales from his private play world may also be a child with AS. The child who never lies, the child who has a razor-sharp sense of right and wrong, the child who would never sneak a cookie from the cabinet may also be a child with AS.

As parents of children diagnosed with AS, we admit that we once viewed our children's unusual AS-related behaviors in terms that eased some of our discomfort about them. When confronted with the less attractive aspects common to AS—the social problems, the tantrums, the sometimes inexplicable behaviors—we tried desperately to balance the books, to take our children's "good" characteristics and use them to offset, to make up for, to diminish, and even to totally disregard the "bad" behaviors and the glaringly unusual deficits. If we were guilty of not facing the situation head-on, we were not alone. We had doctors and friends who assured us that this was "just a phase," educators who were blinded by our children's academic strengths or unusual intellectual abilities, and family members who reminded us of someone else in the family (whom we might now recognize as being somewhere "on the spectrum"), "and look how well he turned out."

Be realistic about your child having AS. The first step is learning to see deficits and problem areas for what they truly are, not what you wish they would be. It helps to learn not to say "My child talks only about earthquakes and has no relationships with peers, *but* he is very bright," but rather "My child talks only about earthquakes and has no relationships with peers, *and* he is very bright."

ASPERGER SYNDROME: SOMETHING TO HAVE OR SOMEONE TO BE?

The strengths of people with AS make them interesting, bright, inventive, curious, and capable of great accomplishments. Many have a great, offbeat sense of humor. As parents of children with AS, we are often faced with the dilemma of determining which AS behaviors to tolerate or encourage and which we should strive to reduce or eliminate. Certainly atypical behaviors that a child with AS might engage in may actually serve a purpose. Some persons with AS, for example, deal with stress by rocking, pacing, turning light switches on and off a set number of times, repeating nonsense phrases, or performing some other activity that appears odd to others. A child might insist on wearing the same shirt every day, violently resist brushing his teeth, or scream every time you start your car. Within the context of AS, these behaviors might "make sense." They might even be comforting. However, that should not stop you from taking a close, objective look at them and asking how they're impacting your child's ability to cope in less socially stigmatizing ways.

While we celebrate and treasure all that our children can do, we should never lose sight of or diminish—in our own minds or in those of others—the things that are difficult for them. It's one thing for a preschool child to have a good attention span; it's something else when that attention is focused on the size, shape, and color of switch plates to the exclusion of virtually everything else. When a child is young, especially, it's tempting to dismiss certain deficits. After all, are catching a ball, having good handwriting, or being able to sustain a brief, polite conversation with Uncle Ed really essential for future success? In and of themselves, the answer may be no. Nevertheless, as parents, it is our responsibility to look ahead and understand that behaviors and deficits are neither discrete nor limited. They have far-reaching implications, which for a host of reasons may result in social stigmatization, isolation, and rejection. They may "set up" someone to be dependent on the presence of objects, routines, and persons that can never be absolutely guaranteed. Perhaps even worse, they may teach a child that because he is now, for example, dependent on a given routine or unable to get dressed independently that he will always be that way. We will talk a lot more about the importance of teaching children independence in their daily lives later on, because this is one area in which we believe parents are not getting the help they need.

One of the most significant predictors for future success and personal happiness for persons with any type of disability is not academic success but social success. A child who cannot catch a ball, for example, stands to lose a lot more than the chance to be a Little League hero. He may not be invited to join in games, may be self-conscious and feel badly about himself, may experience an early lack of interest in anything having to do with physical activity or sports, and may believe that all this is because something is "wrong" with him. However, the child who learns to catch—or ride his bike, play the game someone else wants to play, or dress in an age-appropriate manner—may be asked to join the group and have one less thing to feel self-conscious about.

While it would be unwise, even cruel, to force a child to do things against his will, there is an argument to be made for helping your child expand his repertoire of interests and skills beyond the boundaries that AS can impose. Some of our children need help, sometimes very intensive help beginning when they are very young, to master many of the basic skills of life, and one of the most important skills is adaptability. Some of our children are amazingly resistant and unyielding when it comes to making changes. Dr. Bobby Newman, a nationally certified therapist in applied behavior analysis (ABA), makes the point that the purpose of therapy and intervention is to give people the skills they need so that they will be able to make choices in life.

The child who always wears the same shirt because he has always worn the same shirt and his parents believe he never could wear any other shirt is not making a choice, even though parents and others may see it in those terms. In contrast, a child who has been taught to adapt to change, to be flexible, and to be comfortable with change is one who not only has a better chance of fitting in but is less anxious and stressed. After all, imagine your whole day depending on whether or not the "special shirt" was available. Rather than alleviating a child's stress by providing the special shirt, well-meaning parents actually may be adding to it. Life being what it is, sooner or later something will happen to make that shirt unwearable. Then what?

This is not to say that introducing flexibility into your child's life will be easy. It won't, and not everything will yield to change. But it is essential that you make the effort to expand your child's emotional comfort zone.

THE MOST IMPORTANT SKILL: INDEPENDENCE

Another important way to prepare a child to reach his potential is to teach independence. For children who are more seriously challenged by other forms of ASDs, professionals and parents alike share an urgency about teaching self-help, personal care, and daily living skills. In the best schools, such seemingly "basic" skills as appropriate table manners, folding and putting away clothes, making a bed, handshaking, hairbrushing, preparing a simple meal, crossing the street safely, answering a telephone appropriately, and bathing and toileting are important components of a formal curriculum that is taught systematically to mastery. Ironically, even though among children with AS there is a high percentage who have difficulty learning these same types of skills, most will never cross paths with a professional who can teach them (or, better, teach their parents to teach them). When we fail to teach independence—and independence is a learnable skill, not some mysterious, inherent quality—we limit our children and even define their futures in terms of what they cannot do instead of what they can.

Through OASIS and in talking with parents around the country, we know that there are children with AS who are missing precious experiences as well as social, recreational, and academic opportunities because they lack the "prerequisite" independence to participate. We're talking about the seven-year-old with the social skills to attend a sleepover but who must decline because he is not independent in toileting; the brilliant high school senior who cannot attend the Ivy League school so far from home because she never learned to work a microwave, manage a checkbook, or cross a street safely; the twelve-year-old who is perennially on the sidelines at recess because no one thought someone so bright "needed" to know how to throw a ball or ride a bike.

We have read posts from many concerned parents who see the corrosive effects of being locked in to a cycle of hovering, reminding, nagging, arguing, threatening, punishing, and sometimes worse over the same things every day but have no idea how to stop it. And if a parent feels exhausted, frustrated, and incompetent, imagine for a moment how the child must feel. Remember that no matter what your child's measurable IQ, having an ASD almost always suggests an inability to learn through observation. Most children do not need to be explicitly taught how to dress; ours probably do. Most children are inherently driven to be independent and may even attempt to do things before they are ready. They will soldier through numerous cycles of trial and error to reach their goal; ours probably won't. Most important, and difficult for parents and experts alike to fully comprehend, despite our children's seeming facility with words, there are some skills that just cannot be taught by telling someone how to do it. For most persons with ASDs—regardless of where they fall on the spectrum—acquiring the skills of daily living and independence is more a "show" than a "tell" process.

THERE ARE REASONS FOR HOPE

All parents wonder, and worry, about what the future holds for their children. Parents of children with AS worry, too, but about things other parents never have to consider. If you read other books on Asperger Syndrome, you may be struck by the uncertainty that seems to color discussions of the future for children with AS. If you dig deeply enough into the more academically oriented works, you may be alarmed by case studies involving bizarre behavior, including violence. As you read, and wonder, it is important to bear in mind the following limitations of any current prognostic picture:

• *Most authorities deal with clinic populations; that is, persons who need or desire professional help.* This fact alone skews the sample, so to speak, because for every person with AS who comes under professional care, there are others who are functioning well enough without it.

• *Awareness of AS is too recent and effective interventions too new to be reflected in current prognoses.* Twenty years ago, when the adults with AS whose cases inform the prognosis as we know it were children, AS did not exist, technically speaking. The statistics and case histories available today tell us much about an AS population that, for the most part, did not receive appropriate support and intervention in their younger years.

• *Amid the uncertainty, there is hope.* This generation—our children—will be the first with Asperger Syndrome to have the benefit of understanding, knowledge, research, treatment, and intervention that did not exist even ten years ago. While no one can say with certainty what lies ahead for any child, the small daily victories they can achieve thanks to information, awareness, and the appropriate use of therapies and interventions are glimpses of promise.

Chapter 3

HOW ASPERGER SYNDROME IS DIAGNOSED

For most parents, the process of evaluation and diagnosis is an emotionally mixed experience. There is the sense of relief at finally knowing what "it" is. Having a name for the collection of behaviors and issues opens new doors to information, support, and services. Being able to use that name telegraphs to others that your child's problems don't stem from poor parenting, bad attitudes, egocentricity, laziness, or guile. As a parent, you may come away from the confirmed, official diagnosis with renewed hope and purpose, a focus for your energy, a sense of a new beginning.

At the same time, it's impossible not to see the diagnosis as marking an end to other things: the hope that your child will completely "outgrow" or "learn to cope" with his differences, the possibility that her problems aren't as serious as you had feared or will be only temporary, self-limiting, and easily "cured." In the same moment when you feel pressured to charge down this new road with confidence and hope, you may feel lost, overwhelmed, and disappointed by the realization that you have to be there at all. We devote chapter 4 to the impact of the diagnosis on parents. Here we discuss how Asperger Syndrome is—and is not—diagnosed, and how to sort through the sometimes-confusing terminology professionals use when discussing it with parents.

Much confusion has arisen around the terms *diagnosis* and *classification*. For the purposes of this book, we use the term *diagnosis* to denote the identification of a disease or condition by a medical professional with expertise in the area of developmental disability—a physician, psychiatrist, neurologist, neuropsychologist, pediatrician, and so on. The diagnosis may be reached through any combination of various tests, information on the child obtained from parents and teachers, and interviews with the child.

Classification is a term used by school districts and state education departments to identify types of disabilities for program design and record keeping. A classification is not the same as a diagnosis. Depending on the child and the state in which he attends school, the child may be diagnosed with Asperger Syndrome yet not be classified by his school district as being on the autism spectrum, while another child with AS in a different state would be classified as "autistic." In another example, a child may be classified by his school district as emotionally disturbed and later diagnosed by a psychiatrist as having a psychiatric condition such as obsessive-compulsive disorder (OCD) or Asperger Syndrome. Federal and state special education statutes and regulations offer a limited number of classifications. So while a condition such as OCD is recognized as a disability and is a medical diagnosis, there is no specific classification for AS as far as federal special education programs or funds are concerned.

WHY PURSUE A DIAGNOSIS?

You might be reading this book because you have reason to suspect that your child or someone else may have AS. After reviewing the various diagnostic criteria and doing some homework, you may feel that you've learned enough about AS to make that call. You may even wonder if there is any point to having your child officially diagnosed if you believe already that he or she has AS.

We strongly advise that anyone you suspect may have AS be diagnosed by a professional. Having a true diagnosis is an important first step in accessing the appropriate and most effective services, supports, interventions, and treatments. Your conviction that your child has AS is all but meaningless when you enter the realm of health insurance coverage and coding, and the identification and classification necessary to access special education and/or related services. Failure to obtain an official diagnosis may cost your child coverage and services.

It's also possible that your child does not have AS at all, but one or a combination of disorders whose symptoms appear to the untrained eye to add up to AS (say, for example, obsessive and compulsive tendencies, social phobia, and a tic disorder). Or perhaps your child has AS along with other disorders or disabilities, each of which may require specialized treatment. Even experienced medical specialists can be challenged in trying to determine how best to qualify and address a child's obsessive behavior about how he displays his collection of spark plugs (is this a typical AS special interest? obsessive tendencies? OCD?) or mood swings (is it bipolar disorder? anxiety? stress due to lack of social understanding?). Is a child unable to pay attention in class because he has anxiety? Or is he anxious in class because of an attention deficit disorder that makes it difficult to pay attention? Questions such as these should be referred to experienced medical specialists.

THE PITFALLS OF LATE OR MISSED DIAGNOSIS

Some people feel strongly that "diagnosis doesn't matter," that all it does is "label" or, in the words of a best-selling pediatrican, "pathologize" people. We disagree. Even if a correct diagnosis is nothing more than a compass, pointing you toward the right information and treatment, it is invaluable. Even without diagnosis, your child will still have problems. How you, your child, and those who know and work with him perceive those problems and address them sometimes has everything to do with what we call them. As we discuss in detail in chapter 6 and throughout, some of the rules for intervention and treatment that work for other PDDs, psychiatric disorders, and learning disabilities may have a negative effect for people with Asperger Syndrome. Having a correct diagnosis not only helps you and your child find and receive the most appropriate, effective interventions, it may be even more valuable in terms of helping you steer clear of the wrong ones. According to our OASIS survey, of 514 children ultimately diagnosed with AS, before that, 374, or about 40 percent, were believed to have had some form of attention deficit disorder. Not only did some of these children receive less than opti-mal interventions, they may have missed out on years—in some cases, decades—of the help and understanding that could have made an important difference in their lives.

WHY IS ASPERGER SYNDROME SOMETIMES DIFFICULT TO DIAGNOSE CORRECTLY?

The complex, multifaceted nature of AS and the fact that no two peo-ple with AS are exactly alike in the type and severity of their symp-toms account for some of the difficulty in diagnosing it. Also, AS may share a number of behaviors and characteristics with other pervasive developmental disorders, so-called autism spectrum disorders, learning profiles and deficits, and emotional and psychiatric disorders. In addi-tion, as we've mentioned, a significant portion of persons with AS also have other coexisting, or "comorbid," conditions or disorders.

— • • • —

Comorbidity: Other Conditions That Can Complicate the AS Picture

ADHD

Attention-deficit/hyperactivity disorder, or ADHD, is a neurobiological disorder characterized by pervasive difficulty with or inability to sustain attention or control impulses at a level deemed developmentally age appropriate. Thought to affect between 3 percent and 5 percent of school-age children,[1] there are three types of ADHD:

ADHD primarily inattentive type
ADHD primarily hyperactive/impulsive type
ADHD combined type

Because ADHD and AS share similar features, it's not uncommon for a child to be first diagnosed with ADHD and later rediagnosed with AS. In addition, children may have a dual diagnosis of AS and a form of ADHD.

Anxiety

According to the National Institute of Mental Health, anxiety disorders, which are the most common form of mental disorder, affect over 19 million individuals yearly.[2] Whether the anxiety experienced by individuals with AS is a direct result of their neurobiological makeup, a response to the stresses of living with AS, or a combination of both is difficult to determine, but a significant number of children and adults with AS do experience some form of anxiety disorder at some point in their lives.

Some common anxiety disorders that have been known to affect those with AS are as follows:

Generalized Anxiety Disorder (GAD): Individuals with GAD suffer from chronic and pervasive worry that goes well beyond what would be considered normal responses to daily living. Those with GAD worry excessively about everything, often for no apparent reason. They have difficulty relaxing, are constantly "on edge," and may have problems falling asleep. Sometimes they experience physical symptoms such as trembling, twitching, headaches, nausea, sweating, and irritability. During times of stress, anxiety can increase; and considering that children with AS are under stress most of their waking hours, it's not surprising that they could easily become anxious. Parents of children with AS have frequently mentioned that their kids perpetually see the glass as half empty and tend to look at the negatives rather than the positives. A child with AS who behaves this way could possibly be suffering from GAD.

Obsessive-Compulsive Disorder (OCD): Individuals with OCD experience "repeated and unwanted thoughts and behaviors that seem impossible to stop."[3] OCD is thought to affect 1 in 50 people, or 2 percent of the population, at some point in their lives. Individuals with AS who are also diagnosed with OCD experience ritualistic behaviors and a need for routines that may significantly impact their ability to function. Children with AS who also have OCD face additional educational challenges. Of the 576 families who completed the OASIS survey, 12 percent have children who have been officially diagnosed with OCD, and OCD was suspected in 38 percent of children prior to their diagnosis of AS. However, not every person with compulsive tendencies, obsessive tendencies, or both has OCD.

Social Phobia and General Phobias: Phobias can be defined as "extreme and irrational fears"[4] that disrupt an individual's life. Individuals with AS are often diagnosed with social phobia, an intense fear of social situations that results in anxiety, panic, and avoidance behavior that can be extreme and adversely affect ability to function. Individuals with social phobia may feel incapable of performing in certain social arenas and may avoid interacting with groups of people, prefer to stay with people with whom they're familiar, and be unwilling or unable to seek out new social situations. Because individuals with AS may face profound social difficulties generally, it can be too easy to attribute aversive behaviors to AS. Social phobia does respond to treatment (medication, cognitive behavior therapy, or both).

Posttraumatic Stress Disorder (PTSD): As awareness of AS increases, adults who as children were either misdiagnosed or undiagnosed are being recognized as having Asperger Syndrome. In addition, some of these adults (and children) receive a secondary diagnosis of PTSD. Many grew up misunderstood and, unfortunately, all too often mistreated. Individuals with PTSD often have pervasive and persistent recollections of traumatic incidents, and these memories can be quite debilitating. In addition to depression, loss of sleep, and decreased appetite, individuals with PTSD often feel extreme anxiety. While many become withdrawn and avoid social contact, in the most severe cases individuals can become aggressive and angry. Like many conditions, PTSD ranges from mild to severe.

Seizure Disorders
Having an ASD significantly increases the risk of seizure disorder. According to Dr. Stephen M. Edelson of the Center for the Study of Autism, "About 25 percent of autistic individuals may experience clinical or subclinical seizures which, if left untreated, can lead to deleterious effects."[5] In general, family members of children with AS also seem to have a higher incidence of seizure disorders.

Depression

Depression is one of the most common conditions affecting children and adults with AS. While teenagers who are coming to the realization that they are different from their peers are particularly susceptible, parents need to be aware that depression can occur in an AS child *at any age, even in the very young child.* Parents need to be particularly diligent in looking for clues that a child may be depressed.

Keep in mind that some of the warning signs may seem like typical AS behavior and therefore are not easily recognized. It's important to look for changes in behavior as well as specific symptoms. In addition to watching for irritability and physical complaints such as headache and stomachache, the American Academy of Child and Adolescent Psychiatry recommends that parents be aware of the following signs of depression:[6]

- Change of appetite with either significant weight loss (when not dieting) or weight gain
- Change in sleeping patterns (such as trouble falling asleep, waking up in the middle of the night, early morning awakening, or sleeping too much)
- Loss of interest in activities formerly enjoyed
- Loss of energy, fatigue, feeling slowed down for no reason, being "burned out"
- Feelings of guilt and self-blame for things that are not one's fault
- Inability to concentrate and indecisiveness
- Feelings of hopelessness and helplessness
- Recurring thoughts of death and suicide, wishing to die, or attempting suicide

Bipolar Disorder

Bipolar disorder, also commonly referred to as manic-depression, is a disorder involving episodes of mania and depression, which are cyclical in nature, with mood swings that may cycle from high to low and back again. It is caused by abnormalities in brain chemistry and function. Though it is thought to affect 1 percent to 2 percent of adults worldwide, only recently has attention been given to children with the disorder. While adults with bipolar disorder often experience extreme changes in mood and behavior and energy, children with the condition "usually have an ongoing, continuous mood disturbance that is a mix of mania and depression."[7]

Symptoms include:

- An expansive or irritable mood
- Depression
- Rapidly changing moods lasting a few hours to a few days
- Explosive, lengthy, and often destructive rages
- Separation anxiety
- Defiance of authority
- Hyperactivity, agitation, sleeping little or sleeping too much
- Bed-wetting and night terrors
- Distractibility
- Strong and frequent cravings, often for carbohydrates and sweets
- Excessive involvement in multiple projects and activities
- Impaired judgment, impulsivity, racing thoughts, and pressure to keep talking
- Daredevil behaviors
- Inappropriate or precocious sexual behavior
- Delusions and hallucinations
- Grandiose belief in own abilities that defy the laws of logic (ability to fly, for example)

For more on AS and bipolar disorder, see George T. Lynn, *Survival Strategies for Parenting Children with Bipolar Disorder* (London and Philadelphia: Jessica Kingsley Publishers, 2000).

Tourette's Syndrome and Tics

There are several different tic disorders. The best known, Tourette's syndrome (TS), is a neurological disorder characterized by motor tics, involuntary movements, or vocalizations. Movements are repetitive in nature and may vary in location. Symptoms can be mild to severe and range from simple movements such as eye blinking, throat clearing, and coughing to more complex full-body movements or movements accompanied by vocalizations. This disorder occurs more frequently in boys than girls and almost always appears by the age of eighteen.

Contrary to popular belief, the uncontrollable expression of obscene language (coprolalia) is among the rarest of TS symptoms.[8]

Although children with Asperger Syndrome may have a diagnosis of TS, it is also important that it not be confused with stereotypies (commonly and possibly inaccurately referred to as "stimming"). Since TS is believed to be an inherited condition, it is not uncommon to discover that extended family members of children with AS have TS or another tic disorder.

Oppositional Defiant Disorder (ODD)

Oppositional defiant disorder is a psychiatric disorder that has not yet been widely documented as a condition that frequently occurs with AS. However, our OASIS Survey on Diagnosis revealed that as many children were being diagnosed with ODD as with TS and bipolar disorder. We should also note that many parents indicated that their child had been diagnosed with ODD before being diagnosed with AS, suggesting that for some children with AS, ODD may be an incorrect diagnosis.

According to the American Academy of Child and Adolescent Psychiatry, ODD is distinguished from normal childhood arguing, talking back, and disobedience by its persistence and the degree to which it interferes with daily functioning. Between 5 percent and 15 percent of school-age children have ODD. Symptoms include:

- Frequent temper tantrums
- Excessive arguing with adults
- Active defiance and refusal to comply with adult requests and rules
- Deliberate attempts to annoy or upset people
- Blaming others for his or her mistakes or misbehavior
- Often being touchy or easily annoyed by others
- Frequent anger and resentment
- Mean and hateful talking when upset
- Seeking revenge

Online Sources for Further Information on Comorbid Conditions

CHADD (Children and Adults with Attention-Deficit/Hyperactivity Disorder)
http://www.chadd.org

National Institute of Mental Health
http://www.nimh.nih.gov

American Academy of Child and Adolescent Psychiatry
http://www.aacap.org

Child and Adolescent Bipolar Foundation
http://www.bpkids.org

Tourette Syndrome Association
http://www.tsa-usa.org

For a wealth of information on practically every comorbidity common to children with ASDs, visit Tourette Syndrome "Plus" at www.tourettesyndrome.net/.

ASPERGER SYNDROME: LEARNING HOW TO SEE

If you or others are asking, "Does this child have Asperger Syndrome?" you will be looking for signs, symptoms, and behaviors that match one of several sets of diagnostic criteria. Unfortunately, AS is not one of those disorders whose six most common telltale signs would fit neatly on the back of a brochure. Some of the commonly used criteria refer to behaviors that, arguably, most children engage in to some degree at some time. Many of us whose children have been diagnosed will admit, if we are honest, to having reassured ourselves or others with "Lots of kids do that."

So where does typical behavior end and atypical behavior begin?

- *Tommy never seems to look any adult in the eye.*
- *Roger is obsessed with dinosaurs.*
- *Ashley doesn't really fit in among other kids in her group.*
- *Kurt is unbelievably clumsy.*

Do these children have AS? Probably not, if they are developmentally within the normal range in other important areas.

AS does not describe a single behavior or deficit, but a specific combination or constellation of them that are present to a significant degree.

So, if a single child had Tommy's inability to sustain eye contact, Roger's dinosaur obsession, Ashley's lack of social competence, and Kurt's awkwardness, would that child have Asperger Syndrome? Again, maybe not. Children are very complicated little people, works in progress, with unique profiles of strengths and weaknesses. No single area of deficit "proves" AS. As you consider a child who might have AS, remember to see things in the broad and ever-changing context of the whole child. The importance of a specific skill or deficit depends on what other areas of strength or weakness accompany it. We would most likely be correct in assuming that these children, despite their areas of concern, would not have AS if:

- *Tommy does not make a lot of eye contact but has no trouble fitting in socially among his peers.*
- *Roger is obsessed with dinosaurs but will talk just as readily with his jock friends about baseball and with his grandparents about their garden.*
- *Ashley is shy in group situations but has several close friends.*
- *Kurt, though the proverbial bull in a china closet, has no difficulty with other fine and gross motor skills.*

However, we might be concerned about any of these children if:

- *Tommy's lack of normal eye contact also included a deficit in shared attention (he did not look at what another person pointed to) and frequent misunderstanding of basic facial expression and tone of voice.*
- *Roger's facts about dinosaurs were the first utterances he made to everyone he met whether they were interested or not, whether he knew the person or not, and he became upset every time anyone tried to change the subject.*
- *Ashley's behavior around other children suggested to even an untrained person that she "literally didn't seem to know what to do or say," and playing with other children really consisted of playing her own game alongside them without showing any interest in them.*
- *Kurt's awkwardness was apparent across a wide range of activities that even children we consider uncoordinated on the playing field have no trouble with—handwriting, dressing, grooming, folding, using scissors, and so on—and his facial expressions and communicative gestures seemed odd.*

Do all of these children have Asperger Syndrome? From this small bit of information, neither we—nor anyone else—should say. Our point here is simply to emphasize that when you become familiar with the various diagnostic criteria and begin measuring a child against them, consider not only the presence of behaviors but their frequency, severity, and the degree to which they interfere with other aspects of the child's life.

• • •

Learning Disorders Commonly Seen with AS

Dysgraphia

Dysgraphia is a complex learning disorder of written language that affects a considerable number of children with AS, although many remain undiagnosed. There are three types:

1. Dyslexic dysgraphia
2. Dysgraphia due to motor clumsiness
3. Dysgraphia due to a neurological inability to understand space

Dysgraphia may present differently from one child to the next. One child's handwriting may be messy and impossible to decipher, and the writing of another child may be exceptionally neat with all letters perfectly formed. The first child may rush through an assignment without forming any of the letters correctly, and the second child is not actually writing in the usual sense but painstakingly "drawing" each individual letter, a process so slow that it might take him an hour to finish a one-page assignment.

Dysgraphia is not just about speed of writing and accuracy of the formation of letters. Other processes are involved, including the following: attention; eye-hand coordination; motor planning; memory; fine- and gross-motor skills (weak upper-body strength can make it difficult for the child to position his body appropriately for the task of writing); language; and the ability to process and perform multiple tasks such as listening, looking at a blackboard, and taking notes simultaneously. Proper writing demands that you be able to recall instantly the answer to a test question while forming letters, a feat some persons with AS simply cannot accomplish. For individuals with dysgraphia, the writing process may be mentally and physically exhausting. All too often, their resistance to projects involving writing is viewed as stubbornness, laziness, or perfectionism.

Realize that a child who can draw beautifully, put together small puzzle pieces, or complete other fine-motor tasks with ease may still be dysgraphic. One child who spent hours making detailed drawings struggled when it came time to taking his spelling test. The assumption was that he didn't know how to spell and, because he had a difficult time explaining himself verbally, he was viewed as a child attempting to make excuses for not being prepared. After all, there were stacks of carefully drawn mazes to prove that he was capable of holding a pencil; therefore his refusal to write was viewed as stubbornness and disobedience. Consider having your child evaluated for dysgraphia if you notice any of the following signs:

- Extreme resistance to writing, accompanied by anxiety and acting out and/or saying that writing is "boring" or "stupid"
- Difficulty maintaining a good writing posture (e.g., the child slumps over desk, props up his head with the nonwriting hand, or frequently complains of being tired while writing)
- Unusual or awkward pencil grip that doesn't improve with thicker pencils or pens or other special pencil grip aids
- Complaints that writing is painful or uncomfortable
- Difficulty taking notes in class
- Difficulty completing written tests in the specified time frame
- "Meltdowns" when faced with a writing assignment
- Excessive time needed to complete written homework
- Exhaustion, crankiness, or depression after completing a written assignment
- Difficulty with placement of text on the paper (e.g., math problems appear either in one corner of the paper or are scattered everywhere on the page)
- Avoidance of tasks that require paper and pencil (e.g., he or she refuses to write down a birthday wish list or Christmas list, even though he is capable of forming the letters)

- Comments from adults such as "his handwriting could be neater if he only tried harder," or "he understands the material but refuses to write down the answers when asked"

Dyscalculia

Dyscalculia is defined as difficulty performing and comprehending mathematical calculations. Between 6 percent and 7 percent of school-age children exhibit difficulties in some area of mathematics.[9] Contrary to the belief that most children who are diagnosed with AS are mathematically gifted, significant numbers of children struggle with mathematical computation and problem solving. Dyscalculia is indicative of one or more of the following neurological problems that are often seen in AS children: language processing, visual spatial confusion, difficulties with memory and sequencing, and high anxiety. A child with language-processing difficulties may not understand the questions being asked, and a child who has a weakness in visual processing and exhibits spatial confusion will have difficulty visualizing numbers and situations required to solve math problems. A child who struggles with the organization of information and sequencing will have difficulty remembering the steps to complete calculations.

Even though we tend to think of math and language as "different," the types of difficulties persons with AS may have in terms of language can have a profound effect on their ability to use math.

Dyslexia

Dyslexia is a language-based disability in which a person has difficulty understanding both oral and written words, sentences, or paragraphs. Individuals have trouble decoding and translating printed words into spoken words and struggle with reading comprehension. While 15 percent to 20 percent of the population has some form of reading disability, dyslexia is the most common cause of reading, writing, and spelling difficulties.[10] Affecting males and females equally, it is thought to be an inherited genetic disorder. According to the Learning Disabilities Association of America, in addition to often reversing or improperly sequencing letters within words when reading or writing, individuals with dyslexia may also exhibit difficulties with the following:[11]

- Perceiving and/or pronouncing words
- Understanding spoken language
- Recalling known words
- Handwriting
- Spelling
- Written language
- Math computation

Nonverbal Learning Disability (NLD or NVLD)

Among the newest and least widely recognized learning disorders, NLD shares many of its characteristics and behaviors with AS. According to researchers at Yale University, many of the children who participated in their AS study fit the NLD learning profile. There are many misunderstandings about NLD. One is that it is the "same as" AS. It is not. AS is a psychiatric diagnosis, and NLD is a learning profile. Though many persons with AS can also be said to have NLD, it is possible to have NLD without AS and AS without NLD. Pamela Tanguay, author of *Nonverbal Learning Disabilities at Home: A Parent's Guide*, suggests that parents be aware of the following signs that a child may have an NLD:[12]

COGNITIVE/ACADEMIC

- Generally the child's WISC (the widely used Wechsler Intelligence Scale for Children) VIQ is higher than their PIQ, but not in all cases—particularly during adolescence. VIQ, or verbal IQ, is a measure of an individual's abilities in terms of expressive and receptive language. PIQ, or performance IQ, is a measure of how an individual uses reasoning to plan and carry out actions. PIQ is determined through performance tests that assess fine- and gross-motor skills and visual-spatial and visual-motor function.
- The child has an excellent vocabulary and more than typical verbal expression, starting at a young age.
- The child has exceptional rote memory skills.
- The child has excellent attention to detail but is likely to miss the big picture.
- The child may be an early reader *or* may have early reading difficulties. However, in either case, the child has general difficulty

with reading comprehension beginning in the upper elementary grades, especially for novel material.

- The child has difficulties in math, especially in the areas of computation, word problems, and abstract applications.
- The child may have significant impairment in concept formation and abstract reasoning.
- The child likely has great difficulty generalizing information; that is, applying learned information to new situations.
- The child's strongest learning medium is simple/rote auditory—if he hears it, he will remember it.

PHYSICAL

- Physical awkwardness is quite common; the child appears to lack coordination. As a youngster, she does better in individual than in team sports.
- The child has difficulty learning to ride a bicycle, catch and/or kick a ball, hop and/or skip.
- Physical difficulties may be more pronounced on the left side of body.
- The child's fine-motor skills may be impaired; handwriting may be poor and/or laborious.
- The child commonly has significant problems with spatial perception.

LANGUAGE/COMMUNICATION

- The child interprets information quite literally.
- The child does not normally process or benefit from nonverbal communication; body language, facial expressions, or tone of voice may be lost on him.
- The child cannot intuit or read between the lines, impacting both conversation and reading comprehension.
- The child has poor social skills; he or she will most likely have trouble making and/or keeping friends.

EMOTIONAL/BEHAVIORAL

- In all likelihood, the child has tremendous difficulty adjusting to new situations or changes in routine.

- The child generally appears to lack common sense or "street smarts"; he can be incredibly naive.
- Anxiety and/or depression are common, especially during adolescence. This problem may be quite severe.
- The child may suffer from low self-esteem.
- The child may be withdrawn, even to the point of agoraphobia.
- There is a higher than normal incidence of suicide within the NLD population.

Hyperlexia

This condition is marked by a child's precocious ability to read words at a level far beyond his years and/or an intense fascination with numbers and letters. Hyperlexic children may later exhibit problems with appropriate socialization skills and an inability to understand verbal language. Some may read extremely well, yet be unable to retain or understand what they have read. Hyperlexia is often accompanied by a number of characteristics typical of other learning disorders and particularly AS:

- Selective listening
- Difficulty answering who, what, where, when, and why questions
- Difficulty learning expressive language
- Echolalia
- Perseverative behavior and rituals, such as rocking, repeating words
- Sensitivity to tactile, auditory, and olfactory stimulation
- Specific and unusual fears
- Difficulty with abstract concepts
- Difficulty initiating and maintaining reciprocal conversation
- Self-stimulatory behavior, "stimming" (rocking, pacing, etc.)

Central Auditory Processing Disorder

Central auditory processing disorder (CAPD) is an extremely complex and little-recognized inability to listen to or comprehend auditory information despite having "good" hearing. An individual with CAPD has reduced or impaired ability to identify, recognize, discriminate, and understand what he hears. A child with CAPD may be unusually sensitive to typical noises and/or unable to discriminate between fore-ground and background noise and may respond to each simultane-ously. A child with CAPD can become emotionally overwhelmed by certain sounds and noisy environments, sometimes resulting in with-drawal or tantrums. Those with CAPD have difficulty following com-plex sentences and instructions despite having an average or above-average IQ. Children with CAPD often "mishear" words and sounds and will compensate by attempting to "fill in the blanks," sometimes resulting in a complete misunderstanding of what they heard. (For more, see chapter 6.)

THE "LABELING" ISSUE

Confronting the possibility that a child may have a problem is never easy. We reflexively reject the idea of giving a name—whether it be a diagnosis or even a description—to what we may view as our child's idiosyncrasies, behaviors, disabilities, or problems. On a sub-conscious level, we worry that having a label will render our child less of an individual in the eyes of others, that she will be thought of first as a person with a disability and second—if ever—as the person we know and love.

In just considering seeking a definitive diagnosis, we may be un-derstandably reluctant to seek out what we fear may be bad news. In our protective parent mode, we may deny the behaviors and issues that other family members, friends, and teachers question. Alter-nately, we may have known all along that the problems were real and we now have to present this information to family members and friends. These may have been people who have told us that our child's problems were a figment of our imaginations, or they them-selves may be in denial or grieving the diagnosis. Many parents find the prospect of breaking the news to their child's grandparents particularly difficult and painful. Looking back, we can both see that while we were protecting our children from the judgments of others who we feared would misjudge them, we were also protecting ourselves.

The trail that begins with a parent's first concerns and ends at di-agnosis is rarely a short straight line. Often professionals are stymied because certain behaviors may lead to a different type of diagnosis, because they perceive that those behaviors can be modulated, controlled, or extinguished, or because they believe that since the child is of at least average intelligence (which most AS children are), he will learn to control them himself. The syndrome's relatively recent inclusion as an official diagnosis coupled with the prevailing current view that it is an autism-related disorder may mean that professionals don't recognize it or, if they do, may be reluctant to say so.

WHY PARENTS, DOCTORS, AND EDUCATORS MISS THE DIAGNOSIS

It is not our intention to criticize parents or professionals, but it's a fact that Asperger Syndrome is commonly misdiagnosed or underdiagnosed. Our OASIS survey found that the overwhelming majority of children (67 percent) had received another, incorrect diagnosis prior to AS. For 46 percent, AS was the second diagnosis; for 29 percent, the third diagnosis; for 13 percent, the fourth diagnosis. Even professional organizations admit that gaps in professional awareness on all forms of PDDs remain.

Some parents and professionals simply avoid diagnosis for as long as they can. A nationwide 2000 survey on special education by Roper Starch Worldwide found that 48 percent of parents polled felt that having a child labeled "learning disabled" was more harmful than dealing with the child's problems privately, and that 44 percent of parents had concerns about their child yet waited for a year or longer before acknowledging the problem and seeking help. When parents or others suspect the problem may be something as misunderstood and stigmatizing as autism, the process can be further complicated. Sometimes one parent or close family member is concerned, while another actively resists believing anything could possibly be wrong. Our own OASIS survey found that 49 percent of parents let over two years pass between the time concerns about their child were first raised by others or voiced to them and the time they received a correct diagnosis. Only 20 percent of children were diagnosed with AS a year or less after concerns were first raised.

Parents who do consult professionals may find themselves on yet another circuitous path, for many reasons. Because we may be ambivalent or anxious about having our child "labeled," we may be too easily satisfied with—or, in truth, grateful for—a more palatable, less frightening explanation or diagnosis. Even in the wake of extreme and troubling behaviors, some parents turn first to social workers, educational consultants, and all manner of therapists (including practitioners of alternative treatments, such as homeopaths, nutritionists, chiropractors, energy healers, and so on). The neurologist, psychologist, psychiatrist, or other specialist most qualified to make the diagnosis too often represents the "last resort."

If you are a parent who believes an alternative approach to treatment is best for your child, you should still consider getting a sound medical diagnosis. Receiving a diagnosis from, say, a pediatric neurologist does not obligate you to follow the treatment course this doctor will suggest. Conversely, although the alternative treatment your child receives may prove beneficial to him, the practitioner providing it is probably not trained or qualified to accurately diagnose Asperger Syndrome and/or its related comorbid conditions.

• • •

Say What?

When considering the dozens of descriptions various specialists have been known to apply to persons with AS, we could not help but recall the parable about the blind men and the elephant, in which each man identified the elephant as a different animal depending on which part of it he felt. Often specialists see and identify only the facet of AS that pertains to their area of expertise. Having been identified as having any of these does not exclude your child from having AS.

> One doctor's Asperger Syndrome
> is another doctor's PDD-NOS
> is yet another doctor's high-functioning autism
> is a speech pathologist's semantic-pragmatic disorder
> is an educational consultant's nonverbal learning disability
> is a psychologist's personality disorder
> is an audiologist's central auditory processing disorder
> is an occupational therapist's sensory integration disorder.

Although we have seen an increased awareness among professionals, you may still come across one or more without much experience with Asperger Syndrome. The result can be a diagnosis that correctly identifies one or a few facets of the syndrome but fails to account for the big picture or the interrelationship between different aspects. Some professionals feel that an individual can be diagnosed only if he or she exactly matches the diagnostic criteria. To illustrate this point, let's look at two different doctors and their diagnosis of Johnny at age six.

Dr. A has not seen many children with AS and makes diagnoses strictly by the book. He may see that Johnny presents with severe and pervasive social impairment and an unusual, all-absorbing interest. However, Johnny is also very talkative, and though his conversational style seems a little bit odd, he forms full sentences, uses pronouns properly, and has an amazing vocabulary for his age. Johnny may also have fairly good gaze moderation. In addition, Johnny has other factors that help explain some of his problems. He is an only child who, due to chronic asthma, did not attend nursery school or preschool (perhaps explaining his social difficulties). As for Johnny's intense interest in astronomy, Dr. A finds it precocious and somewhat overwhelming, but he also suspects that Johnny is an overindulged child who is resorting to a familiar topic because he is uncomfortable in the doctor's office. Dr. A regards the one instance of literalism he sees—Johnny looking apprehensive when Dr. A's nurse remarks, "I'm running to lunch now. I'm so hungry I could eat a horse"—as mildly amusing. Dr. A sees nothing unusual in Johnny's motor clumsiness: "After all, not every child can grow up to be an Olympic gymnast," he tells Johnny's mother. "And once he's in school and starts writing and drawing more, he'll pick it right up."

Like almost all pediatricians, Dr. A likes children and appreciates them as individuals. Based on what he learned during his training, Dr. A is averse to "alarming parents unnecessarily" and subjecting children to tests and evaluations they may not need. In his many years of practice, he has seen children with similar or even more troubling behaviors who grew up "just fine." He has also seen patients whose behaviors were treated inappropriately with negative results, so he tends to err on the conservative side. Although at Johnny's mother's behest, he reads the diagnostic criteria for AS and admits that Johnny's behaviors fit some of them, he believes that there is enough about Johnny that either does not fit or is not addressed by the criteria that he cannot make a diagnosis. "Johnny is still very young. Let's just wait and see."

Johnny's parents believe in second opinions, so they take him to see Dr. B.

Dr. B, who trained at a major university hospital, now treats a number of children diagnosed with AS and serves as a consultant to several local school districts on cases such as Johnny's. Unlike Dr. A, Dr. B knows from experience that the strict diagnostic criteria as presented in DSM-IV-TR do not tell the whole story. Dr. B is less concerned with the individual symptoms and behaviors Johnny shows than with the overall pattern they form. In contrast to Dr. A, Dr. B takes into account Johnny's motor clumsiness and literal-mindedness (neither of which is stated in the DSM-IV-TR criteria but are common among persons with AS). Unimpressed by Johnny's expressive language skills, Dr. B sets up toys in his office and engages him in a couple of play activities to test his theory of mind. He asks Johnny to describe what a friend is ("Someone who does everything that I want to do and loves dinosaurs") and what someone means when they say "hop in the car" or, if he were older, "kill two birds with one stone." Based on what he sees, Dr. B makes the diagnosis of AS and/or refers Johnny for further neuropsychological testing, which will expose the language and communication deficits behind Johnny's precocious use of language as well as pinpoint the nature and extent of his motor skills deficiencies.

We all approach the diagnostic process differently. Parents whose children have already been properly diagnosed often feel that Dr. B is the hero. However, in that twilight time between first suspecting a child has a problem and the final confirmation, some parents might find Dr. B too "aggressive," too willing to "pathologize" unusual but "normal enough" behaviors that Johnny may well grow out of, given more time around other kids, more practice with motor skill tasks, and maturity. Some parents may actually prefer Dr. A to Dr. B, because he seems more understanding, more accepting of Johnny as he is.

Patty recalls how thrilled she was when a pediatric neurologist assured her that all Justin needed to overcome his problems was occupational therapy. "Even though I suspected that there was much more to Justin's problems than OT could ever address, I couldn't help clinging to some of the terms the doctor used, like *outgrow* and *catch up*. I'll never forget saying to a friend, 'If the doctor did not give him a diagnosis, how bad a problem could it possibly be?' " She saw in her "Dr. A" someone who was more optimistic about her son's possible prognosis than she expected another doctor might be. Looking back now, she considers Dr. A seriously uninformed.

In contrast, Barb's early attempts to discuss her child's difficulties with professionals, family, and friends met with well-meaning suggestions to either "relax," "stop looking for problems," or rethink her parenting approach. It's not at all uncommon for families who visit OASIS to describe how they knew something was amiss but couldn't convince anyone that there was a problem that couldn't be resolved by changing how they parented their children.

Even those of us who acknowledge there is a serious problem often hope that another explanation exists. Carolyn, whose child eluded correct diagnosis, recalls how she subconsciously welcomed teachers and doctors who made comments to the effect that her son's problems all stemmed from her "poor parenting skills." "I don't want to say that I was pleased to hear that, because I wasn't. However, as long as I believed that, it meant that there was nothing really wrong with Stephen," she says. "Knowing that if the fault lay entirely with me, I could change, things could get better."

Particularly in the early years, some of us may see our child's differences and idiosyncrasies as just that. We interpret any suggestion that he or she "should be more like the other kids" as misguided pressure to conform for the sake of conformity. "Whenever someone remarked on Evan's obsession with trains, I remember thinking to myself, *Well, at least he isn't into that violent Power Rangers stuff, like the other kids,*" Marie recalls. "What I didn't understand then was that people weren't really commenting on Evan's preference for trains but the unusual quality of it."

ALL IN THE FAMILY?

Finally, we know that children with AS often come from families in which other members have AS or AS-type traits. Many experts now believe that there exists what is known as a broader autistic phenotype (BAP)—essentially, autistic tendencies that are milder, less numerous, or have less adverse impact on the individual's ability to function than those of autism itself. (See chapter 1 for a discussion of the genetics of autism.)

If you have read up on AS and started questioning some of your own behaviors or those of other family members, you are not alone. It's not unusual for a parent to be diagnosed as having AS or a related disorder in the wake of a child's diagnosis. Some experts suggest that a parent or other family member having AS traits or AS itself can be a unique source of support and understanding.

You, your spouse, or other relatives may share some of the same characteristics your child has. If your child counts among her relatives a grandfather who is emotionally distant but a brilliant mechanic, a cousin whose single-minded interest in dinosaurs landed him a scholarship and a plum job at a major museum, or an uncle with an odd yet refreshing *Monty Python*–esque take on the world, you may be less likely to be alarmed by similar behaviors in your child, or, for that matter, in yourself or your spouse. Mark, whose son wasn't diagnosed until age twelve, despite the fact that his problems were obvious from age five, explained why he delayed diagnosis: "What was the point of having my son tested and labeled? He was doing okay in school and he spent all his free time on the computer—just like millions of boys his age, and exactly like his uncle Ivan. True, he didn't have any friends, and his tantrums grew worse over time. But as my mother keeps reminding me, I was a lot like that myself. I just couldn't understand why he had to have a label. Elliot was just Elliot. What was it going to change? We knew who he was and what he was about."

On the other side of the table, there are professionals who may be reluctant to press you to pursue a diagnosis, albeit for very different reasons. Teachers, pediatricians, therapists, and others who have had the unenviable task of informing a parent that they believed a child's behavior or development warranted further evaluation may be reticent to broach the subject. They tell of parents who become angry, hostile, and even abusive.

IS YOUR CHILD'S PEDIATRICIAN OR FAMILY DOCTOR ABLE TO MAKE A DIAGNOSIS?

If your child's doctor was in training anytime prior to the mid-1980s, he probably learned that autism was extremely rare, and he probably had never heard of AS. If he was in medical school a decade later, he still might not expect to see more than a handful of cases of autism in his career. Depending on your doctor's age and the particulars of his training, he may have learned many things about PDDs, autism, and Asperger Syndrome that we now know are untrue. He may still assume that autism spectrum disorders (ASDs) are "rare," the product of poor parenting, essentially untreatable and hopeless, and easily identified. Don't be surprised if your child's pediatrician or your family practitioner tells you she has never heard of Asperger Syndrome.

If you have concerns about your child, resist the temptation to read your child's doctor's seeming lack of concern or her suggestion that you "wait and see" as an all-clear signal. It may not be. A physician may have concerns about a child's behavior or development, but it's hard to press for an evaluation if, for example, a parent insists that everything is going pretty well in kindergarten or that little Jessica is screaming because she just "hates" going to the doctor (as many kids do). Also remember that the doctor's office is a place that many children associate with unpleasant events such as injections and illness. Children with AS, ASDs, and sensory integration issues may be particularly tense, anxious, upset, prone to tantruming, quiet, loud, or generally misbehaving simply because they're reacting to the smells, sounds, lights, and textures they experience there. However, they may appear to be responding not that differently from typical children.

If your child's doctor does raise concerns with you, take them seriously. Some doctors will press forcefully for an evaluation at the first sign of unusual behavior. However, some doctors see things differently. These doctors may be more comfortable (some would say too comfortable) taking a "wait and see" approach. Others may feel that even some widely accepted conditions such as attention-deficit/hyperactivity disorder (ADHD) "pathologize" behaviors that they believe should be considered within the broad range of normal childhood development. Others may truly believe that your child will outgrow a sensitivity to being touched or to the smell of fresh eggs. Finally, your doctor, like Dr. A in the earlier example, simply may have been undertrained in this particular area.

If you feel that your doctor isn't taking your concerns about your child seriously, continue to press the issue. Insist on a referral for private evaluation, or contact your school district about having your child evaluated, even—and especially—if the doctor is unwilling to cooperate. Change doctors, if necessary. Whatever you do, don't give up.

IN SCHOOL

Chances are that most teachers at regular nursery schools, pre-schools, and kindergartens do not have training in special education issues. There, teachers routinely deal with children who experience problems with separation anxiety, crying, tantrums, reluctance to share with peers, difficulty following directions, parallel play, and poor socialization skills. Most children will learn to adjust to a class-room environment, although there are always late bloomers, and any experienced, knowledgeable teacher will make allowances for them. Under these circumstances, many teachers are reluctant to voice their concerns about a particular child's behavior or responses, but if they do so, you should listen.

Today we know that the pre- and early school years are prime time for identifying Asperger Syndrome and starting appropriate interventions. Ironically, this is also the period in a child's life when he is least likely to be viewed as having a serious neurologically based problem and most likely viewed as "socially immature" or having a "behavior problem." Young children often behave very differently at home, sur-rounded by parents and family, than they do outside of the home. The fact that day care or school is for them a "new environment" makes it easy for everyone, but especially parents, to attribute any problems to that. Parents know that some children arrive at certain developmental milestones later than others, and that sometimes it just takes certain children a little longer to "grow out" of a behavior. There is also the prevailing notion that boys are developmentally and emotionally "be-hind" in some areas simply because they are boys. You may have seen this with another of your children or perhaps even yourself. It may be difficult to sort out which behaviors warrant further attention.

Children in public school settings have a small advantage, in that even if their teachers lack special education training, they have ready access to special education teachers, administrators, and therapists within their district, and probably even within the school building, who do.

Sometimes the problems teachers raise don't strike parents as serious. One parent recalls, "I remember listening to the preschool teacher and thinking to myself, *Is it really such a big deal that he hates to touch finger paints or finds the kiddie music they play during snack time so annoying he has to cover his ears?* I thought she was overreacting." Another parent says, "I knew she couldn't use scissors or write very well at age four, compared to the other kids. But my wife and I talked it over, and we thought of all the things we had done late as kids, and concluded that perhaps this prekindergarten program was a little too goal-oriented and competitive for our daughter."

A woman who has worked for over a decade as a special educator offered this insight into why teachers may not be totally candid in discussing their suspicions with parents: "For some parents, the very suggestion that their child be evaluated is enough to set off a flurry of unpleasant letters to the teacher, the principal, the superintendent, and the entire board of ed. Sometimes their attitude is 'If you were doing your job teaching, she wouldn't have these problems.' Other times, it's 'Who are you to say that there's something wrong with my child? Look at [name another child] and his behavior.' One parent even said, 'How can you say that? You're not a child development expert.' And my answer to that was, 'You're right. I'm not a child development expert. And that is why I feel that your son should be evaluated by someone who is.' "

— • • • —

Warning Signs and Inadequate Diagnosis

Has your child been adequately evaluated? Are the results obtained and conclusions drawn about your child accurate? Here are some warning flags to watch for as you go through the process:

• *Professional lack of experience with AS.* You may encounter professionals who either have never heard of AS or who have had little or no experience with people who have it. An evaluator who fails to ask about your child's social behavior or who dismisses your concerns about stereotypies, noise sensitivity, or literal-mindedness probably will not provide the best assessment. You could provide him or her with selected publications, papers, videos, as well as information on respected AS-related Web sites, including OASIS. On the other hand, given the fact that for initial diagnosis you really do want someone with expertise, if it is practical, it might be better to simply move on.

• *A diagnosis or description of your child that either does not fit or fails to account for certain behaviors and symptoms.* Many of the behaviors and symptoms that accompany AS can look like other conditions or disorders. If you believe that those evaluating your child are going off track, have materials on hand and be prepared to point out how you believe your child's symptoms differ from, say, ADHD, or how a diagnosis may be a comorbid condition but does not explain other behaviors and deficits. If your evaluator seems to be ignoring the symptoms and behaviors that don't fit the diagnosis he seems to have his heart set on, press him on why he believes those behaviors are inconsequential or should not be considered.

• *An attitude that reveals a lack of understanding of autism spectrum disorders.* People with Asperger Syndrome can be difficult to "read" for someone unfamiliar with the syndrome. As you surely know by now, it's not easy for people unfamiliar with AS and other PDDs to appreciate the degree to which some of our children's behaviors and symptoms are literally beyond their control. Often, our children appear to be "too bright" or "old enough to know better." If you believe that the person evaluating your child simply doesn't get it, consider stopping the evaluation and requesting a different evaluator and/or team. Signs that this may be the case include the evaluator indicating that behaviors that you know are beyond your child's control are willful ("I know he could do a better job of writing if he just put his mind to it"; "He needs to learn to ignore the noise from outside"), the result of poor parenting ("I guess he's used to getting his way at home"; "She's too old to be sucking her thumb"), or manipulative ("I guess he knows that if he screams long enough, Mom will come running").

• *Stating or indicating that Asperger Syndrome is not a "legitimate" diagnosis or that it is the diagnostic equivalent of the flavor of the month.* Signs of this include inappropriate editorializing along the lines of "Ten years ago, we never heard of this. Suddenly everyone seems to have it"; "I guess parents just like this label better than autism"; or "You know lots of people consider some PDDs a sort of 'trashcan diagnosis.'" If your evaluator makes these kinds of comments, find another one.

• *Beating around the bush, pussyfooting, offering prognoses that are either extremely positive or extremely negative, inability to describe in detail resources available to you.* Because Asperger Syndrome is related to autism, professionals unfamiliar with the range of interventions and treatments available may opt to "spare" you the emotional trauma of a "hopeless" diagnosis. Some will say that they don't believe in labeling children early or that they feel that as long as the problems are being addressed, "it doesn't matter what you call them." Others may prefer the "wait and see" approach. Finally, there are those who honestly feel that a child who does not ring every diagnostic criteria bell is better described as having "Asperger-like tendencies," "PDD-type issues," or some such non-diagnosis. You may be able to circumvent this by letting these professionals know that your top priority is getting your child correctly diagnosed—no matter what that diagnosis may be—and getting the appropriate treatment as soon as possible. Tell them that you are aware that AS and PDDs are related to autism. Also let them know that you are counting on them for the correct and direct diagnosis that will spur the appropriate treatment and intervention your child needs now.

• Remember also that Asperger Syndrome cannot always be fully "diagnosed" through the type of evaluations commonly conducted by school districts. Asperger Syndrome is a medical diagnosis, not a learning disability or profile. Although a psychoeducational evaluation can reveal a range of problems common to AS—problems with semantics and pragmatics, fine- and gross-motor skills, non-verbal learning disability, and so on—there is no single test for AS. If your child is being evaluated through your school district, the evaluations should be conducted by a team of experts from all relevant disciplines. (See box "School District Evaluations," page 94, and chapter 8.)

STARTING THE PROCESS

Your goal is to find at least one professional who knows Asperger Syndrome. How do you find someone with that kind of experience? While we cannot tell you exactly where to find such a person, we can give you some tips on increasing the likelihood that you will. A university-affiliated teaching hospital will probably have on staff more doctors specializing in pediatric psychology, neurology, and psychiatry than your local community hospital. Your access to these people and institutions may be compromised or restricted by geography, your health insurance coverage (or lack thereof), and other factors. We would argue that this might be one area where it would be worthwhile to travel for a consultation or pay out of pocket for an "uncovered" evaluation.

Given how much depends on an accurate diagnosis, try not to think of it simply as another consultation or doctor's appointment but as an investment in your child's future, the cornerstone upon which everything else will be built. Regardless of the diagnosis you receive, you, your spouse, your family, your school district, and the other professionals working with your child will be expending time, resources (financial and otherwise), and energy on your child's behalf. Through it all, probably no one will work harder toward those goals than your child. A diagnosis will not only help you visualize your child's destination, it can help you choose the best, safest, and easiest route to get there.

•••

School District Evaluations

The federal Individuals with Disabilities Education Act (IDEA) demands that every school district identify and evaluate every child within its jurisdiction from age three to age twenty-two suspected of having a disability. This includes children who are still too young to attend school and those who currently attend private schools, parochial, or religious schools, or are home-schooled. Under IDEA, autism and related disorders are considered disabilities. These evaluations are free of cost to parents, and most doctors, educators, and other professionals who share their concerns about your child will suggest you contact your school district. Don't be surprised if the person recommending you contact your school district knows little about the process from that point forward.

Some parents are understandably hesitant to approach their school district's special education office. They worry that their child will be "labeled," for example, or that their child's disability will become part of her record or become public knowledge. You may opt to postpone alerting your school district and requesting a district evaluation until after you've had your child assessed privately. However, IDEA requires school districts to provide special education and related services to disabled children. Provision of such education and/or services will be determined by an evaluation your school district performs. In other words, your child probably will undergo a school district evaluation sooner or later anyway.

The quality of school district evaluations, like that of special education programs generally, can vary from district to district. Initial evaluations should involve a multidisciplinary team and produce independent written reports outlining each evaluator's general impressions of your child, the tests administered, and the resulting scores. These reports will also include information on the child's behavior and demeanor during the evaluation and some general concluding remarks. You have a right to read and receive copies of all evaluations and to correct errors of fact you may find in them.

Parents are sometimes surprised to learn that these evaluations do not offer medical diagnoses or always outline specific recommendations. An evaluation may conclude with a recommendation that "occupational therapy is indicated," but it will not say, "Sally should have four half-hour sessions of occupational therapy with Mrs. Smith." School district evaluations are obviously limited in making determinations about a child's neurological and psychiatric issues, and they cannot produce an official medical diagnosis. Some school districts hire outside practitioners, special education schools, or other institutions to conduct their evaluations; other school districts have the evaluations done by school or staff psychologists or special education teachers.

School districts differ on their policies, and state special education laws also vary. Your location may necessarily limit your options in terms of where your child can be evaluated initially at school district expense.

We also find that some school districts are more reasonable, flexible, and generous than others. For more information on IDEA and schools, see chapter 8.

Where to Start

Ask the doctor, teacher, or school district administrator who is recommending that your child have an evaluation for a referral to a specialist. Note their suggestions, but be prepared to research other possible candidates. Unless you're told that the person being recommended to you specializes in PDDs and/or AS, you'll have to keep looking. This is especially important if you believe that, beyond the core symptoms of AS, your child also has problems that suggest other disorders or learning disabilities. When you receive a recommendation, ask the following questions:

- Why do you feel this is the best person to evaluate my child?
- How long have you been referring patients/students to this person?
- Can you tell me what you know about this person's qualifications or expertise in PDDs, ASDs, and AS?
- Can you tell me anything about this person's manner and how well he relates to children like mine?
- Have you referred other children with issues similar to my child's to this person?

Don't be entirely surprised if you find out that the person making the recommendation knows little about the professional he is recommending. Some doctors and school district personnel use one or a few evaluators because that's simply how they do things or there are few alternatives in your area. Your doctor may have to limit referrals to those professionals who participate in your health insurance plan. Your school district administrator may be obligated to provide you a list of possible evaluators but be prohibited from steering you away from those who do substandard evaluations or have less experience in a particular area. If you feel confident that the professional being recommended to you is the right person, your search can end. However, even with a glowing recommendation in hand, you may still wish to seek out other options or learn more about the professional you have already decided to use. It's time to broaden the search.

You may feel as if you are the only person in the world coping with Asperger Syndrome. You are not. Chances are, there are other parents in your county, your town, your school district, perhaps even your own neighborhood who have a child with AS or a related disorder. Other parents are a great resource, because they've been where you are right now. Most people you will contact through disability-related support organizations, Special Education PTA (SEPTA), and online resources are parents of a child with a disability as well. Chances are good that these parents and groups can provide useful information on the different practitioners, institutions, and resources in your area. Further, they may be more forthcoming and candid than professionals in their assessments of possible evaluators.

Who to See, Where to Go

Psychologist, psychiatrist, neurologist, neuropsychologist, developmental pediatrician, pediatric psychologist, pediatric psychiatrist, pediatric neurologist, pediatrician, family doctor, psychotherapist—what they all have in common is that they are all, theoretically, qualified to diagnose Asperger Syndrome. Anyone in any of those fields, with the right education and experience, should be able to recognize AS. That said, there are important differences among each of these specialties in terms of education, training, licensing requirements, and the types of interventions and treatments the specialists are most likely to recommend. If a pediatrician and a pediatric psychiatrist, for example, can both diagnose, how do you decide which might be most appropriate for your child? Here are the players.

Pediatrician or general family practitioner. A pediatrician is an M.D. who specializes in the care of children from infancy through the teen years. Most pediatricians are general practitioners. Generally, a pediatrician refers to other specialists patients who have or are suspected of having more serious or chronic problems. Although pediatricians are experts in normal child development and most do some developmental screening in the course of regular care, several recent studies have revealed that they do not generally receive adequate training in recognizing signs of developmental disorders. At the same time, a benefit of the increasing prevalence of AS and related disorders is that there are pediatricians who are known within their communities for being better informed and more attuned to working with children and families facing these disorders. Ask other parents you know for recommendations; you may indeed find a "specialist."

Pediatricians can prescribe psychoactive (mind-altering) medication, but treating AS-related symptoms can involve new medications, some of which may not be FDA-approved for pediatric use and/or may have potentially serious side effects. (For more on prescription psychotropic medications, see chapter 7.) Unless your pediatrician specializes in treating children with AS and related disorders or has a number of such patients in her practice, you might consider consulting with a neurologist, psychiatrist, or other medical specialist when it comes to medication decisions.

Developmental pediatrician. A developmental pediatrician is a pediatrician who specializes in child development. If you've never heard of this relatively new subspecialty, you're not alone. There are about one thousand of them throughout the United States, but if possible, you might consider a developmental pediatrician for your child's primary care. In addition to the three years' training in general pediatrics, developmental pediatricians devote an additional two or three years to training in the evaluation and care of children with developmental issues, so they're more familiar with different forms of therapy, intervention, and special education options.

Neurologist, pediatric neurologist. Neurology is the medical science devoted to the study and treatment of the nervous system (which includes the brain). Pediatric neurologists are neurologists who specialize in children. Neurology is a physical science in the sense that it is concerned with the actual "hardware" of the brain as opposed to behavioral issues and interventions. Among the specialists listed here, neurologists are the most qualified to evaluate problems involving motor skills, balance, vision, speech, cognition, and adaptive behavior, among others. They are trained in diagnostic technology, such as electroencephalography (EEG), computer-assisted tomography (CAT scan), and magnetic resonance imaging (MRI), to name a few tools that are not yet routinely used in Asperger evaluation but might be indicated to rule out other possible problems (seizures, tumors, etc.). A neuropsychological evaluation (or *neuropsyche,* for short) can combine standardized assessment with psychological screening and diagnostic medical testing to create a multidisciplinary profile. Because only a complete neuropsychological workup can identify underlying and complicating problems (for example, seizure disorder, dyslexia, problems with motor skills, congenital neurological problems), it's considered the gold standard of diagnostic testing.

Psychologist, pediatric psychologist, neuropsychologist, pediatric neuropsychologist. In most states, a psychologist holds a doctorate degree in psychology or a related field. Pediatric psychologists specialize in children. Neuropsychologists focus on the relationship between the brain and behavior. Unlike psychiatrists and neurologists, psychologists and neuropsychologists are not M.D.s. They aren't trained to administer or interpret diagnostic medical tests, nor can they write prescriptions. Some psychologists do make recommendations regarding medication and may work with a consulting psychiatrist who actually writes the prescription and monitors the child periodically. Psychologists can see children for ongoing psychological therapy and provide guidance in helping children cope with emotional issues and, in some cases, socialization skills. They can also perform psychological evaluations, and some are trained to administer standard educational assessments. Such evaluations can be very useful, and school districts commonly refer children to psychologists and pediatric psychologists. However, because Asperger Syndrome is a complex neurological disorder, a purely psychological or educational evaluation may not capture the full diagnostic "picture" or identify or rule out neurological issues. Neuropsychologists, because of their extensive training in noninvasive means of determining neurological function, may be preferred. A neuropsychologist may perform a neuropsychological evaluation and refer the child to a neurologist if medical testing (e.g., MRI, EEG) is indicated.

Psychiatrist, pediatric psychiatrist. A psychiatrist is an M.D. who specializes in emotional and psychological disorders and mental health. A pediatric psychiatrist specializes in children. Perhaps to a greater extent than any other specialty, psychiatrists combine an understanding of the biology and the psychology behind thinking and behavior. Psychiatrists can order and interpret medical diagnostic tests and write prescriptions.

Psychotherapist, therapist, social worker, mental health counselor, family therapist, etc. These professionals all hold a graduate degree in the mental health field. Because licensing requirements vary widely from state to state, it is difficult to make a general statement about their qualifications. However, in most cases, any of these professionals can see private clients and offer counseling in much the same way a psychologist would. They cannot order or interpret medical tests; nor can they write prescriptions. If you are considering having your child evaluated by someone in these professions, you should find out precisely what training he or she has received in conducting evaluations.

BEFORE THE EVALUATION

It's not always easy to have your child evaluated. The first, natural impulse is to do all you can to make your child look, perform, and behave as well as he possibly can. However, there is no way to "prepare" your child for this type of testing beyond making sure that he is well rested and comfortable. In order for children to qualify for special education services, they must demonstrate a substantial deficiency in one or more areas related to education. Typically, children with Asperger Syndrome present a mixed picture because of their normal to high IQs and seemingly well-developed speech. Unfortunately, these strengths combined with an evaluator's inexperience and failure to test for or take into account typical Asperger-related deficits (such as problems with semantics and pragmatics or sensory and fine-motor problems) may result in an evaluation that does not identify the real issues. (See boxes in this chapter on "Comorbidity" and "Learning Disorders Commonly Seen with AS.")

Prior to an evaluation, you may be asked to fill out forms on your child's medical, developmental, and educational history. You may also be asked to complete a standard assessment questionnaire designed to elicit information on your child's behavior and development. There may be additional copies enclosed, with instructions that one be completed by your spouse and, possibly, your child's current teacher. If you and your spouse are each asked to complete separate questionnaires, do so independently, without consulting each other until you're finished. You will probably want to "compare notes" once you're done, but resist the temptation to change your answers later. Even a seeming discrepancy in your answers—say, you answered that your son's tantrums were "often violent" and your husband qualified them as "sometimes" so—can provide useful information.

Your child's developmental history is important to any diagnosis. Be prepared to consult your child's "baby book" and perhaps your home video collection and family photographs for accurate information on developmental milestones and other behaviors. Another critical source is your child's pediatrician, who will have kept a full, contemporaneous record of your child's developmental progress, screening results, illnesses, and disorders. This is an excellent opportunity to request a copy of your child's entire file from her pediatrician. A letter or written report from your child's pediatrician is also useful. If you aren't specifically requested to provide one, consider asking your pediatrician for one anyway. Any input from other professionals who know or have worked with your child, including teachers, should be welcomed by the person or team who will conduct the evaluation.

Although you may not be asked to provide it, consider also getting letters about your child from previous teachers, if possible. Especially if your child is older, such retrospective reports from teachers or caregivers over time can give the evaluator a more detailed (and perhaps more objective) picture of your child's development.

You may also want to write a letter—with salient points boldfaced for easy reference—outlining your child's history and the progress of his problems as you have seen them. Unfortunately, the evaluation process is focused on identifying what is "wrong"; you can write about the positive aspects as well. Write briefly about your child's interests, successful social interactions, what he enjoys doing, his general temperament, and his personality. You may want to include a photo in the file. If your child is currently in school (including nursery school or preschool), collect in a three-ring binder copies of written work, drawings (particularly if your child seems to have motor skills issues), a list of books he's reading (if applicable), and anything else you believe will be helpful.

In the best of all worlds, the people who conduct these sensitive and important evaluations would avail themselves of the opportunity to observe each child in his home and in his school or day care environment. We know that children with Asperger Syndrome can behave quite differently from one situation to the next. Much could be learned by simply contrasting a child's emotional closeness with his family to his social isolation among his peers, for example. While some professionals do venture out to gather this information, many do not. If you think it is important that your child be observed at school or at home as part of the evaluation, say so.

CONFIDENTIALITY CONCERNS

During the evaluation process, you may be asked questions that are quite personal regarding the family history of emotional or psychological problems, learning disabilities, alcoholism, substance abuse, suicide, arrests and/or convictions, and so on. In most cases, these questions will concern not only you, your spouse, and your child's siblings but aunts, uncles, cousins, and grandparents on both sides of the family. Legally, this information must be kept confidential. However, for various reasons, you may not feel comfortable revealing personal information, particularly concerning other family members' personal lives. If that is the case, or if you fear someone's reputation, employment, or insurance status may be compromised or threatened by such revelations, don't answer those questions in writing. When you meet with the evaluator, explain your concerns and be prepared to let the evaluator know orally, without giving names, if there is a history of learning disability, autism, Asperger Syndrome, autism spectrum disorders, Tourette's syndrome, epilepsy or seizure, depression, anxiety disorder, obsessive disorder, compulsive disorder, obsessive-compulsive disorder, violence, alcoholism, drug abuse, or some conduct disorder.

Some parents feel more comfortable sharing this information with a private practitioner than with a school district evaluation team. One mother we know found a pediatric neurologist whose written report was informative without being needlessly revealing. She explained orally to the doctor her family's history of alcoholism, depression, violence, and that one of the child's uncles had an extensive juvenile record. Having recently moved to a small community, she was concerned that this information was prejudicial, especially in light of her son's sometimes violent tantrums. In his written report to the school district, the neurologist merely acknowledged that "family history may be a factor" without offering any further detail.

PREPARING YOUR CHILD FOR THE EVALUATION

Your child's evaluation may be conducted in a quiet room at his current school by a special education teacher or school psychologist in just an hour or two. It may involve several days of tests at the pediatric or child development or neurology department of a local hospital or university medical center. Your child may be diagnosed on the basis of parent and teacher questionnaires, extensive interviews with you and your spouse, and a few play-therapy sessions. Or your child may be observed at home and/or in school in addition to being tested. Whatever the circumstances, there are ways you can help your child and yourself to feel more comfortable.

• Get clear directions and make a "test run" days before the first appointment to be sure you know where you'll be going.
• If you think it may help your child, arrange for him to visit the testing place ahead of time and, if possible, meet the person or people who will administer the tests.
• Find out beforehand how long each session will run, what kinds of materials your child will be asked to work with (blocks, patterns, puppets, dolls, board games, beads, etc.), and what he may be asked to do (hop, tell a story, listen to a story or to a tape and then answer questions about it, remember words, count, read, build, etc.).
• If at all possible, find out the sequence of the tasks your child will be asked to perform and where the testing will occur. Your goal is not to "prepare" your child for the test; that is impossible. But you will circumvent much of your child's anxiety by being able to say, "First, you and Dr. M will work with blocks, and then she will ask

you to listen to a short story. . . ." If you're not sure what will happen, say so, but add, "These people are really nice, and they will show you lots of cool new things and ask you to play with them, or hear some nice stories." If your child is old enough to associate the terms *test* and *evaluation* with tests given in schools, be sure to explain that these are different because there are no right or wrong answers. You might explain that the person who gives these tests is really trying to "see how you do things in your own way."

• Find out where you'll be during the tests. In the same room? In an adjoining room watching through a two-way mirror? In the waiting room? Discuss with the evaluator beforehand what will occur if your child asks for you, panics, or has a tantrum. Be sure that the person conducting the evaluation understands the warning signs for extreme distress or meltdown. Also be sure that everyone understands that if your child asks for you, you will be allowed to see him.

• Find out if your child will be allowed to have water, juice, or a snack with him, if you think he may need it.

• If at all possible, schedule the testing for when your child will be fresh, well rested, and not hungry. (An exception would be certain medical tests, such as an EEG, for which your child may need to be sleep-deprived.)

• For most children, morning works best. You know your child's limitations. If you know he won't tolerate a three-hour testing session, request that it be broken into two separate sessions. Also be aware that even if your child is not especially stressed or exhausted by the testing (for most, it's actually fun), it's a novel situation. Consider keeping your child home for the rest of the school day or going out for a special outing or treat afterward, especially if there will be further testing and he emerges from the first round a less than happy camper.

• Make the evaluator aware—orally and in writing—of anything that might affect your child's performance: medications (including over-the-counter products such as antihistamines, cough syrup, and of course prescription medication), recent or current illnesses (cold, flu, tummy ache, etc.), chronic health problems (asthma, etc.), or any changes in sleep schedule.

• Make the evaluator aware—orally and in writing—of your child's sensory issues: problems with noise in general, particular sounds, fluorescent lighting, particular smells, textures, or types of environments. If your child is fascinated by or obsessed with Thomas the Tank Engine, coins, black crayons; is repulsed by the texture of clay, or the smell of Play-Doh or felt-tip markers; or gets panicky in large, uncarpeted, "echoey" rooms, let your evaluator know. This way, the evaluator can modify your child's tests so that, for example, he does not become upset when asked to relinquish the treasured black crayon.

Plan to give yourself and your child plenty of time to arrive on the day of the evaluation with some time to spare. As anxious as you might feel, try to exude an air of casual confidence and be loving and attentive toward your child. Answer all of his questions, no matter how many times he asks. If it will short-circuit a brewing tantrum, give in to his needs, if the issue isn't a serious one. On the other hand, if your child wakes up not feeling well or having had a bad night with little or no rest, consider canceling for that day and rescheduling.

WHAT TYPES OF TESTS WILL BE GIVEN?

There is no one single standardized test for AS, though there are now a number of scales available for helping determine whether a person might have AS. Even if there were a single test for AS, anyone suspected of having AS would still require further evaluation for common problems such as learning disabilities, graphomotor problems (having to do with the physical act of writing), processing deficits, and psychological issues, to name only a few of the possibilities. A thorough evaluation will explore every area of concern. The publishers of standardized assessment instruments are constantly releasing new instruments and revising those currently available. It would be impossible to list every single test that might be administered to your child. However, the tests administered should address the areas listed here. We also list a few examples of each type of test. These are not necessarily the only tests of this type, nor are they necessarily the most appropriate test for your child. That determination will be made by your evaluator(s). Also note that most of the test examples listed are designed for school-age learners.

In assessing your child, evaluators will probably focus on these main areas:

Intelligence: an assessment of your child's ability to learn and to behave adaptively, or in response to situations of daily living. The best and most widely used intelligence tests assess and measure a wide range of abilities and deficits. Contrary to popular misconception, IQ is not necessarily a measure of "how smart" someone is, though it is reasonable to assume that someone with a normal IQ of 100 probably learns more easily and is better able to apply what he learns than does someone with an IQ of 80. It is helpful to view IQ testing and the resulting scores as an indication of a person's ability to learn, and learning requires skills in perception, memory, recall, organization, and generally making sense of what one experiences. So a good IQ test assesses and measures "social judgment, level of thinking, language skills, perceptual organization, processing speed, spatial abilities, common sense, long- and short-term memory, abstract thinking, motor speed, and word knowledge."[13] In addition, most comprehensive IQ tests generate scores in subsets, which are usually divided between those that assess verbal skills and those that assess nonverbal skills. Some subtests for verbal skills in the Wechsler test include arithmetic, sentences, and general information; for performance (or nonverbal skills), some examples include picture completion, object assembly, geometric design, and mazes.

Some of the most widely used IQ tests include Wechsler Scales of Intelligence (WISC; there are special tests designed for specific age groups), Stanford-Binet Intelligence Scale, 4th Edition (SBIS-4), Kaufman Assessment Battery for Children (K-ABC), and Kaufman Brief Intelligence Test (KBIT).

Academic achievement: an assessment of your child's academic progress, or what he has learned, skills he has acquired. Academic achievement tests can be designed to assess specific skills or areas (such as those listed below), or they can cover several academic areas.

• Reading skills: Gray Oral Reading Test–3 (GORT-3), Slosson Oral Reading Test–Revised (SORT-R), Woodcock Reading Mastery Tests–Revised (WRMT-R), Test of Reading Comprehension, 3rd Edition (TORC-3)
• Math skills: Stanford Diagnostic Mathemetics Test–4 (SDMT-4), Test of Early Mathematics Ability–2 (TEMA-2)

- Written language skills: Test of Early Written Language–2 (TEWL-2), Written Expression Scale (WES), Test of Written Expression (TOWE), Writing Process Test (WPT)
- Spelling: Test of Written Spelling–4 (TWS-4)
- Comprehensive Achievement Tests, tests that assess several areas of academic achievement at once: Test of Academic Achievement Skills–Revised (TAAS-R)

Behavior/psychological: an assessment of your child's behavior; this may include psychological tests and scales to assess conditions such as ADHD. There are literally hundreds of tests available, but among those that are commonly used for individuals on the autism spectrum is the Vineland Adaptive Behavior Scale (VABS), which many experts in the field consider a required assessment. Depending on your child, she may also be evaluated for possible comorbid conditions such as ADHD (the Conners' Parent and Teacher Rating Scales is a popular instrument). Your child may also be asked to draw pictures, tell a story, or play with toys or dolls or puppets.

Perceptual abilities: an assessment of your child's visual and auditory perception. There are dozens of tests in this category.

Speech and language: assessment of your child's ability to physically create the sounds of language (speech) and to use language (verbal, nonverbal, written) effectively. Some of the more commonly used tests include the Peabody Picture Vocabulary Test–III (PPVT-III), Test for Auditory Comprehension of Language–III (TACL-III), Goldman-Fristoe Test of Articulation.

OTHER AREAS THAT MAY BE ASSESSED

Even if there is no "apparent" reason to suspect a problem in a particular area, IDEA (Individuals with Disabilities Education Act) requires that your child's evaluation address not only obvious areas of concern but "all areas of suspected disability." So, for example, a child who appears to have normal expressive language should still be evaluated for speech and language.

THE RESULTS: WHAT DO THEY MEAN?

Several weeks may elapse between the completion of the evaluation and your receiving the results. You should receive a written, detailed report and, ideally, have a chance to discuss the findings with someone who took part in the evaluation. You should ask to see a draft of the final report before it is submitted to your child's school district. If your child was evaluated by a team, there should be written reports from each evaluator and, in some cases, a general summary of all the reports as well. The reports should include:

• General narrative of your child's history, including date of birth, complications of pregnancy or delivery, major illnesses, developmental history, relevant family history, current behaviors, and issues that prompted the evaluation.

• A narrative description of your child as the evaluator found him during the evaluation. Don't be offended if your child is described as "uncooperative" or "inattentive." That type of information will help those who read the evaluation to put the child's performance into context. That may be important if, for example, there is a substantial difference between your child's performance during a session in which he seemed tired and cranky and another session in which he seemed relatively content and cooperative.

• A list of all medical tests run and standard assessment instruments used, including information on which parts or subtests were used, the scores (both raw scores and percentiles), and if appropriate, some narrative description of anything remarkable in your child's behavior during those tests. For example, an evaluator may note, "Danny performed well for the first half of the block design test, but once his concentration was broken by the appearance of a bird on the windowsill, his performance on this test diminished markedly." Interpreting the numerical scores of standardized assessments can be confusing. Ask the evaluator to explain what the numbers mean in terms of your child.

• A narrative conclusion that gives the evaluator's overall impression of the child and further interprets the test scores. This is important, because when it comes to Asperger Syndrome or any PDD, it is not simply symptoms, behaviors, strengths, and deficits that matter individually but their pattern. So, for example, an evaluator might note that the discrepancy found between your child's verbal IQ and his performance IQ is "seen commonly with Asperger Syndrome."

• A diagnosis, depending on circumstances. If your evaluation was done by your school district or by a professional or facility paid by your school district, you may not receive a medical diagnosis. If your evaluation was conducted by someone who could make a diagnosis, that may be included in the report. However, if you arranged for a private evaluation, you may instruct the evaluator not to include a specific diagnosis in his report.

• Recommendations for appropriate intervention. How specific these recommendations will be depends on several factors, including who conducts the evaluation and how familiar she is with special education and related services in your area. Some professionals who conduct evaluations write their reports with the understanding that they will be used primarily by educators to craft an IEP (Individual-ized Education Plan), Section 504 accommodation plan, or other education plan. (See chapter 8.) This type of report is often very detailed in terms of its recommendations. Others produce reports that are less specific and, frankly, not as useful to you as a parent in procuring services for your child. If you receive such a report and feel that it offers you little specific guidance, consider seeking a second opinion and/or hiring an educational consultant experienced in AS to review the test results and make more concrete suggestions for intervention and therapy.

WHAT DO THE SCORES MEAN?

Part of the joy of parenting is getting to know and enjoy the uniqueness of each child. When your child seems a little bit more unique, perhaps you feel even more protective of what makes him a true individual. By the time most of us reach the formal assessment stage, we may feel we've been defending, explaining, and making sense of our kids for some time. So it can be a bit unsettling to encounter the terminology, if not the very premise, behind the standardized assessments and the scores they yield. You would not be a parent if you could read terms such as *low average* or *significant delay* about your child without your heart sinking. Perhaps understanding something about where the tests and the terms come from will help.

Standardized tests are the tests evaluators use because they have been shown to be *valid* (meaning they measure what they claim to) and they are *reliable* (meaning that similar test takers with similar levels of skills and deficits will come within reasonable range of the same score, regardless of other factors). These are vastly oversimplified explanations, but essentially all most parents need to know. The most important aspect of standardized tests is that they have gone through a process called *norming*. Prior to publication (and, ideally, periodically through the years to come), a standardized test is given to a carefully chosen group of individuals like those for whom the test has been designed. If the norm group is well chosen, their scores when distributed should reflect a *normal, or bell, curve*. As a parent, it's important to understand that standardized test scores and the descriptive terms that explain them are neither arbitrary nor based on the opinions of the test's author. They don't tell you how your child scored on a particular test or subtest (that would be the *raw score,* which in and of itself tells a parent little) but how your child scored when compared with the test's norm group and, by extension, with other children of similar age, grade level, or (in some cases) disability.

Let's look at a standardized assessment most of us know: the IQ test. The normal distribution of scores for a test such as the commonly given WISC-III places the *mean score* (the average score; or the total of all scores divided by the total number of scores) at 100. In other words, if 5,000 children took this test, and we added all of the scores, then divided the sum by 5,000, the result would be 100. It's important to understand that this doesn't mean that most of those children obtained a score of 100; in fact, it's possible that none of them did. Another important (but very complicated) statistical concept is the *standard deviation*. The standard deviation results from a sophisticated mathematical formula and tells us how the scores are spread across the normal curve. Standard deviations are important for another reason: Some states and school districts may dictate "cutoffs" for eligibility based on standard deviation scores.

For the WISC-III, for instance, the IQ scores are distributed as follows:

IQ SCORE	STANDARD DEVIATION	PERCENTAGE OF SCORES IN RANGE
55	−3 SD	0.13
56–70	−2 SD	2.14
71–85	−1 SD	13.59
86–100	0 SD	34.13
101–115	0 SD	34.13
116–130	+1 SD	13.59
131–145	+2 SD	2.14
≥146	+3 SD	0.13

As you can see, the vast majority of scores—68.26 percent—fall within 86 to 115 points. Within that range is the normal IQ of 100 and what some may refer to as "high normal" (above 100) or "low normal" (below 100). Meanwhile, less than 1 percent of scores fall at or below 55 (severely mentally retarded) or 146 (gifted). Another way to read scores such as these would be that an individual with a score of 146 or greater on this test scored higher than 99.87 percent of other test takers, or, conversely in the case of a score at or below 55, then 99.87 percent of test takers had higher scores than 55.

For required reading on understanding test scores, go to Wright-slaw.com and download their "Tests and Measurements for the Parent, Teacher, Advocate & Attorney" at www.wrightslaw.com/advoc/articles/tests_measurements.html.

WHEN THE DIAGNOSIS IS NOT CLEAR

Sometimes, especially when children are young or when their cases seem unusually complex, the results of the evaluation and the diagnosis may seem to be unclear. You may be told that your child has "autisticlike behavior," "possible Asperger Syndrome," "atypical autism," "high-functioning autism," or any of several other terms. Even among professionals, the boundaries between different ASDs and certain learning disorders (for example, AS and nonverbal learning disability) are the subject of much debate and ongoing study. Despite increasing awareness of all PDDs, you might encounter doctors, therapists, and educators in whose minds the distinctions between them are blurry to invisible. While a rose is a rose is a rose, an ASD diagnosis can be one of several things, and it will be different for every individual.

There are differences between AS and other ASDs. We know, for example, that most people with AS respond only to those incentives and rewards that "make sense" to them. This is why for some people with AS token reward systems may not be sufficiently motivating to influence behavior. If you are dealing with a school district or an educator who believes that "it doesn't matter what you want to call it, all ASDs are the same," you should be prepared to explain specific aspects of your child's diagnosis. Also consider how the diagnosis may influence interventions, educational placement, and the professionals who may be working with your child. A teacher or program geared toward dyslexia may not be the most effective for your hyperlexic child. Some of the standard proscriptions for engaging the student with ADHD are precisely the opposite of what many with AS need. Teachers whose only experience with ASDs is with nonverbal, cognitively challenged students may not know how best to approach your child with AS.

TAKING IT ALL IN

Literally hundreds of different assessment instruments are available today, and the lists of percentages and scores, as well as the parade of acronyms, are often enough to make parents feel totally out of their depth. After you've had time to read and consider the report, make time to discuss your response and your questions with the person who wrote the report. Don't be afraid to ask questions about terms you are unfamiliar with (and there may be many) and, even more important, what they mean for your child in "real-life" terms. Ask your professional to do the following:

- Explain what the skills or deficits are indicative of (neurological, psychological, emotional, physical problem).
- Describe possible treatments and interventions.
- Discuss the implications of any given skill, deficit, or diagnosis in terms of possible impact now, in the near future, and in the distant future.

- Explain how possible treatments and interventions work and give you some idea which are more effective.
- Help you begin prioritizing skills to develop, deficits to address, behaviors and other issues that may need attention.
- Offer a list of local and national resources, as well as the names of at least a few local professionals, organizations, schools, and other agencies or groups that might be helpful.

If your child has received a diagnosis, ask questions about that, too. You might want to know how that diagnosis was arrived at, and what was first ruled out (and why). If, for example, your child's behavior is suggestive of an attention deficit, ask the evaluator to explain what results led her to conclude that attention deficit is not an issue. You may discover that despite all the testing, there remain some open questions about your child. Find out what they are and ask questions until you are satisfied that you understand, why, for example, the evaluator thinks that your early, precocious reader is hyperlexic (see page 81) and has low comprehension, or what evidence led to the conclusion that your child may also have a comorbid condition, such as obsessive-compulsive disorder (see page 69).

SHARING THE DIAGNOSIS WITH OTHERS

Once you know your child has AS, you confront the question of who to tell, when to tell, and what to say. There are no hard-and-fast rules here. While some choices may be obvious (grandparents, mature siblings, teachers, doctors, close family friends), others fall into a surprisingly wide gray area. Even if you feel strongly about being open and honest about your child's diagnosis, you must be realistic, too. Not everyone you think should know will use the information the way you would hope. Some people—including family members and close friends—may be insensitive or unable to fully understand the implications of AS. One basic rule of thumb might be to consider educating anyone whose misunderstanding could cause your child embarrassment or stress. One mother told people about her son's AS only when she felt that *her son* would benefit from their knowing.

There are pros and cons to any approach. We strongly urge you to consider your child first, as an individual whose right to privacy should outweigh any compulsion on your part to "enlighten" the world at large. If your child is old enough to have an opinion in this matter, it should be heeded. Obviously, with younger children, the matter is entirely up to your discretion. Remember, though, that kids do grow up. Five years from now, would your child feel comfortable knowing that the next-door neighbor you barely speak to or the dry cleaner knows she has AS?

While your child's grandparents will probably be eager to learn all about the diagnosis, the mother of the kid next door probably does not need to know much beyond the fact that your child may experience certain difficulties in play situations. One benefit of the increasing media attention is that you can collect basic articles and tapes of television programs that you feel provide a good introduction, lend them out, and let the media do the talking.

• • •

What to Say

When you least expect it, you may find yourself having to explain your child's behavior. Try to keep it brief and relevant to what's happening at the moment. If your child is tantruming in a restaurant, for instance, there simply isn't time to get into a detailed explanation. You might say something like this:

"My son has a neurological disorder that sometimes makes it impossible for him to control his behavior. It's kind of like what happens when an older person suffers a stroke or Alzheimer's disease and it becomes difficult to respond appropriately to stressful or confusing situations. Right now I'm helping him by removing him from this situation [or hugging him or letting him pace for a few minutes or whatever it is you are doing]. He'll be all right in a few minutes. Thanks for your concern."

Other families have printed up business cards to hand to strangers that say, "Thank you for your concern. My child has been diagnosed with Asperger Syndrome, a neurological disorder. For more information on Asperger Syndrome, contact OASIS at http://www. aspergersyndrome.org [or any other resource you wish to list]."

As parents, the two of us have taken completely opposite approaches in our respective communities. Barb's son was diagnosed at an older age and never required special education. His related services were provided privately. Over the years, the focus of her AS-related activism has been through the relative anonymity of OASIS. Locally, she has been open and honest about her son's AS to those people she feels will help him, including school personnel, medical professionals, family, and most friends, and she has been more than willing to share her experiences with other families of children with AS who might benefit. His AS is by no means a secret, but decisions about whom to tell are made individually and according to the particular circumstances. Additionally, now that he is a teenager, he is allowed considerable input as to who is told beyond these essential persons. In contrast, Patty's son was diagnosed at a much younger age, does require special education, and over the years has been involved in numerous disability- and AS-related therapies and interventions. Because she is active in local community special ed and autism organizations and has spoken publicly on behalf of both, many people outside the first circle of family and friends know that Justin has AS. While she believes that this has helped raise awareness about the disorder and increased understanding of her son, she is much less open as he grows toward adolescence. She has also had some unpleasant experiences as a result of the disclosure. Once, on a playground, an obviously inebriated woman shouted that "a kid like [Justin] shouldn't be let out of the house."

We could all use a little more support, but your aim in telling should be to increase understanding of your child, not pity for him or for you. If your words or manner reveal that you are anxious, embarrassed, ashamed, or upset about the diagnosis or your child's behavior, listeners will view AS and your child as things to feel anxious, embarrassed, ashamed, or upset about. If you can talk about AS and your child in a relaxed, confident, matter-of-fact way, you will be telling others that AS is nothing to be afraid of. Through your words and your actions, let people know that your child is a person beyond his diagnosis. Limit the amount of information you offer to what's relevant to the situation at hand, and always consider your audience. Have your own little "spiel" always at the ready.

SHARING THE DIAGNOSIS WITH YOUR CHILD

One of the most difficult decisions we face as parents is how to present information about Asperger Syndrome to our children. We worry that our child's self-esteem will suffer. We're concerned that our child may become severely depressed by the "official" confirmation that he is different from other children. We wonder if telling will give our child an "excuse" to fail, act out, or simply give up making the effort therapies and interventions demand in order to be effective. Although parents and professionals seem to agree that children with AS do realize that they are different from other children and are sometimes painfully aware of how much they struggle, there is no agreement on when or how to share the diagnosis with them. It is imperative that children understand that they are not bad or evil, and most certainly that their struggles are not their fault, but it is equally important that they be told of their Asperger Syndrome or differences in a positive way.

Sixty-four percent of the families who responded to the OASIS survey who told their child about their AS did so within a year of learning of the diagnosis. The majority of families who have shared the diagnosis with their child feel that it has resulted in a positive impact on their child's self-esteem. One parent wrote: "My son is aware that he is not like other kids. I think it has been helpful for him to have a reason that explains why some things are hard for him. Also it gives him a greater sense of pride in his accomplishments, since he knows that he has to work harder for them because of the Asperger's." Of the parents who reported that telling their child was a negative experience, nearly all mentioned that at one time or another their child has used the diagnosis as an excuse not to do something that would be considered within their range of abilities. A few parents have reported that their children became depressed and angry that they were different from other children.

Later, on page 337, we talk about how mistakes persons with AS make in attribution—essentially explaining the cause or the nature of what occurs to them—can result in misunderstandings and a distorted, negative self-concept. When a child who doesn't know he has AS concludes that everything that seems to go wrong in his life is his fault, the burden is overwhelming.

Here the experience of adults with AS provides some guidance. Nearly all of the adults with AS who completed the OASIS surveys confirmed that they would like to have known about their diagnosis earlier. Unanimously, they recommend that parents share the diagnosis with their children. Looking back, they wished they had had an understanding of why they were so different from others, because most of them were terribly misunderstood or mistreated.

— ● ● ● —

What Adults with AS Say About Telling Children

We asked adults with Asperger Syndrome, "Do you feel that being told about your AS would have been helpful to you as a child?" Here are some of their responses.

"I feel that it would have been very helpful. In particular, it would have helped to have been told that it was understood that I couldn't read facial expressions or body language and that I was bothered by bright lights and loud voices. It would have been nice to be told that this is because my brain is different and it was not my fault."

"Because I was nearly four and not yet speaking, my parents were certain I was retarded. Though hyperlexic and ultimately identified as gifted, the early 'label' affected me. Because of my social difficulties (especially being bullied), I was viewed as unlikable by adults and peers. Had I been told, and had my parents been told that my problems were related to a developmental disorder, I think I and they would have been more accepting of my uniqueness. Instead, I grew up feeling inadequate, unliked, odd, and was often depressed."

"Ideally, the child would be diagnosed young enough that Asperger's and/or autism could just be used casually all the time so there wouldn't be any big 'telling' at all—just natural questions and answers as they come up."

We also asked adults, "State how you feel about the importance of children learning about their diagnosis."

"I think it is extremely important. AS children usually realize that they are different, and they get told so by other people in not-so-nice terms (*lazy, crazy, arrogant, impolite, stupid,* etc.). Learning about the diagnosis also means to get rid of those wrong labels and self-accusations. It is (or can be) an important step in learning to accept oneself the way one is. It's also very important because you can start to search for others with the same diagnosis."

"Knowing that one is neurologically different at least gives some explanation for the behaviors other people find odd; it also suggests that compensation strategies may work to make one 'fit in' a little better—if one so desires."

We discovered differences of opinion among the experts when it came to when and how to discuss a child's disabilities with him. Some believe that giving children a name for their differences will empower them and help them to see having AS in a positive light. They point to the advantages of thinking "the Asperger way" and mention the dozens of famous scientists, musicians, writers, and other creative thinkers who probably had AS. Others believe it's preferable to talk to the child in terms of his strengths and weaknesses. They feel that the term *Asperger Syndrome* may be meaningless to a child, and the word *syndrome* reinforces the idea that the child has "something wrong" or a "disease." Carol Gray, who has worked with hundreds of children with AS, expressed the opinion that children need to be told before they approach the natural emotional and hormonal fluxes of adolescence. The combination of learning you are "different" at a time in life when peer acceptance is so important coupled with an AS-related risk of depression is probably one best avoided, if possible.

The question of what and when to tell your child has no one right or wrong answer. You will want to factor in the temperament of your child. Is your child more easygoing or does he tend to be explosive? Is your child depressed? Do you think it is likely that your child will misunderstand what it means to have AS? Before you do anything, it is imperative that you understand the diagnosis and have reached some level of acceptance. If you aren't sure that the AS diagnosis is correct or you have not yet come to terms with the disorder, it may be more difficult to explain it to your child. If you are anxious and sad, your child may sense this and interpret those feelings as being directed toward him rather than the fact that he has the disorder.

Take your child's age and developmental level into consideration. An older child will likely be more able to absorb and understand information than a younger one. Sitting down with a list of diagnostic criteria and talking about it with your six-year-old might not be the most appropriate way of bringing up the diagnosis. However, if your thirteen-year-old is inquisitive, she might wish to investigate on her own, either by reading books or looking at information from Web sites. Several teenagers with AS have found online support, and many are very involved in their treatment and participate in educational decisions such as attending IEP meetings.

Present a united front. Even if one parent or caregiver disagrees with the diagnosis, it's important that the two of you present a united front. If one parent is still dealing with denial or simply refuses to accept that there is any kind of problem, you may not be at the best point for informing your child.

Call on your professional team for advice. No one else can make this decision for you. That said, it could only help to have the input of those who know your child—teachers, therapists, doctors, and others—on the matter. You may find, for example, that your child asks her teacher "What's wrong with me?" several times a week, or someone else may weigh in with why they think now may not be the time.

When to consider telling your child. Your child might be ready to know about AS when

- she starts to ask questions or express concern such as: *Why am I different? Why do I have to go to speech therapy? Why don't I have any friends?*
- she begins making comments about other children who may have AS or a related disorder, such as: *Why doesn't Joseph look at*

me when I talk to him? Why is it hard for Daniel to hear the school bells? Why doesn't Cindy play with the rest of the kids at recess?

- she seems to be attributing her difficulties to the "fact" (in her mind) that she is "dumb," "stupid," "lazy," "worthless," and so on. For the sake of her self-esteem, we would say that anytime the challenges of AS take a toll on your child's sense of self-worth, you should consider telling.

Once you've made the decision to tell your child, try to read at least one of the several books, workbooks, and articles that have been especially created to help a child learn about her AS or related disorder.

● ● ●

Recommended Reading: Telling Children About the Diagnosis

GENERAL

Catherine Faherty, *Asperger's: What Does It Mean to Me?: A Workbook Explaining Self-Awareness and Life Lessons to the Child or Youth with High-Functioning Autism or Asperger's* (Arlington, TX: Future Horizons, 2000).

Carol Gray, "Pictures of Me: Introducing Students with Asperger's Syndrome to Their Talents, Personality, and Diagnosis," from *The Morning News* (Jenison, MI: Jenison Public Schools, fall 1996). You can order back issues at www.thegraycenter.org.

———, "The Sixth Sense," from *Taming the Recess Jungle* (Arlington, TX: Future Horizons, 1993).

Plan your talk. Think carefully about the message you want to send. Will you use the actual term *Asperger Syndrome* or speak in terms of "brain differences" and individual strengths and weaknesses? Will you talk about other people who have been known to have AS (including yourself or family members, if relevant) or will you focus only on your child? Will you discuss how it affects your child in school or socially or both?

Ideally, you'll plan the appropriate time to tell your child. Remove any distractions, allow plenty of time to ask questions, and have a place for your child to escape to, such as his room, if things become too intense for him. You might plan this for a weekend or holiday or other day when there are no other commitments. If possible, pick a time when things in school and elsewhere are going relatively well. Try to avoid telling your child about his diagnosis in the immediate wake of a tantrum, a difficult period, a failure in school, a social disaster, a bad medication reaction, or any other event that could cause him to associate the news with a bad memory.

Plan as you might, however, that ideal moment may never come, so at least have an outline of what you would like to say in the event your child beats you to the punch and asks before you are ready to tell. If your child catches you off guard, say, in the car (isn't that where everything important seems to happen?) or when you are running out to a business meeting, do the best you can. Ignoring the question will probably make your child more anxious, so try to say something that validates his question and makes it clear that you will talk to him more about it at a specific time, preferably as soon as possible. If, for example, your daughter says, "Somebody at school told me that I'm different because there's something wrong with me. Is that true?" you might respond, "In one way or another, everyone is different from everyone else. There is nothing 'wrong' with you. You sound like you might have some questions. Let's make a special time tomorrow afternoon after school, and I'll answer all of your questions."

Next decide who will do the telling. Will you do this alone, with your partner, or as a family, including perhaps siblings, grandparents, favorite relatives? Will your child's doctor or therapist be involved? You might wish to include other people who you know have a special rapport with your child and with whom you know he would feel comfortable. Needless to say, anyone whose presence may be disruptive (young children, for instance) or distracting (the grandmother who still has not accepted the diagnosis) should not be included.

When you do discuss the diagnosis, pay careful attention to how your child is responding to the news from moment to moment. You better than anyone will notice the first signs of stress or distress in your child's general demeanor. Many children with AS do better if they get information gradually and informally. You may have already told your child more than you realize in the course of explaining why, for example, the noise at the indoor pool bothers her or she has trouble catching a ball. Give your child time to absorb what she is being told and to ask questions. If you find that your child is becoming upset or doesn't seem to understand, end the discussion. Try again when your child indicates that she is ready or curious.

Trust your instincts. If you feel that your child isn't ready to talk about the diagnosis, you're probably correct. If the time doesn't feel right to you, don't be pressured into discussing the diagnosis before you and your child are ready. Years from now, your child may feel that he would like to have known earlier or never known at all. This is simply a risk you have to take. You will know when the time is right.

Accept your child's response—no matter what it may be. How well your child will be able to understand the implications of his diagnosis depends on his age, level of maturity, and general awareness about the social world around him and his place in it. Give your child the time, the space, and the emotional support he needs to process the information and come to terms with it. Remember your own reaction and that of others close to your child. Be prepared to deal with more questions and a host of emotional responses, including anger, depression, anxiety, and sadness. Know that this will take time, patience, and no small dose of wisdom.

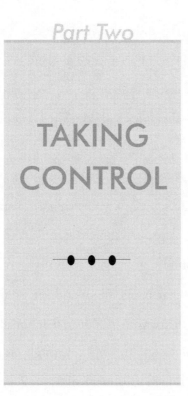

Part Two

TAKING CONTROL

● ● ●

INFORMATION is power. So is having the right attitude. You may discover that you have become the "resident expert" on your child and on Asperger Syndrome. Becoming an expert on AS, however, is only the beginning. If you thought you were juggling too many hats before, add these: detective, advocate, ambassador, psychotherapist, education specialist, and socialization director. And wear them all proudly.

Invariably, you will encounter a professional, another parent, or a resource with information that seems to contradict what you learned someplace else. Everyone has an opinion, and parents and experts can disagree strongly. Sometimes our kids' problems have no clear answers, and trial and error (and, we hope, success) become our way. Making the job ever more daunting is the lack of information on the exact causes of AS and long-term outcomes for everything from specific therapies and educational approaches to medication.

It is a challenge, but it is one that loving, informed parents can rise to. Consider the source of your strength. Part Two of this book is devoted to helping you assemble the tools you need to do the best you can for your child.

It falls to parents to change the world for a child with AS. Without realizing it, perhaps, you are doing that already simply by caring and taking the time to see the world through his eyes. The therapies and interventions, the educational techniques, and the various other ways in which you help your child grow toward independence, self-awareness, and understanding are essential. But so is changing the understanding of AS and your child for everyone your child knows, and maybe some people he or she does not.

Chapter 4

CAN THIS BE MY CHILD?

Accept the gift that is your child. Give your child
the gift of you.

—An OASIS parent

• • •

OASIS Members Speak

We asked OASIS members: "If you were to sit across from a
parent who had just learned that his or her child has AS, what
would you want to tell them?"

"Don't close any doors. Keep your dreams for your child and a
belief that he can achieve them. Place no limitations on your child
and don't let others place limits on him, either."

"Your child is no longer a problem child. He or she is now a child
with problems, and you can work with those problems and around
them. A better understanding of your child will lead to your child
feeling better understood. And your child will be a much happier
child for that. After all, we all want to be understood."

"These children are incredibly courageous and strong people.
They have so much to deal with every day and almost every

moment of the day. And they just keep battling. My son is one of my heroes. I have the utmost respect for him and what he has to do just to conform to our neurotypical world."

"Talk! Talk! Talk! Reach out for help, advocate for your child, read everything you can. Try to get people interested and educated about AS. Don't ever be ashamed. Try to accept what has been dealt to you. Accepting it doesn't mean you have to like it, but accept it. You will if you love your child."

"When the shock wears off—and it will—you will realize that this is the same child you have nurtured and loved since birth."

"Don't ever put yourself in a trap of wondering why your child isn't normal. Your child is as normal as your child can be. I started to get caught in that trap, and my pediatrician once said to me, 'How do you know your child is not normal?' In other words, what truly is 'normal'? You will find your own definition of normal in everyday life—your version of it."

"I might caution them not to hang on to the 'high-functioning' idea too tightly. The social disability may make the high IQ useless. Then again, it may not. That's the hard thing. You just don't know. Maybe the best advice would be to stay very much in the present. Enjoy the small victories. Enjoy who the child is and don't waste time on hoping for someone who is not here now. My biggest mistake was probably hoping for something that didn't happen. Imagine the message that must have given my child. Remember that building self-esteem means addressing reality, which includes dysfunction. When your child reaches adulthood, you will definitely wish you had taught him or her the meaning of limits. Don't make excuses because of AS for antisocial or negative behaviors. Our kids need to learn how to behave even more than everyone else. However, it is also important that you teach them skillfully and according to their ability. It can be a real tightrope."

"Get support and select your friends carefully. Don't be around people who will negatively impact your ability to be there for your child."

"Hang in there! Keep reminding your child that God loves him and so do you, that you will always forgive him and you will never leave him. This way he will know that no matter what, he can always trust you."

"Let yourself feel bad for a while, without showing your child. Your family is probably not going to be what you thought it would be, and you need to let yourself grieve for that vision of a perfect little family that you have to let go of now. Eventually you'll be able to see that what replaces it can give you just as much joy as that ideal in your head would have."

WHEN we set out to write this book together, we promised ourselves and our families that it would be a book about Asperger Syndrome, not about us or our sons. The longer we looked at this material and thought about what we wanted to say in this chapter, the more we realized that it would be impossible not to touch on our own experiences here.

BARB'S THOUGHTS

This is a journey that takes time and patience. In reality, just as our son has developed and grown and changed over the past eleven years, so have we. And so has our acceptance of Asperger Syndrome. Give yourself time to mourn and time to accept that things will likely be very different from what you had planned or dreamed for your child. Most important, though, realize that while your dreams and hopes may have changed, your child remains the same child you loved even before the first moment you saw him. What has changed is that you now have a name that best describes your child's strengths and weaknesses. In having that, you now have a means to help him better understand the world.

With your love, understanding, and guidance, with appropriate supports and intervention, chances are good that he or she will do well. This is not to say that there will be no moments when you feel as if everything is going backward. It is important that you learn to look carefully at your child's abilities and do your best not to compare them with those of other children. The very best piece of advice came from someone who reminded me that I should never measure my son's progress against typically developing peers. Instead I needed to look at where he was and where he is now. Your child may seem to take giant steps backward or even sideways before achieving a milestone. It is essential that you remember that your child is still a child—someone who deserves to be loved, appreciated, and understood.

Do your best to make sure that you allow yourself, your family, and your child time away from therapies and the diagnosis and worries about the future. Remember to take time to enjoy your child and try not to see everything through "Asperger eyes." I can recall more than one occasion when I attributed some behavior to Asperger Syndrome, only to realize later that it was just normal kid behavior or something entirely unrelated to AS.

Parenting a child with AS can be frustrating and difficult, and at times overwhelming, but it can also be just as joyful as raising any other child.

THE JOURNEY CONTINUES

Learning to accept, live with, and grow through parenting a child with Asperger Syndrome is a deeply personal and at times difficult journey. We each began at different points on the road, with children with different symptoms, under completely different circumstances, and we may end up at different destinations. Barb's son was diagnosed at age nine after many doctors, tests, and other explanations, before Asperger Syndrome entered the *DSM-IV,* at a time and in a place where knowledgeable professionals were scarce and access to interventions limited (in part because many had yet to be developed or disseminated). Patty's son was diagnosed at five, by the second doctor he saw, after Asperger Syndrome entered the *DSM-IV,* at a time and in a place where there were several experts in AS nearby and many interventions and therapies available locally. She also had access to books, support groups, and OASIS.

In some ways, it might seem that our experiences could not have been more different. Yet if you consider only what it means to love a child with AS, there is so much that we share, not only with each other, but with every family whose life has taken this unexpected turn.

Just as no two people with AS are exactly alike, neither are any two parents or caregivers, including spouses and partners. Parents seem to fall into several different and distinct camps in terms of how they view AS and the impact it has on their lives. And how they feel—about the experience, about their child, and about themselves— may change over time, because the role AS plays in your child's life—and in your own—can change. The one thing that you can expect when your child has AS is the unexpected.

WHEN THE LANDSCAPE SHIFTS

All parents hold expectations and assumptions about their children. Often this seems such a natural thing to do that we give it little conscious thought. Most of us never realize how much about our children we take for granted until something like the AS diagnosis suddenly throws all of our assumptions to the wind. Depending on how we come to understand that our child has AS, those old dreams either drift away quietly, one by one, or get blown to bits in a single hurricane. Either way, when it's over, the landscape of childhood and parenthood is forever changed.

In our OASIS survey of 372 parents of children with Asperger Syndrome, we asked, "Immediately upon realizing that your child had Asperger Syndrome, which of the following describes your reaction?" We asked parents to indicate all the emotions that applied and were not surprised to find that most experienced several at once.

How Other Parents Feel

Relieved	63%	Guilty	22%
Sad	54%	Angry	19%
Anxious	47%	Disappointed	18%
Overwhelmed	44%	Surprised	17%
Fearful	34%	Energized	16%
Hopeful	29%	Hopeless	14%
Confused	27%	Shocked	14%
Depressed	26%	Disbelieving	13%
Alone	22%	In denial	11%

When we asked these parents how their feelings had changed over time, it was interesting to discover that 36 percent felt as hopeful or more hopeful than they had in the beginning, yet 29 percent felt as overwhelmed or more overwhelmed than they had initially. Generally, feelings such as disbelief, anger, shock, denial, depression, hopelessness, confusion, and guilt diminished over time. Perhaps reflecting the roller-coaster ups and downs of coping with AS, sadness, anger, and feeling overwhelmed stood out as the most persistent emotions.

Even though two-thirds of our respondents had been dealing with the diagnosis for three years or less (and nearly half of them for a year or less), 80 percent of all respondents answered yes to the question "Would you say that you have come to terms, reached a point of resolution, or gained acceptance of your child's Asperger Syndrome?"

WHY THIS "LOSS" IS DIFFERENT

Most of us are familiar with the psychological stages of coping with major life crises: denial, anger, bargaining, depression, and finally acceptance. Although usually associated with bereavement, these same responses are noted in parents of children who have disabilities. At some point, we must come to terms with the loss of the child as we imagined he would be. Some experts say that what some of us mourn is the death of our own dreams for our child, the demise of the expectations we probably gave little thought to until they were threatened. Certainly there is some truth to that, but with the passage of time, the loss we feel is in many ways far more profound and less easily resolved.

That is because Asperger Syndrome seems to strike at the very heart of what we who are neurologically typical assume to be prerequisites of basic human happiness. Understanding, friendship, community, love, family, parenthood—the very fabric of life—can be taken for granted for your child, unless he has AS. Patty always thinks of the day Justin was diagnosed as the moment when all of the whens of his future turned into ifs.

It's only natural to grieve over the possibility that your child's AS may stand in the way of these experiences. However, remember that the individual with Asperger Syndrome may not see her situation in exactly the same light. Here and in almost every other aspect of parenting these children, we must, as autism educator Carol Gray (the creator of the popular social skills technique Social Stories) so wisely advises, "abandon all assumptions." There is no question but that experiencing AS from the inside out, as our children do, can probably never be fully understood by those of us on the outside peering in, no matter how well we know or how deeply we love them. To presume otherwise is to risk further misunderstanding and to risk making decisions based on erroneous "conclusions."

Barb remembers her son commenting that while he liked having friends and enjoyed their company, he did not "need" friends in the same way that she did. Initially, she found this concept frightening but later came to understand that he was being truthful. He wasn't judging relationships or saying that he didn't have feelings for people or lacked a desire for friendship, but rather that he was capable of enjoying his time alone in a way that perhaps most people do not. In his early elementary school years, Patty's son had an active social life and a number of close friendships but was baffled as to how she could possibly enjoy the time she spent with most "other people" who were not him or his father. As a preteen, he gets along better in casual relationships but is more comfortable spending his after-school hours alone rather than having a friend over.

What most of us do wish for our children is that they be graced with whatever it takes to live the lives they wish for themselves and to be comfortable being who they are. Every therapy, every intervention, everything that you will do for your child from this point on is geared toward giving her the tools, the skills, the secrets of what Dr. Diane Twachtman-Cullen describes as "the hidden curriculum" of daily life. However hopeful we may be and however successful our children may be in adapting to this world, many of us will encounter situations in which their differences remain glaringly clear. Having some philosophical and emotional "foundation" about this experience is crucial.

For parents of children with AS, the feelings of loss and sadness ebb and flow over time, depending on numerous factors. There will be setbacks. Twenty-five percent of respondents who were asked to describe how their attitude toward their child having AS had changed over time agreed with the statement "My attitude changes so drastically from day to day, I find it difficult to generalize." However, it is reassuring to know that 49 percent said that they felt "more optimistic," and only 9 percent said that they felt "less optimistic."

BLAZING A NEW TRAIL

Even when you feel like anything but the brave, intrepid explorer, that is really what you are, clearing the trail your child may follow to his own goals and dreams. Even during those times when the way seems clear, most of us still hear the loud humming of the wide, smoothly paved superhighway of "typical" life we have detoured from. As one mother put it, "For one day, I would just like to feel what it's like to know that my daughter will not scream if the cupcakes have pink rather than blue wrappers or that when a classmate greets her, she will respond appropriately. I see other kids going through life just being typical kids, and from where I stand, everything they do that their parents take for granted strikes me as a small miracle. I would just like to feel that my daughter would not need a miracle to have an uneventful, good day."

This process also entails revising our ideas about what it means to be a parent and a family. For example, parents of only children find themselves second-guessing themselves, wondering who will feel obligated to care for or at least care about their child with AS once they are gone. Parents of larger families may worry that unaffected siblings are not getting enough attention today and may wonder whether those siblings will be there for the child with AS tomorrow. Some of us face the prospect of having a child who will always be more dependent on us or on others, or a child whose social isolation seems the antithesis of childhood. There may be moments when we feel very much out of the loop. The "small" things we take for granted that "all" children experience mean something different when it's your child who isn't invited to the birthday parties or who has no place in the whirl of extracurricular activities that other parents good-naturedly complain of having to chauffeur their kids to. At the other end, many of us know the guilty feeling of reassuring ourselves that our child is "not as bad off " as another we saw in the doctor's office, on the playground, or at the store.

Will there ever come a time when you don't look back over your shoulder to what might have been—and who your child might have been—were it not for AS? Probably not. Coming to a point of resolution or acceptance doesn't necessarily exclude a continuing sense of loss, nor does it require you to deny the very real disadvantages this disability confers. Resolution may entail living with a more fluid attitude and the freedom to embrace both the positives and negatives. As we mentioned previously, one of the insidious things about AS is how easily its strengths give rise to weaknesses and vice versa. A skill or tendency that served your child well in elementary school (such as an encyclopedic knowledge of Beanie Babies) may spell social disaster in his teen years; on the other hand, the obsession that drives you batty in middle school may be the foundation for the career of your child's dreams. When you do look back—and you should—keep your eyes on the path you have traveled, not the one you left behind. Gauge your child's progress—and your own—by where you have come from, not by how far you may have yet to go or where you might have been had you taken that other road.

Start sketching your own map, knowing there will be many false starts, dead ends, trails erased and retraced. Our advice: Don't go it alone. Find support and never hesitate to take advantage of someone else's willingness to listen, advise, or console. Try to be there for the next parent who follows you.

— • • • —

How to Find or Start a Local Support Group

The past few years have seen a dramatic increase in local support groups, which provide information and support to both families of children with Asperger Syndrome and adults with the diagnosis. Some are sponsored by universities, hospitals, or national organizations (such as the Autism Society of America), but the great majority have been created by family members or adults with AS. The Internet is an excellent source for locating local support groups, and the OASIS Web site as well as other AS-related Web sites offer listings of existing local support groups. In addition, you can contact the Autism Society of America, the Learning Disability Association, United Cerebral Palsy, the Easter Seals Society, and just about any other major disability-related organization. Ask if they have information on support groups that would be appropriate for families of individuals on the autism spectrum.

Unfortunately, local support is still nonexistent in many parts of the country. If this is the case where you live, consider starting a group yourself. Although this may seem a daunting task, please understand that it was families who were interested in contacting others who organized 99 percent of the existing local support systems.

Your local support group can be whatever you want it to be: small or large, formal or informal in structure, devoted to fund- and awareness-raising efforts or simply a place to offer parents a true community of understanding. An initial meeting can be held at a local bookstore where a few parents share coffee and swap stories, or it could be held in a local church, library, or mall meeting room. Starting a support group doesn't require a great deal of special skill or talent. Once you've chosen a location to meet, the next step is to advertise for either an informal get-together or an organizational meeting. Contact your local newspaper and ask to have your meeting time and place listed in the Community Service section. Call your children's doctors and ask them if they'd be willing to post a notice in their offices or share the information with other families of AS children. Contact OASIS and ask that your group be listed in the support group area. Notify the special education department of your school district and ask if they'd be willing to pass along information about your meeting. Once people start to hear about your group, you may be surprised at how quickly the word travels and how supportive people can be.

Once you have several families gathered, you'll be able to determine the course you would like your group to take. Some groups have expanded into state or regional support networks and hold regular monthly meetings, sponsor conferences and workshops, and provide services such as social skills training or play groups, while other groups remain informal and meet only a few times a year to socialize.

In addition to contacting parents, you might want to talk with one of the professionals working with your child and ask if he or she would be willing to help sponsor a local support group. If you believe it would be helpful, consider inviting doctors, therapists, teachers, and others who are knowledgeable to join your group, perhaps as advisors or regular speakers.

For more information: A wonderful source, "How to Start Your Own Local Group," can be found on the Web site of the PDD/Asperger Support Group in Fairfield, Connecticut, www.pddaspergersupportct.org.

Perhaps most important, give yourself time, space, and a break. At one point or another, most of us feel we haven't lived up to our own expectations. There may be moments when, as one mother told us, "Despite the fact that I loved my daughter so much I would die for her, there were times when I began to question if I could ever love her enough to get us both through the tantrums, the obsessions, and the compulsions. I never could give myself credit for long stretches of patience, for the days when I managed to deal with every potential crisis 'by the books.' In that one moment when my patience snapped, I knew that I was the worst mother on the planet and feared that all the good I'd put forth until then had been totally undone."

THE STRESS OF PARENTING A CHILD WITH AS

Parenting a child with AS can be difficult. You are not the only parent in the world who has spent over $1,000 on your child's special interest, questioned your ability to parent your other children effectively, or felt that coping with AS has stressed your relationship with your spouse or partner.

Getting the Diagnosis

According to our OASIS survey, many parents lived with questions and uncertainty for months and, more often, years before obtaining a diagnosis and direction. Only 20 percent indicated that they had received a correct diagnosis and treatment within a year of first having concerns about their child. For the majority, the period between first worries and diagnosis spanned years. We asked, "How much time passed between the time concerns were first raised by others or voiced by you about your child and correct diagnosis and treatment?"

1 year	20%
1 to 3 years	29%
4 to 6 years	27%
7 to 9 years	15%
10 years or more	9%

Parents' Marriage and Relationships

There's no question that the demands of parenting a child with special needs can affect a relationship. Our 327 respondents were split exactly 50-50 on the question of whether their relationships with their partners had or had not grown stronger since their child began displaying symptoms of AS, although 70 percent said that dealing with AS had created additional stress in their relationship. Forty percent said they had more arguments with their partner than before, and 63 percent indicated they felt that dealing with the child's AS "significantly reduced the amount and/or quality of time" the couple spent alone together. Fifty-nine percent agreed with the statement "Since our child began displaying the symptoms of Asperger Syndrome, I feel that I am less emotionally available to my partner than I was before." Interestingly, only 40 percent indicated they felt their partner was less emotionally available to them, and 58 percent said their partner was their "most important source of support."

The responses to several other questions in our twenty-five-question survey for parents on their relationships indicated that the vast majority—79 percent—agreed with the statement "When it comes to major decisions about our child, my partner and I usually see things eye to eye." However, even when parents did agree, it was clear that in most families, one parent took the lead when it came to learning about interventions and treatment and dealing with school-related issues.

We feel it's also important to note that our survey confirmed the findings of other studies about parents of children with AS and PDDs regarding the presence of neurological disorders. Of our respondents, over a third indicated that they themselves have been diagnosed with (in order of prevalence) depression, Asperger Syndrome, ADHD, bipolar disorder, and autism, among others.

Other Children in the Family

It's not uncommon to hear parents say that their other children are the "best thing to have happened" to their AS children. True, AS demands much of a parent's attention and energy, and children with less immediate and pressing needs can sometimes be overlooked. However, often it is the siblings who help teach and reinforce the much-needed social skills for their AS brothers and sisters. It is also important to realize that the lessons learned are not mutually exclusive—it's not just a matter of what the neurotypical child teaches the AS child, but also what the AS child teaches the sibling. Though many sibs of AS children do at times feel left out, embarrassed, or humiliated, many of those same children grow up to become caring and compassionate adults.

Although parents aren't generally comfortable talking about it, many do find their parenting skills validated when there is more than one child in the household. Not only do they have "proof" that they are in fact good parents, they also have a frame of reference to measure what is "normal" development. This seems to be particularly true if the AS child is not a first child. It's also reassuring to look to the future and know (or hope) that there will be "family" who will care for our AS children if this becomes necessary.

There is no question but that siblings of children with AS are often required to make sacrifices and assume responsibilities most other children do not. From convincing Sister to give up the last waffle for the sake of the peace to rushing out of Brother's basketball game because of an AS sensory meltdown, in ways great and small, other children feel—and, in truth, sometimes are—cheated. They may be teased or made to feel uncomfortable about having a sibling who's "different," whom they may be forced to defend. Understandably, siblings can feel that the child with AS "gets away with" more than they do or doesn't receive equal discipline or punishment.

These issues should be discussed with the siblings of AS children, and just as the child with AS requires assurance that it isn't his or her fault, so does the sibling. As time needs to be set aside to nurture adult relationships, time should also be allotted for siblings of children with disabilities. Parents also need not feel guilty if they fully enjoy the successes of their non-AS children. One mother expressed that it took her several years to accept strangers' compliments about the behavior of her younger, neurotypical daughter. Every time someone said something nice about how well she behaved in the grocery store, she was reminded that these same sorts of people were the type to judge her parenting of her AS son.

While we all recognize how AS changes the way we parent the affected child, our surveys suggest that it also colors how we parent our other children. Forty-two percent of our respondents agreed with the statement "Dealing with our child's Asperger Syndrome has significantly reduced the amount and/or quality of time we spend with our other children." Only 22 percent felt they and their partner managed to divide their time and attention equally among all of their children.

It's common for parents of children with AS to question and doubt their parenting skills. We were surprised to learn to what degree that shaken confidence extended to their parenting of their other, non-AS children. Understandably, many parents felt that dealing with AS in one child had an effect on how they viewed their other children's behaviors and development. While 36 percent said they "did not worry at all about my other children's behaviors," 23 percent agreed with the statement "I seem to be always on the lookout for AS behaviors in my other children." Fifty-five percent indicated "At times I have difficulty determining what are 'normal' childhood behaviors." This is made even more difficult by the fact that it's not at all uncommon for a sibling to have what has come to be known as a "shadow syndrome," and in some cases there may be a sibling who is diagnosed with AS, autism, speech delay or other language disorder, NLD (nonverbal learning disability), or a related disorder.

Financial Matters

Having a child with AS can have a profound effect on a family's financial picture. Some families find that there's literally no end to the amount of money they could spend on treatments, interventions, special programs, and professional services. In addition to the obvious costs for medical care and therapies, AS has its own "hidden" costs in the form of purchases related to special interests (11 percent say they spend over $1,000 a year); special-needs camps, day care, and after-care; special clothing; and specialized legal counsel for matters related to special education and estate planning.

Compounding the financial stress for a significant number of families is the fact that having a child with AS either prevents one parent (usually Mom) from working or restricts where and how much she can work. Conversely, having to meet the added expenses has also forced a number of mothers who would rather be at home back into the workforce.

One common theme we noted from the 120 parents who took time to write to us on the topic was regret over the services and activities they knew their child would benefit from but that they could not afford. The fact that most health insurance policies don't cover lifelong developmental disabilities—including AS and PDDs—is an outrage. Only 4 percent of our respondents indicated that their child's AS-related medical costs were fully covered. Sixty percent said that their child had to forgo consulting a professional or undergoing a recommended treatment or therapy because the cost was prohibitive.

Several parents mentioned that they had paid for diagnostic testing and services before they learned that their child may have been eligible to receive these services free of charge through their local school district. (See chapter 8 for more on this topic.)

DAY-TO-DAY PARENTING STRESS

Unfortunately, often by the time most parents learn about AS, their competence has been questioned if not undermined by family members, friends, educators, doctors, and strangers. We all want to be "good parents" for our children. Sometimes parents doing their best for a child with AS don't look like good parents to those unfamiliar with AS. Sometimes they don't feel like good parents, either. As many parents who post on OASIS's message board note, to say that "no one understands" is putting it mildly in some cases.

You will strive for the consistency and the "right" response prescribed by experts (most of whom, it is only fair to point out, do not live with children with AS). You will live out the little secret few of us would ever admit to our child's teachers, doctors, or even ourselves: sometimes moms and dads melt down, too. Tempers flare, despair crashes down, and patience shorts out. Through all of that, however, you can still be the best parent for your child if you remember that no one is perfect. Look around and see how other parents behave around their children, then ask yourself who you know who could do a better job of understanding, fighting for, protecting, and loving your child than you. Chances are, no one.

AS dramatically raises the parenting stakes. Just being the "good enough" parent of reassuring child psychology books will never be good enough again. Nothing about your child having AS will magically make you more patient, more tolerant, more understanding, or more forgiving. However, having a child with AS certainly will give you far more opportunities to develop these qualities and practice these skills than most other parents get. By the same token, you also will have more opportunities to come up short. Whether you believe that this experience results from the will of a higher power or a biological fluke, there will be lessons learned.

REASONS FOR HOPE

Even if you feel that the world has ended, it does begin again. Now, however, it is a new world. You may be surprised to discover how well prepared you already are for this journey. As one mother told us, "You will understand that basically you have been coping pretty well with a difficult situation. When you look back, you will find that over the years you have instinctively developed coping mechanisms and have been doing the right things." For example, you may have "learned" not to tell your child the specifics of an upcoming outing, because you know how he will react if the plans change, or you may have naturally developed a way of speaking in short, direct sentences. Many of us look back and see that the things we did that most often drew criticism and derision were in fact the right things to do.

Yes, there is much to gather from "outside" in the form of information and support. Always remember, though, that you have several resources that can never be replaced and that in the end will mean more to your child's happiness than any other: your love, understanding, and acceptance.

Chapter 5

BUILDING THE FOUNDATION
FOR SUCCESS

No intervention or therapy is 100 percent effective or appropriate for every child. No one has yet devised the guaranteed, one-size-fits-all treatment and intervention plan that takes into account all of your child's needs, your family's values and lifestyle, your resources. Dr. Ami Klin of Yale University has often stated that if you put one hundred individuals with Asperger Syndrome into one room, you will discover that no two are exactly alike, that each of them may be more different from one another than they are the same. What works for one family and one child may not work for another.

You may be facing situations like these: Your child's school has a general education plan for him but expects you to provide most of the socialization training. Or your child's occupational therapist has the right approach for attacking those motor skills problems but not a lot to offer in terms of guidance for adaptive physical education. Or your child's psychologist or psychiatrist has some attractive suggestions for reducing classroom anxiety, but your school district lacks the personnel, the experience, or the will to implement them. You, the parent, may be the bridge between what should be done and what does get done.

WHERE DO PARENTS FIND
THE INFORMATION AND SUPPORT
THEY NEED?

In our OASIS survey, we asked, "When you think back to the first few months after you realized that your child has AS, what do you believe helped you the most to cope and to help your child?" Of the 84 percent who responded who had access to the Internet, 46 percent said that the Internet was "the single most important thing." Another 36 percent said it was "one of the most helpful things." Tied for second place as the single most helpful resource were participating in an online message board and participating in an online chat room. Those who were able to make contact with a parent in their area considered it an essential resource—for 16 percent, it was "the single most important"; for another 22 percent, it was "one of the most important." This suggests that local support—through existing organizations such as special education–oriented parent-teacher organizations, AS-dedicated formal groups, or informal networks of parents—could play a much more important role. (On page 134 we offer tips for finding or starting your own support group.)

When asked which resources were among the most helpful, the vast majority—68 percent—chose "information found in books, magazines, newspapers, and other media." Forty-three percent included "information from doctors, educators, or other professionals" and 43 percent indicated "information from national organizations."

Ironically, though it may seem that vast deserts of ignorance dominate the landscape, once you find that oasis (yes, pun intended), you could drown in the amount of information there is to read, absorb, and apply. It's important for you to determine for yourself what you need to know versus what it would be nice to know. They are not the same. The past few years have brought an explosion in media interest about all autism spectrum disorders. There are more Web sites, more message boards, chat rooms, and Listservs, more books, more organizations, more newsletters, and more coverage in professional journals and all forms of mainstream media.

In stark contrast to the situation a decade ago, the amount of information available today can be overwhelming. Although it may not be obvious, the fact is, anyone can write a book, put up a Web site, circulate a newsletter, and even write or produce a major piece for a respectable news organizations. There is no guarantee that anything you read or see will be accurate or even helpful. Our advice is to be selective and ask questions. Read critically. Guard your time. Better to find five tried-and-true sources you feel you can return to as you need than to deluge yourself with dozens of sources, none of which is "complete."

BE THE EXPERT ON YOUR CHILD

If your child is newly diagnosed, you have only begun to amass what can easily become a mountain of reports, letters, and other important papers. It is wise to start laying down the paper trail you will need when dealing with your school district, your health insurance company, and just about everyone else who comes into your child's life.

- Set aside one place in your home—perhaps a desk tray, basket, or large manila envelope taped to the wall—for all important papers, including receipts for therapy, medication, and transportation to and from appointments. Periodically sort through and file it all.
- Set up a filing system that makes sense to you. You can use a file cabinet, file box, or a large loose-leaf binder. The loose-leaf binder has the advantage of being portable enough to travel with you to doctors' appointments and IEP (Individualized Education Plan) meetings. Use clear plastic sheets to hold smaller papers or anything you refer to or copy often.
- Start keeping important phone numbers in your personal address book, home address book, organizer, Rolodex, and anyplace else you might need them. Program the most important—your child's school and doctor—into your phones, if possible. The inside cover of your binder is also a good place for phone numbers.
- If you find a good comprehensive article or pamphlet that you think explains your child well, consider getting several copies made to hand out to grandparents, teachers, coaches, baby-sitters, and others you believe need to know.
- Consider making a second "general information" binder to share with your child's school and teacher. This binder will include a

few pamphlets and general information papers on Asperger Syndrome, a list of recommended reading, and a short description of your child and his needs. In the "Education" area of the OASIS Web site and on page 403 of this book, you'll find a sample letter you may compose about your child.

FINDING HELP: YOUR CHILD'S TEAM

Why Have a Team?

Not everyone will need a "team" of professionals to help them. Each child with AS is unique. Some may not require special education classification or services, or need to have an ongoing relationship with a child psychologist, psychiatrist, or mental health counselor.

When you're just starting to get your bearings and adapting to new approaches for school, behavior, and other important issues, it's a good idea to have a professional in your corner. For most children, AS changes, so it's wise to look ahead. Many parents recall behavioral tactics and interventions that worked like magic for a while and then lost their power, and sudden, inexplicable changes, for better and for worse. It's not unusual for a very young child with AS to become moody and difficult once she realizes that she is different from other children or that socialization is difficult for her. Any life event that can trigger problems for a typical child—emotional trauma, moving, loss of loved ones or family pets, divorce, an old friend who suddenly "outgrows" the relationship, the arrival of a new sibling, an unsympathetic teacher—can have equal but unpredictable effects for the child with AS. That moment of crisis may not be the best time to start looking for a professional. It may be wiser to meet with or at least have recommendations of a doctor or therapist you could turn to in an emergency.

Beyond that, there are often more mundane situations that call for a professional's intervention. One of the most common is school, particularly when it comes to making decisions about placement, the most appropriate classroom situation, and the need for other supports, such as one-on-one aides, or paraprofessionals. Through OASIS, we've heard from many parents who are distressed because their child's teacher or other district personnel are "recommending" medication for the child in lieu of providing appropriate supports. In situations like these, the opinion of your child's doctor can tip the balance in your favor.

Who Is on Your Team?

Your team may be just one person whom you and your child trust and feel comfortable with, or it may be three, four, or more. Either way, be the "captain," the person who makes sure that each team member gets relevant test results and other important information from the others. There's no hard-and-fast rule about what kind of professional is "best" in every case. You may find a teacher or a counselor who has a great rapport with your child and an instinctive understanding of AS. On the other hand, you may find that your local ASD expert is someone whose advice is invaluable but who does not see patients regularly. You may need to patch together what you need from an array of sources. Your child may see a counselor or therapist for socialization work and an occupational therapist for sensory integration issues weekly, while she sees an M.D. for medication management only several times a year.

One of the biggest challenges for parents in many areas of the country is lack of access to professionals familiar with AS and related disorders. Often the solution is to find a sympathetic doctor or therapist and help that person become as well versed in AS as you are. Granted, this isn't an ideal situation, but it may be well worth the effort, particularly if you anticipate resistance from your school district or any other situation that might require some professional backup. If you and your child can build a relationship with such a professional, particularly one not averse to consulting with other specialists outside your immediate area, all the better.

WHEN PARENTS AND PROFESSIONALS DON'T AGREE

In dealing with professionals, parents sometimes find themselves in the uncomfortable position of disagreeing with recommendations or observations. As much as we wish it were not so, the fact is that everyone who deals with your child has the potential to make a mistake. As a parent, it is your right—your obligation—to question the professionals working with your child. Though ultimately you decide the course, any disorder as challenging as AS is a hotbed for second-guessing. Don't feel compelled to follow outside recommendations solely because they come from professionals. This sword cuts both ways, however. A potentially successful intervention is just as easily undermined by the parent who opposes a particular behavior modification plan on principle or by the teacher who halfheartedly trains the paraprofessional she doesn't believe your child truly needs.

Professional training, federal mandates, state regulations, and best-practices standards of treatment are only as good as the people charged with applying them. You may feel that you have more than enough to juggle without having to worry about how the people who are supposed to be helping your child feel about you or your partner personally. In a moment of frustration or disappointment, it's not always easy to think beyond the immediate problem. However, try to remind yourself that with each encounter (or confrontation), you are laying down a piece of road that you and your child may be traveling for years to come. This is not to say that you should simply go along to get along, or be more concerned with being liked than being listened to. It does mean, however, that approaching advocacy as a form of negotiation can be more effective and less stressful for everyone involved.

There are times when you may have to temper your natural parental response to become your child's most passionate, most vociferous, and most aggressive advocate. We parents often feel like we're "fighting" for our child, but in fact we're really negotiating—for services, for understanding, for support from those who may not agree with our decisions. Ultimately, we are working toward building, brick by brick, a place in the world for our child.

When most of us think about advocacy, we immediately think of school and special education services. But advocating for your child with AS often means laying the groundwork for understanding, becoming your child's ambassador to the world. You may find yourself asking others to make allowances and accommodations for your child that can range from asking a neighbor to turn down a radio to demanding that your school district hire a full-time specialist to help your child in class. Learning the basics of negotiation can ease your stress, build goodwill, and, most important, get you and your child where you want to go.

Try to See the Other Side

If a professional is recommending something for your child, try to understand why he or she is doing so. While it is true that no one knows your child better than you do, you may encounter (if you are fortunate) at least one professional—be it a doctor, a teacher, a therapist—who has seen a number of children who share at least some behaviors, traits, deficits, or skills with your own. Patty admits to being taken aback years ago when upon meeting a teacher who would end up working successfully with her son for many years, the teacher remarked, "I may not know your son that well yet, but I know autism." "I remember thinking, *Who do you think you are?*" she recalls. Now as a teacher herself, she admits that while she would never utter those words to a parent, she understands what that teacher meant and that it was, in fact, true.

Like parents, good teachers and other professionals also see our children as individuals, but they do see them differently. However, it is a history of experience with a number of individuals and professional knowledge of the disorder that gives them this alternative viewpoint. Good teachers—and doctors and therapists—want to see children and their families grow and succeed. What they are that most parents are not are witnesses to the big picture of how the disorder and challenges may play out in a child's life, both today and tomorrow. They also have the advantage of the professional distance to suggest and even carry out interventions, behavior plans, and therapies that a child may be less than happy about. If we are honest, we know that sometimes other professionals can teach or coach our kids through things that we know we could never do on our own. You owe it to your child—and yourself—to give them that chance.

Parents ourselves, we are reluctant to state the obvious, but here it goes: Parenting a child with a disability often demands being more protective and more defensive than we might be of a typical child. By the time you've received a diagnosis or come into contact with professionals, you may have had a lot of practice in feeling that it's just you and your child or you and your family versus the world. Yes, it hurts to hear someone speak of your child's deficits, and it's not unusual to feel you're being criticized when even the most well-meaning professional suggests things we might do differently. It's difficult to push a child you feel needs protection. It's almost impossible to expose to risk and possible failure someone you believe has not gotten a fair shake. After all, you might wonder, if so many things are so hard for him, is it really right to demand that he learn to do things that may be difficult or at which he may fail?

The answer is yes. Remember, your child is not a "done deal"—not by a long shot. You do not know everything he is capable of achieving or overcoming—no one does. One thing professionals may have a clearer view of is a child's potential or the value of trying, of taking a chance. Where a parent might see the possible pain of total failure at, say, participating in a gym class or learning to ride a skateboard, a teacher might see instead the value of a small victory in the attempt, the pride that follows the one little step that works.

As parents, we have to face the fact that we probably are not the most objective observers of our children. We can't be. It is important that we learn to listen calmly and rationally to what professionals say. Before thinking or saying, "Not my child," or "He doesn't really need that intervention," ask the professional what the recommendation is based upon, why she is making it, what results she hopes to see, and what present or future problems she hopes to solve.

SETTING THE AGENDA

No matter how young your child is when you realize he has AS, you probably worry over the time you've lost, the signs you missed, the opportunities for intervention that seem to have passed. This is natural but ultimately unproductive. If you're looking back (and we all do it), do not overlook the right things you did as well. All that you can control, and all that really matters, is what you can begin doing today.

The big question many of us confront is not so much "Now what?" but "What next?" And even more agonizingly, "What first?"

Chances are, your child will receive more than one form of intervention. If your child qualifies for special education, some of these—academic help, occupational therapy, speech and language therapy, for instance—will be provided in the course of the school day. Even so, many parents feel the need to do more. Special education is designed to help students with issues that pertain directly to their ability to learn. You may be surprised to learn that socialization therapy isn't always a top priority for school districts, even though it is probably the single most important intervention for AS.

Because children with AS are usually relatively high functioning, they don't routinely receive the training in daily living skills that lower-functioning students do. A surprising number of parents report that their ten-year-old math whiz is still not brushing his own hair or tying his own shoes. Though the role of self-help skills in education might be debatable, the importance of children learning the basic skills of independent living is not. Many parents find that they need extra help.

SETTING PRIORITIES

Which is more important? Socialization skills taught and practiced in a group or one-on-one therapy? Participation in a small group that shares your daughter's special interest or having the experience of being part of a modified or regular Girl Scout troop? Which behavior should be addressed first—the tantruming or the refusal to do homework? How much time should be spent on OT to strengthen handwriting muscles? How much on structured play dates? How much on academic work?

Through it all, remember that you can effectively target and address only one behavioral issue at a time. Inevitably some problem behaviors or issues will have to wait their turn. In some cases, change will come slowly, and that can be frustrating for everyone. Now is a good time to talk with your partner and perhaps your child's doctor and teachers to pinpoint the most pressing needs. While it would be nice if Seth's handwriting were easier for him, it may be more important that he learn to ask for help when he is confused or use some relaxation technique when he begins to feel stressed. Bear in mind that your priorities may not be his teacher's or your partner's. Try to talk it out and reach a compromise. Especially if you're working on changing behaviors, it is essential that everyone be on the same page. Do your best to present a united front and be consistent. Your conflicting demands and changing expectations coupled with your child's struggle to change are a recipe for frustration, low self-esteem, and less willingness to "get with the program" in the future.

Even if your child hasn't been told of his diagnosis, if he is old enough he should be included in your plans for intervention. People with AS are known for their "immunity" to the motivational tricks that work so well on most of us. However, one great thing about children with AS is that it is often easy enough to discover what will motivate them: access to the special interest, an opportunity to participate in something they enjoy, a chance to talk about a topic they really care about. Still, every person is different. Knowing that occupational therapy may make handwriting easier or that speech therapy will simplify listening to directions can give the child a goal, a reason for the many hours of hard work ahead. In a loving, nonjudgmental way, discuss the areas in which you will all be working toward improvement, and specifically how you will help your child. Have a plan that involves you, your partner, and others close to your child, so that he doesn't feel he's going it alone. And never miss a single opportunity to praise your child specifically, lavishly, and generously for his efforts.

BE A DETECTIVE

One sound strategy is to begin with an inventory of challenges, problems, and deficits you and your team believe should be addressed. It is relatively easy to pinpoint the necessary prerequisite skills for academic success. If, for instance, a child were struggling in most of his subjects and was behind grade level in reading, we would almost automatically focus on improving his reading. Unfortunately, identifying the pivotal prerequisite skills or compensatory strategies for an individual whose profile may be complex is not so simple. Start by talking candidly with a select group of those who know your child well; this may include professionals, family members, people you trust. What do they see as the most pressing issues? As a parent, you may have become inured to something like constant run-on talking or even tantruming. For example, many of us have lived with—and learned to accommodate and "live around"—tantruming for so long that we may not fully appreciate the impact it has on your child's social opportunities among his classmates or its disruptive effect on others. Of course, the final decision as to where you will concentrate your efforts is yours, but getting input from others can be very helpful. If, for instance, your spouse, your child's teacher, and her socialization therapist all consider improving frustration tolerance job one, then you can proceed as certain as you can be that you're on the right track.

You might want to spend a week or two collecting data on your child's behavior. See page 424 on how to do this. It might help to list the behaviors or challenges and then note which of these are self-contained or isolated (e.g., frustration over missing a favorite television program before going to school) and which have a strong negative effect on other areas (e.g., sensory sensitivities, problems with social skills). As you learn more about AS, it will become easier to trace problems back to their not-always-obvious root causes. For example, difficulties with transitioning and changes in routine are not behavior problems in the usual sense. They often result from a basic anxiety and misunderstanding that can be allayed with visuals like calendars, pictures, and schedules; Social Stories (see chapter 6); and routines.

Sometimes the most pressing problem is obvious—frequent outbursts, for instance—but the best intervention may not be. Though three children's meltdowns may look very much the same, they may each have a different cause. For one child, it may be an anxiety disorder, for another a sensory integration issue, for a third, simple fatigue and stress from the classroom environment. Determining the true cause often requires detective work. For parents, that means never taking any behavior at face value and never projecting how you would feel in your child's situation. Think back to all of the times you responded to your child's crying or smiling with a remark that essentially told him what (you thought) he was feeling: "I'll bet you're mad that your bike tipped over," "You must have had a great/rough day at camp," and so on. Some of us do this because a child lacks the ability to express himself or herself, and observations like these can help open up a conversation. However, particularly with a child who has AS, the emotion behind the expression is not always easy to read. Children with AS who have had a good day at school may become difficult once home simply because they *can* be difficult at home, where people are more understanding. It's always better to ask questions or otherwise get to the crux of the issue before offering "guesstimated" observations.

Once they know about AS, most parents can look back on specific incidents and behaviors with new eyes. You may realize, for instance, that your daughter's screaming fit at the department store makeup counter had everything to do with the bright lights, the crackle of the store PA system, and the ambient noise of a crowd of people talking in a large space with marble floors. Once you learn how to pinpoint the underlying problems, it becomes easier to see how large a role a condition like sensory integration disorder or the basic inability to process social information may be playing in behaviors or responses that otherwise would be easily misread.

Often, we and the professionals we consult are so focused on what is "wrong" that we lose sight of or forget about what goes "right." This is especially true when you're tracking the precursors to undesirable behaviors and reactions. However, you can learn almost as much from paying close attention to those situations and moments in which your child functions the best. It might help to begin keeping a journal that also includes incidents that occurred in the past. Let's start with a particular behavior; for example, a seeming inability to hear when spoken to. List on a piece of paper when and under what circumstances you notice the behavior most frequently and/or in its most extreme form. Include in your notes details about the environment: the size of the room, the number of people, the noise level, what kind of noise it was, the reason your child was there at that particular time, what else was going on (whether or not he was engaged in a pleasurable activity, for instance), and so on. Also think back on the day: Was there another incident or situation that preceded this incident, even if it occurred hours or days before and seems, on the surface, unrelated? Was your child rested, ill, or coming down with something? Did the place or the situation have a "history" for your child (for example, the doctor's office where she got a shot, the mall where he heard a fire alarm go off)? Did your child have expectations of what it would be like there? Were there unexpected changes?

Next, list the places and situations where the behavior does *not* occur. What do they have in common? How are they different from the problem situations? Consider your child, time of day, environment, and so on.

GATHER INTELLIGENCE FROM ALL YOUR SOURCES

Ask teachers for their input, too. Each person who deals with your child will have his or her own opinions on the causes and the possible interventions. For some children with AS, environment is an important factor in behavior, and different environments can spark or tamp different behaviors. In addition, some of our children can be extraordinarily sensitive to different personality types. Your child's doctor or teacher may not observe behaviors or reactions that you consider serious. One child we know had a fairly serious motor tic involving his hands, yet a pair of occupational therapists never saw it once in nearly a year of twice-weekly sessions. Another child, whom his teacher considers "a joy to have in the classroom," drives his mother to distraction with his constant whining and frequent outbursts. Conversely, teachers may report behaviors that parents never witness, including some that they simply do not believe their child capable of, such as hitting, screaming, and acting disrespectfully.

Children with AS often respond differently to different situations. The classic example is the child who manages to hold it together during the school day only to come through the front door upset, on edge, or furious. Or, because she cannot apply to one situation what is learned in another, your child may have wonderful table manners at home but not at her grandmother's.

Not everyone will understand the influence of AS on your child. Not everyone who makes an observation or a recommendation about your child will be correct. Sometimes educators, doctors, and other professionals bear news that is disappointing or makes us feel self-conscious about our child's condition or our parenting skills. However, if your child hit someone in school, you'll help yourself and your child by focusing on solving the problem behind the behavior rather than arguing about whether it happened or whose fault it was.

MANAGING THE DAY-TO-DAY

Be Your Child's Protector

If you are neurotypical, you are probably better able to anticipate problematic situations and trouble than your child with AS can. As a result of their inability to rapidly process many bits of social information around them, people with AS are often easy to intimidate, take advantage of, or otherwise hurt. Parents of children with AS are usually instinctively protective, even overprotective. To a greater degree than most people can even comprehend, much less understand, we are our children's shelter.

Sounding more like a Secret Service agent assigned to protect the president than a mom, one mother of a child with multiple sensory sensitivities describes a typical outing to the local ice-cream shop. "Before we even park, I look at the parking lot and try to determine how crowded it is inside. If there are too many cars, we go someplace else. Once inside, I automatically run through what we call the 'Eric Inventory': loud music, crying babies, balloons that threaten to pop, blenders, what Eric calls 'noisy' air-conditioning—which none of us can hear. Before the waitress seats us, I'm scanning the room for the 'right' table or booth: far from the hubbub of the kitchen and the front door, away from the cash register, out of the full sun, and away from birthday parties or other noisy groups. I also make it a point to get a look at the dessert case, just to be sure I limit Eric's choices to flavors that are available that day. They know Eric at this place, so I let him place the orders, because it's good socialization practice. Once our orders arrive, I ask for the check immediately and pay it, just in case we have to suddenly rush out of the place when one of the hundred things that could possibly go awry does. I enjoy Eric's company so much, and I love taking him places. But from the moment the front door closes behind me, I feel like we're all on high alert."

A large part of helping our kids cope with AS is anticipating problems that might arise and having a plan for avoiding, containing, or escaping the fallout. As time goes by and wherever possible, though, we want to focus on teaching our children to improve their own detection systems and their coping skills. For most parents, necessity—and a few memorable scenes—forces the development and constant refinement of our ace troubleshooting skills. That living "on high alert" has become second nature doesn't make it any less stressful or tiring. "I had no idea how much thought I put into just going out with Lisa until my sister-in-law offered to take her out for the day," one mother said. "My 'little list' of dos and don'ts ran fifty items long and included everything from 'avoid the candy aisle at the supermarket' to 'no ice in cold drinks.' When my sister-in-law saw it, she made some comment to the effect, 'Don't you think you're over-doing it?' When she brought Lisa, who had had a wonderful time, home that night, however, she said one of the nicest things anyone's said to me since Lisa was a baby: 'I don't know how you do it.'"

Looking back, most parents report that as their children grew, their ability to cope with difficult situations increased. Sometimes the change occurs as a result of deliberate, intensive intervention; other times, children seem to "outgrow" certain sensitivities and re-actions. In the meantime, it helps to have in place your own personal protocol for potentially volatile situations. Avoiding or protecting your child from overwhelming or uncomfortable situations or stim-uli is not babying, coddling, or spoiling. It's being smart and caring. Depending on the circumstances (where, when, with whom), an in-stance of sensory overload or acting out can be devastating for your child. Forcing him or her to tough it out—which may be appropri-ate for a neurotypical child—probably won't help and, if anything, might be counterproductive, giving rise to future phobia-level fears, anxiety, and avoidant behavior. We have yet to see much hard re-search on this, but we have heard from countless parents and know firsthand the remarkable staying power of unpleasant memories. Sometimes an older child will be willing to attempt a historically dif-ficult situation—a noisy mall, for instance—if he knows for certain that he has a way out. The child who tells you, "I think the noise is starting to make me nervous" or "It's too crowded here for me" is not whining, nor are you "spoiling" him by responding. He is learn-ing to monitor his own behavior and to advocate for himself. As an adult, he alone will be responsible for his own crisis avoidance and rescue. You can reinforce that behavior by responding appropriately. If he needs to leave this time, you leave, though it would not be un-reasonable the next time to encourage him to stay a little bit longer. Patty has found that for Justin, just knowing that he will be taken out of a situation if he needs to be has resulted in his willingness to ven-ture into new situations.

While some AS behaviors may remain unpredictable, a lot of what strikes us as inexplicable and bizarre is actually easily explained. If you can predict or anticipate a reaction, you may have the power to avoid or ameliorate its consequences. Of course, life is full of surprises: the car alarm that sounds two feet from your child's ear, the scent of fresh-baked apple pie that leaves him gagging in the bakery. Some parents balk at having to put so much planning into simple activities such as grocery shopping or buying new clothes for school. Try to remember, though, that AS compromises your child's ability to feel comfortable and in control. Structure, scheduling, and routines help address some of that. But out there, in the world, your child depends on you or another caring person to foresee the potential trouble spots that she cannot and to establish a "zone of control" where none exists.

Be Your Child's Teacher

True, every parent is a teacher. But what we're talking about here is looking at what you can do for your child in a slightly different light. Even those children whose schedules are full of interventions and therapies still have a lot of "downtime" outside the therapeutic "net." While it would be impossible for a parent to spend every waking moment expressly teaching, there is a comfortable middle ground. In later chapters, we discuss specific things parents can do to help teach social skills, among other things.

While you can never ignore the fact that your child is your child, when you decide to teach a particular skill—let's say better table manners or how to follow a schedule—it can help to adopt a more neutral posture than what might be natural to you as a parent. If you have decided that you are going to teach your son to get up, get dressed, and arrive at the breakfast table within ten minutes of being awoken, consider beforehand what will most effectively teach him the independence you wish to instill. Doing most of the things that come a little too easily to some of us as parents—making multiple trips upstairs to "check" on his progress, reminding and nagging from downstairs, and finally lecturing him sternly, venting your frustration, or punishing him when twenty minutes pass and he's still under the covers—do not constitute teaching, nor do they encourage independence. (After all, if they did, you wouldn't have this problem in the first place.) Instead, you might take a more teacherly approach:

• Make your demands and the consequences (for both completing the task and not) crystal clear beforehand.

• Be sure your child has all the skills he needs to accomplish the task in the time allotted. (Can he manage his buttons and zippers? Is he showering independently? Are there distractions in his room that sidetrack him and should be removed?) If he does not, teach him those skills *first*.

• Remove yourself as a prompt or cue. Instead of you personally monitoring him, set a timer for ten minutes and let it run. Say nothing and let the timer determine if your child has accomplished the task.

• If your child succeeds—arrives downstairs completely and neatly dressed, hair combed, teeth brushed, etc.—praise him and reward him as promised.

• If your child fails, leave your anger, frustration, and nagging out of it. As calmly as possible, outline the consequences for the failure to complete the task (no video games after school, perhaps), ask your child what might help him to do better tomorrow, and work on that, if necessary. Then move on.

Be Your Child's Advocate—and His Ambassador

One of the hardest parts of dealing with AS is learning to deal with some of the behaviors and reactions that come with it—including our own and those of others. Ideally, school district personnel, doctors, friends, family members, and strangers should always treat him—and you—fairly and with respect. Unfortunately, not everyone is capable of or interested in rising to the occasion. Some situations are sadly common: the friend who loses interest, the family members who refuse to make allowances, the stranger who loudly asks, "What's wrong with him?"

We will probably never escape the persistent belief that somehow parents are at least to some degree responsible for who their children are or how they behave. No matter what you're doing, there may be someone in your child's world who feels that you should be doing something more or something less, something different or something the same. It's also human nature, it seems, to offer up those opinions—whether they are solicited, informed, or fair. There also seems to be some cultural compulsion to talk at or about anyone who appears somehow different, as if they weren't there or were incapable of understanding what was being said. If you have ever returned from an outing wishing you could never leave your house again, you are not alone.

Build Your Child a Road to the Future

The good news is that as you learn more about AS and more about your child, the unhappy scenes and the stressful moments become easier to avoid and easier to cope with when they do occur. With information and understanding in hand, you can become empowered. Though we may be veterans of show-stopping tantrums, nasty glares, and racing hearts, few of us ever become hardened enough. It may be that you will still spend many occasions trying to locate the quickest route out of a department store, but you'll also have many opportunities to see your child experience a great success. Throughout all of this, you may find that you are a much stronger and steadier person than you ever imagined yourself to be. Develop the right combination of understanding, patience, and courage to try something new, for you and your child.

It may be difficult for you to believe that things may not always be this way, that one day your child may be able to go to a movie without panicking, enjoy having a friend over to play, or attend a high school dance. We—and our children—are shaped by our experiences, and failure, disappointment, and fear can make it difficult to push ahead and to try again. We know firsthand how hard it is to instill confidence in a child when deep inside you fear the worst. It takes a healthy dose of courage to pave the way and then gently push your child beyond where he is comfortable. It also takes practice—practice to find the factors that contribute to success and practice recovering from failure.

Despite all this, we urge you and others who care about our kids to look to their future. True, there are some things about having AS that can never be changed. However, there is much that can be done to expand your child's zone of comfort and to teach him skills for coping outside of it.

Chapter 6

OPTIONS AND INTERVENTIONS

THE first question most parents ask once they know their child has Asperger Syndrome is "What do I do now?" The answer, of course, depends on your child. Although experts and practitioners in different fields may disagree, the fact is, no single intervention, treatment, or therapy works every time for every child. And no single intervention, treatment, or therapy alone will address every concern. The challenge for you is deciding which to pursue, when, and how. It's only natural to feel somewhat overwhelmed.

"I'll never forget those first few weeks after Kevin was diagnosed," his mother, Adrienne, said. "Every time I turned around, it seemed that someone was recommending a different course of treatment. Kevin's psychologist thought that regular 'talk' therapy would help, while the person who evaluated him at school suggested occupational therapy and speech. A few weeks later, he was seen by a neurologist, who raised the issue of medication. Then someone I met through an online chat group claimed that ABA [applied behavior analysis, which we'll discuss shortly] had changed her son's life. When I turned to my 'crew' of experts, the psychologist admitted she didn't know much about ABA, the school's occupational therapist warned me that in his opinion medication was never 'the answer,' and the neurologist bluntly said, 'There's no science behind occupational therapy.' My head was spinning. I was so afraid I would make a mistake and that Kevin would not get the help he needed, or worse, be harmed or set back in some way by the wrong therapy."

Ideally, the professionals who know your child could offer you a comprehensive plan of action that would outline the best choices for your particular child and provide some sound statistics on the effectiveness of each. Unfortunately, the current state of treatment for Asperger Syndrome does not allow for that. For now, it's largely a matter of trial and error, for parents, practitioners, and children, too.

There are some studies, but their practical use to parents is often limited by the size of the study or the profile of the children included. Evaluating the validity of studies of persons with AS is further complicated by the fact that different researchers may apply different diagnostic criteria to determine which potential subjects are included or excluded. In addition, the criteria themselves, as so many experts have pointed out, are not always sufficiently clear. One study may include among its subjects persons another study would exclude. Or one study may exclude persons with AS who had early speech delay, while another would include them.[1]

Relatively few families have access to a professional with extensive experience with AS *and* the wide range of effective interventions. As a result, most parents rely on anecdotal evidence based on the personal experiences of other parents and professionals. It's not a perfect situation, but there are steps you can take to make informed decisions and avoid those interventions from which your child would be least likely to benefit.

Step back, take a deep breath, and remember that even though time is of the essence, you don't have to decide anything today. Listen to what everyone involved has to say. Learn to hear beyond their words and to think critically about the options. Learn to trust your judgment. In most cases, when something works, you will be able to see a difference. Positive changes that result from some interventions (for example, socialization programs, auditory integration training [AIT], or sensory integration therapy [SIT]) may not be obvious until your child has been on the program for several weeks or months. If, after giving an intervention a fair trial, it doesn't seem to make much difference, exacerbates old problems, or sparks new ones, talk with the therapist or practitioner, then consider taking a break from it or simply stopping.[2] You can always try it again at another time (say, for example, over the summer vacation rather than during a busy school year) or with another practitioner.

A MIRACLE? A CURE?

Sooner or later, most of us hear or read about the child who was miraculously "cured" and today shows absolutely no trace of AS or a related diagnosis. We welcome the long-overdue surge in public awareness of AS, but there's no denying the sometimes under-informed, biased, and sensationalistic package many of these stories come in. Parents are understandably drawn to reports of the child who is dramatically improved, even "cured" of AS or ASD. How did they do it? Specific therapies, diets, vitamins and other nutritional supplements, educational programs, massage therapy, homeopathy, acupuncture, experimental use of medications—there's no end to the number of interventions that may have shown amazing results for at least one child with an ASD. And therein lies the problem for parents who may be desperate to help their child. When hope clings by a thread, it's difficult to hear such stories without wondering, "If that child, why not mine?"

Remember, no one knows the cause of AS or any other ASD. It is possible that ASDs, like allergies, come in many forms with many different causes, or even a combination of causes for each individual. The picture emerging from research suggests strongly that there is a strong genetic component and that ASDs affect numerous neurological components and processes. Just because your child and my child both have a special interest or engage in hand flapping does not mean that they do it for the same reason or that the same intervention will produce the same result for both. There is no question that many children have benefited from following a casein- and gluten-free diet. Does this mean that some deficit in how the body handles these molecules "causes" autism in everyone? No. There are children whose attention has been improved by AIT or SIT. Does that mean that auditory processing problems or sensory integration difficulties "cause" AS? No. For every child who has benefited from any given treatment, there are some—sometimes many—who have seen no change. Does this mean that those who advocate this or that intervention are "wrong"? No, again. Is an intervention worth trying? That's something parents must decide.

As a parent, it will fall to you to weigh the options and make the hard decisions. Most parents would do anything for a child. Unfortunately, few of us are in a position to do so, no matter how our hearts feel. For most of us, there's the service the school district denies, the doctor your insurance company will not cover, the therapy that is, literally, five hundred miles away. There is also the matter of time. Our children will not remain children forever. The sooner they begin to learn to be independent, to monitor and regulate their emotions, to understand and make themselves understood by others, the better. For that reason alone, it might make more sense to start off with those interventions that are the most widely used and promising, and save the less established for somewhere down the road.

LEARNING TO WEIGH OPINIONS

Practitioners, educators, and parents can be enthusiastic and persuasive about treatment options they believe in or have been trained to use. They can also be equally opinionated about those they do not believe in or are unfamiliar with. We've heard from many parents who are troubled and confused by the sometimes strong, even emotional, opinions expressed by the professionals they would like to feel they can rely on for unbiased, factual information. Unless you find a specialist who has seen hundreds of cases of AS or a related disorder, your professional may base a recommendation for your child on his or her experience with a mere handful of other cases. Those other children with AS may have widely varying profiles, ages, symptoms, and histories. The parents of girls with AS are doubly challenged in this area, since girls make up a fraction of AS diagnoses, and their symptoms and behaviors can be quite different from those seen in boys.

Under these circumstances, it's probably wise to question anyone—professional or layperson—who makes sweeping generalizations about any form of treatment, pro or con. It's important to discriminate between a statement like "Vitamin B_6 really reduced my son's tendency to tantrum" and "Everyone knows that vitamin therapy is the only way to go" or "There's no evidence that vitamins do anything; don't waste your time." One valuable service the OASIS on-line message board provides parents and others is the ability to poll, albeit informally, hundreds of other people about their experiences with different therapies. Granted, the results are anecdotal, but a parent who posts to ask about, say, sensory integration therapy stands a good chance of hearing from more parents who have tried it than the number of children your child's doctors and teachers may have seen in a decade. Always remember: Posts on message boards are opinions, and it's up to you to sort through the biases.

Sometimes the less orthodox, least studied interventions are those that seem safer, less invasive, less expensive, or just generally more attractive than some others. Each of us has our own internal scale on which we rank potential interventions from "first resort" to "last resort." Understandably, most parents have no qualms about occupational therapy, for example, but are conflicted about the prospect of their child taking psychotropic prescription medication. We have to recognize our own biases to evaluate what's best for our child. You may have a hard time coming to terms with the idea that your child requires a self-contained special education classroom or that he may need to be on medication. Try not to waste time in seeing the solution or the intervention as the problem. The real problem is what brought you to this possible solution. Patty recalls the day she first saw the self-contained special education classroom Justin would join. "I cried later at home," she remembers. "But within a week, I realized that this was a happy place, a place where he could—and did—learn, thrive, and make some wonderful little friends."

It would be unconscionable to suggest that parents "get over it," "get with the program," or "move on" while we're learning to negotiate this new world. Let's be honest: You may never become totally objective about your child's diagnosis or its implications for his life. However, you can work toward separating those strong, complex, and understandable emotions from the important decision making you must do.

How we view our child's treatment reflects not only our experiences and beliefs about AS and the role of intervention but our ideas of what a childhood should be and how AS affects it. You may find it helpful for you and, if applicable, your partner to discuss and establish at least a tentative framework for your approach to intervention. In two-parent families, some couples are equally involved in researching options and communicating with the professionals in-volved. Most, however, find it more practical for one parent to assume most of those responsibilities, although they make important deci-sions together. Yet others find that one parent, due to other demands or an emotional difficulty with accepting the diagnosis, is essentially uninvolved. If you're a single parent, you may have to assume this re-sponsibility alone. You might consider involving a caring, trusted family member or a close friend. It's always good to have someone to bounce ideas off of. Depending on your situation, you will also have to consider access to professionals and services, financial resources, insurance coverage, and other details.

Remember that how AS manifests in your child will change over time, sometimes dramatically and suddenly. You should try to gain at least a basic knowledge of *all* the intervention options, including those you have filed under "last resort," so that you'll have a head start in making important decisions you may confront in the future.

Finally, don't limit yourself to considering resources tailored spe-cifically to AS. Most of the interventions listed here were either de-signed initially for persons with autistic disorder and other PDDs or were developed by persons whose background and training involved persons with autistic disorder. You may find that resources with the terms *autism* and *PDD* in the title are also geared to or can be adapted for AS.

LEARNING MORE ABOUT EACH APPROACH

Later in this chapter we'll review the therapies and interventions that are most widely used in AS. In considering these (or any other therapy), ask professionals and practitioners the following questions.

What specific symptoms or behaviors does this therapy ad-dress, and how? No therapy or treatment can address every issue your child might have. Sometimes parents are disappointed when they learn that a promising intervention helps them manage prob-lems one through six but stops short of eliminating or reducing number seven. Ask your professional to describe the limitations of what a specific therapy can achieve. What, you should ask, is the theory or the research behind this approach? Does that theory make sense to you? Does the research seem credible? If there is little or no research available, ask why. If a professional truly believes that the disorder or dysfunction their approach addresses is at the root of most if not all AS symptoms, ask why. Bear in mind, however, that the best scientists and researchers are still working on this question.

Effective treatments for AS come from a variety of disciplines, each with its own terminology. Sometimes jargon can be helpful, as when it describes a novel concept or process, such as sensory integration disorder. Other times, however, the overuse of highly technical terms will just confuse you. Since you probably will be called upon many times to explain your child or the treatment course you have chosen, it's important to be comfortable in your understanding of it. You don't have to become an expert, but you'll feel more confident if you can explain in plain English, for example, the basic concept of proprioception (essentially, body awareness, or the unconscious awareness of where your body is in space and what different parts of your body are doing) to the grandmother who still asks, "Shouldn't a nine-year-old be buttoning his own shirts?" If your therapist overuses jargon, ask for a translation.

You might want to bring a notebook with you to therapy sessions or appointments, at least in the beginning. Write down questions you have, terms you'd like explained, and anything you've observed in your child that might be relevant. Request any print material that is available and ask for recommendations of books, articles, and Web sites. Don't be shy. If you have a question, ask. If the answer you get doesn't clarify the matter, ask again or ask for an example of how a particular problem may manifest in real life for your child. For example, if the therapist says your child has problems with praxis—or motor planning—you need to know that that may make handwriting difficult and impede his ability to solve jigsaw puzzles or construct structures out of building toys such as Legos.

How long can I expect this treatment to last? There's no single quick fix. Except for therapies with a specific timetable, treatments are open-ended. No one will be able to predict how long your child will need it. For many children, speech and language therapy, occupational therapy, social skills training, and other interventions continue for years. Considering how many different issues can impact on others (for example, how sensory integration issues may affect dysgraphia or attempts to follow a particular diet), it's not always easy to sort out what's working and what's not. In some cases, the improvement can be dramatic and quick; in others it may be more like a steady series of nearly indiscernible changes that culminate in what may appear, weeks or months later, as a newly acquired skill or ability.

What can I do at home, and what can his teachers do at school, to enhance and reinforce the work you are doing with my child? Once you have a basic understanding of what a particular therapy strives to achieve and how, you can help your child expand and build on what he learns "in session." For example, in occupational therapy, seven-year-old Jordan has been working on learning to discriminate visually between objects that are similar but subtly different. On trips to the grocery store, Jordan's mother gives him the task of picking out a carton of his favorite ice-cream flavor from the freezer case. Not only does it reinforce an important skill, but Jordan has one more practical accomplishment to feel good about.

Most professionals working with school-age children are well aware of the challenges their patients face in the classroom. While special education teachers probably will be aware of steps they can take in the classroom to help your child with specific issues (for example, assigning the child with attentional difficulties the seat nearest her), most will welcome reasonable, practical suggestions conducive to a more positive, productive classroom experience. Therapists, doctors, and other professionals can have great insight into behaviors that fail to respond to other interventions. Unfortunately, solutions and strategies that are easily implemented in smaller specialized classrooms or the local weekly socialization class may not always translate smoothly into the regular classroom. No one knows the classroom or your child in the classroom better than his teacher. Strategies that make perfect sense to your behavior consultant or your child's psychologist, for instance, may be simply impractical to carry out in a regular classroom without extra help. Do what you can to help set up situations for everyone's success. Advocate for the smaller class size or the extra help your child's teacher may need to implement that strict behavioral program or the one-on-one support your child needs to protect his emotional health.

Help everyone to see beyond the obvious. Ten-year-old Ethan always became upset and sometimes even verbally aggressive when invited to present a math problem on the blackboard. Because his teacher knew that he knew the answers, she interpreted his reluctance as a behavior problem and responded by giving him time-outs and restricting his access to the computer during free period. The mystery of Ethan's "bad" behavior was solved when his occupational therapist realized that he literally could not touch a piece of chalk without drooling and feeling his stomach churn. Once his teacher understood this, she gave him a small dry-erase white board. When it was his turn to present a problem, he wrote on his board and placed it against the blackboard on the chalk tray, alongside his classmates' board work.

The more children move into mainstream and inclusion classroom settings—and away from the constant presence of educators with special education backgrounds—the greater the need for suggestions and strategies from "outside" therapists. Therapists may suggest classroom activities that will reinforce skills, such as assigning a child with low self-esteem the task of showing a new class member the ropes, or giving a child who is developing better motor planning skills the job of pouring juice at snack time. A child who seems to benefit from short breaks outside the classroom might be used as a "messenger" between the classroom and the principal's office or as an "escort" for other children.

PARENTS AS "THERAPISTS"

Not all interventions lend themselves to a do-it-yourself home approach. However, a dedicated parent can learn enough about Comic Strip Conversations (see page 198), Social Stories, social skills training, and certain forms of behavior modification to use them effectively at home. Occupational, physical, and speech and language therapists can show you tips and tricks to help your child "exercise" new skills and behaviors.

As any trained therapist or professional will tell you, though, there's a lot more to it than knowing the information or the technique. Professionals are trained to be objective and professional, and the success of some kinds of therapy depends heavily on their ability to remain emotionally calm, regardless of what occurs during therapy. Parents, on the other hand, are emotionally invested in both their child and the outcome. It is a rare parent who can achieve a totally "professional" demeanor, and it's probably not desirable, anyway. To work successfully with your child at home requires patience, tenacity, and an ability to check your emotions. It may be difficult to stick to a program if your child becomes easily frustrated or emotional. And, to be honest, it does take time and commitment to implement any program effectively. Some parents believe that most moments spent with their AS child are "therapy"-oriented as is and prefer not to add to that burden. If a specific approach seems suited for you and your child, we urge you to give it a try.

WATCH FOR BURNOUT

Parents whose children receive several types of intervention, concurrently or over a period of time, report experiencing "intervention burnout." No matter how effective or helpful a course of treatment may be, there is no denying the practical toll it can take on you, your child, and the rest of your family. Whatever treatment you choose, learning about it, implementing it, and keeping appointments all take time. You could spend two hours driving each way to an hour-long session with a distant specialist. As one father put it, "It sounds terrible, but there were times when we'd be sitting in yet another doctor's or therapist's waiting room and I'd think, *My daughter should be home playing right now.* The funny thing is, what we were doing was really working. Still, we were constantly juggling our schedules and the other kids'. The therapies and appointments were literally running our lives. There were times, I admit, when I'd almost wish something wouldn't work so we could cross one more weekly commitment off the calendar."

Be on the lookout for signs of burnout in your child, other family members, and yourself. A child who is chronically cranky, tired, overwhelmed, and on edge may be doing too much. Speak with your practitioner about this. Chances are, he or she can suggest techniques for getting around it. Changing the time of the appointment or the order of activities within each session can make a surprising difference.

Remember, parents burn out, too. You may find yourself thinking or saying things critical of the therapy or the therapist, downplaying your child's progress, and/or exaggerating the lack of it. Talk with your practitioner first and discuss your concerns. Ask others who know your child well—grandparents and other family members, teachers and other professionals, adult friends—if they see any improvement or progress. This is particularly important when your child is having trouble accomplishing the goals you and his practitioner have agreed on. Most children enjoy doing things they have some degree of mastery over and may naturally avoid those they do not. One result is that children and their parents are more likely to drop out of therapies that address the areas in which the child needs the most work. Before you decide to quit a therapy, try to be objective.

When therapy becomes stressful for whatever reason, you risk reaching a point of diminishing returns. Rather than stopping altogether, ask the therapist to consider cutting back on the least essential intervention, at least temporarily. Consider the "therapeutic" benefits of activities that are not interventions per se. For instance, you may weigh the socialization benefits your son derives from participating in a flexible and understanding Scout group against what he might gain from joining a more formal socialization group. Or you may opt for a weekly swimming lesson that includes all the children in your family over a second or third weekly physical therapy session. We are not suggesting that there are "nontherapeutic" substitutes for effective interventions, or that less specialized activities are of equal therapeutic value. Realistically, however, parents may find themselves forced to make choices.

THE MOST IMPORTANT MEMBER OF YOUR TEAM: YOUR CHILD

Finally, remember that the person who is working the hardest in all of this is not the parent racing from one appointment to the next or the therapist with the patience of a saint. It is your child. Even when something is really working and the improvements are obvious, it can be challenging, sometimes frustrating work for your child. During a period of "therapy rebellion," Patty's son asked, "Why do I have to do all these things that are so hard for me?" Once children reach a certain age, they may realize that not everyone has to forgo ice cream, take medicine, or have several appointments a week.

Children are smart enough to realize that you don't have to fix what's not broken. They may get a sense that they are doing these things because something is "wrong" with them and they may feel, justifiably, that it's not fair.

When you consider the emphasis parents and professionals place on rewarding improvement, as we should, it's easy to see how a child might wonder how we feel about him when he cannot do things as well. It's important to recognize, encourage, and reward accomplishments and new skills. However, it's even more important to remind him of what you love about him that has nothing to do with that improved pencil grip or better frustration tolerance. This includes particularly AS behaviors that may be rechanneled or reduced but probably never eliminated. Remember to praise your child liberally and lovingly for the abilities and talents that he values within himself. That may be a natural ability with math, music, or photography, an encyclopedic knowledge of streetlights, a prodigious memory, a kind heart, or a willingness to try.

FINDING AND PAYING FOR THERAPY

In our OASIS survey, we found that a substantial percentage of parents had forgone treatment or intervention because they lacked access or the ability to pay.

Most health insurance companies—90 percent to 95 percent, by one estimate—don't cover expenses related to pervasive developmental disorders.[3] Traditionally, disorders viewed as being psychiatric in nature and/or having little or no hope of improvement (which, unfortunately, is what autism and autism-related disorders have been in the past) have never had parity with "medical" disorders that result in similar symptoms, such as trauma, stroke, neurodegenerative diseases (Alzheimer's, Parkinson's, etc.), brain cancer, and so on. Even though it has been established that disorders like AS have a biological basis, the insurance companies that do offer coverage often do so under their mental health benefits. Ironically, the same occupational therapy that a company would cover if a patient suffered severe head injury due to an accident would not be covered if it was to treat a patient whose problem resulted from a pervasive developmental disorder. Some insurance companies refuse to cover diagnostic testing and therapy on the grounds that school districts are required to provide those services. Even those insurance companies that do provide benefits for "traditional" therapies for PDDs may refuse coverage for some treatments or limit the number of doctor visits or therapy sessions they will cover. Another issue for some families is simply finding a doctor or a therapist with extensive experience and a good reputation only to discover that she either does not participate in their insurance plan or does not take any insurance at all.

There is no simple answer to these problems, though parents have come up with any number of creative solutions, including persuading cooperative physicians to submit claims for other, covered treatments. (This "creative coding" is illegal.) We certainly don't recommend you break the law, but why not work to change it? As time-consuming and frustrating as the process may be, you should challenge every denial for coverage with an arsenal of documentation regarding the biological basis of AS and the resulting symptoms requiring treatment and a letter from your child's physician that clearly and compellingly explains the need for a specific treatment. Contact your state insurance commission and learn the commission's position on coverage of pervasive developmental disorders for the type of insurance policy you have. This is important because different types of insurance may fall under different state regulations. Some states have passed legislation that forces insurance companies to treat PDDs exactly like any other biologically based disorder. This is a crucial piece of information, since state insurance laws and regulation supersede anything in your insurance policy.

•••

Steps for Dealing with Denial of Benefits for Autism

The Autism Society of America suggests the following actions for dealing with insurance problems.[4]

- Obtain a written copy of the entire health plan (not just the benefits overview) from your employer or directly from your carrier.

Read the package carefully, including all information regarding exclusion and limitations on the policy. Keep the copy for your records.

- Obtain a written response from your insurance carrier stating the basis for either complete denial of coverage or curtailed benefits.
- You have the option of appealing your insurer's decision. Obtain written guidelines outlining your company's policy regarding the appeal process.
- Should you require legal assistance, you may wish to contact an attorney familiar with the insurance regulations and coverage in your state. A local ASA chapter or public interest law group may be able to assist you in this matter.
- If you have specific questions as to your state's health insurance laws and regulations, contact your state insurance commissioner's office. Usually located in the state capital, your state's insurance commissioner's office is listed in your telephone book.
- Some services for which you are seeking insurance reimbursement may be provided by your local educational agency (i.e., your school district) if they are an educational necessity. For information on your child's educational rights, contact your state parent training information agency and protection and advocacy organizations in your area.

If you cannot afford treatment, be honest with your practitioner. Inquire about the possibility of paying a reduced fee based on your income. Look into other places that may offer the treatment at reduced cost or free through teaching hospitals, colleges and universities, training programs, research centers, and studies. If you know of other children whose parents might be interested in, say, social skills training, consider forming a group and then approaching a practitioner about working with the group for a reduced fee. Contact your local AS-, autism-, or other disability–related advocacy or support group. Sometimes these organizations offer treatment and intervention programs and training for parents in topics such as behavior modification at reduced fees or free of charge.

INTERVENTIONS AND TREATMENTS

Listed here are the interventions for persons with AS that OASIS members expressed the most interest in. (We cover psychotropic prescription medication separately in the next chapter.) These are the interventions parents are most likely to hear about and, according to our OASIS surveys and years of watching the message boards, those that parents are most likely to consider and to use. There is a wide range of opinion among experts on how appropriate or effective some of these may be. You will find experts who are convinced that auditory integration training is useless or that applied behavior analysis (ABA) is incompatible with AS. Our own experiences, and those of hundreds of other parents, however, say otherwise. We cannot emphasize enough that no treatment is guaranteed to be effective for every child. Much depends on the child, the expertise of the practitioner, and the willingness of parents to carry through and reinforce these approaches in all environments, not just a practitioner's office or the classroom. Our purpose here is simply to help you make informed decisions.

APPLIED BEHAVIOR ANALYSIS (ABA)

What It Is

Broadly speaking, applied behavior analysis is a scientific approach to behavior that has been used in a wide range of fields beyond psychology. When the term *ABA* is used in the context of ASD, it usually refers to the method made famous by Dr. O. Ivar Lovaas at the University of California at Los Angeles in the 1960s to teach children with autistic disorder.[5] It is a specific, highly structured technique for analyzing the causes and effects of behavior, with the goal of teaching socially appropriate behavior, self-help skills, academic skills, and speech and language through promptly and appropriately reinforcing desired responses and behavior. Contrary to another popular misconception about ABA, the point is not to teach students to "parrot" behaviors but to learn how to learn and generalize the skills they do acquire, two things that persons with PDD cannot always do naturally on their own.

It sounds good, so why all the controversy? First, let's look at some of the arguments against ABA generally. Catherine Maurice, the mother of two children with autism whose progress through ABA therapy is recounted in her book *Let Me Hear Your Voice,* urges ABA therapists to do a better job explaining to parents what the method is *not.* "It is not training for compliance. It's not turning kids into robots. It's not feeding them candy all day so that they behave." These are, Maurice, says, "negative stereotypes,"[6] and, to the untrained or uneducated eye witnessing some types of ABA sessions, the technique might appear to be any or all of those things. If you are a parent interested in ABA for your child with AS, you may hear others describe ABA in similar terms, or worse. Some people have a problem with behaviorism generally, because they believe that there is "more to" why people, including children, do what they do than just what behaviors are reinforced or discouraged. Yes, it is true that the underlying principles of behaviorism and ABA were first observed and demonstrated through work with animals. But that does not make ABA "animal training for kids," as we have heard critics call it.

That said, parents may be uncomfortable with some aspects of ABA therapy if they do not understand the larger context or the principles underlying the approach. Let's look at a very simple case. Four-year-old Lucy cannot watch a favorite video without jumping up and down on the couch. This behavior is not only disturbing to others but potentially dangerous. You might find some parents and even some professionals who would argue that this is okay because Lucy craves some form of sensory stimulation, and she should be allowed to engage in this stereotypy in the privacy of her own home. Mom might believe that it would be "cruel" to take the video away. The last time Mom tried, Lucy "screamed for twenty minutes and hit me several times" before Mom gave in, put her on the couch, and turned on the video. After Lucy started jumping on the couch, she "really calmed down," Mom says.

Enter the ABA therapist. Remember, ABA concerns itself with observable behavior. From an ABA perspective, we have no way of knowing with certainty why Lucy is jumping on the couch. Here's what the ABA therapist sees (and records): Lucy is watching the video; Lucy is jumping. So what we know is what we see (and perhaps take some baseline data on): Lucy prefers this video (she chooses it every day); it is acting as a reinforcer; Lucy has access to this reinforcer while engaging in the jumping behavior (which occurs only with this particular video); Lucy has also learned that she can obtain the video by engaging in other inappropriate behavior (the screaming and hitting). From observing Lucy for a few days, the therapist knows that the shortest period of time Lucy sits appropriately is now thirty seconds (this will be the minimum interval for the treatment).

The ABA therapist wants to teach Lucy appropriate behavior while watching the video by systematically manipulating the situation and establishing reinforcers for appropriate behavior. This could be done through allowing Lucy access to the video once a day, sitting her on the couch and, using the remote control, not starting the video until she is sitting appropriately. The therapist could then start the video and perhaps offer oral praise, pats on the back, and a preferred edible every thirty seconds that Lucy is watching TV appropriately (every thirty seconds would be considered a "discrete trial"). The second Lucy starts to stand on the couch, the therapist might stop the video, remind Lucy to sit down, perhaps physically prompt her (touching her shoulders in a downward motion, for instance), and praise her when she is again seated. The video goes back on, and the process continues for a previously determined period (perhaps, to start, ten trials of thirty seconds each). The therapist would record data for each trial and when Lucy had demonstrated an ability to watch appropriately for nine or ten out of ten daily trials, the period might be increased to forty-five seconds or a minute. When that criterion was met, on to ninety seconds, two minutes, and so on, until Lucy demonstrated the ability to watch her video appropriately for its thirty-minute length.

Now here come the aspects some parents might find objectionable. Although Lucy's parents certainly did not set out to do so, they inadvertently reinforced inappropriate behavior that must now be addressed. No parent really likes hearing that responding to her child in a way that she feels reflects her understanding of her child's challenges (the "Lucy jumps for sensory reasons" argument, the video makes Lucy so happy) has contributed to the problem behavior. Parents sometimes find it difficult to see (or hear) their children crying, screaming, or tantruming. We want our children to be happy; if something makes them unhappy, our first impulse may be to make it go away. Unfortunately, these noble motives can reinforce behaviors that range from mildly inappropriate to dangerous, especially for children on the spectrum, who do not learn in the same ways that typical children do. Children tantrum and protest for many reasons, but generally they do so to achieve escape from an undesirable situation, attention from adults (both pleasant and unpleasant), or access to desired objects or activities. In the ABA world, when Lucy tantrums for her video, the way to extinguish tantruming is either to not give her the video or to ignore her behavior (and they mean really ignore; no repimands, no explanations, perhaps not even a glance, provided the child is not in danger), or both. For as long as this behavior has persisted, every time Lucy's mother gave in to a tantrum, she demonstrated to Lucy that tantruming "worked" as an effective strategy for getting her desires met. (No wonder Lucy's preschool teacher is reporting that Lucy now hits her classmates.)

In Lucy's mother's case, following through with the ABA therapist's recommendations may be uncomfortable (if she believes that Lucy's primary issue is sensory) and trying (what parent wants to experience a child's screaming and hitting?). There may be other conditions of this particular intervention: For example, Lucy may not be allowed access to the favorite video outside of the ABA therapy until she has learned to watch appropriately. If, say, Hershey's Kisses are the preferred edible reinforcer, the therapist may ask Mom to deny Lucy access to Kisses anytime except during their sessions. This might mean that Lucy's brothers do not have Kisses, either, when Lucy is around. If Lucy's mother feels that Lucy's behavior is tolerable, that it's "unfair" or "mean" to deny Lucy her video or her chocolate Kisses whenever she wants them, that not giving in to Lucy's demands for the video is "cruel," and that—despite Lucy's observable behavior—she's "smart enough to understand why her behavior is inappropriate," ABA will probably not work.

However, if Lucy's mother followed through with the ABA intervention consistently, the odds are very good that within, say, a month, Lucy would no longer be jumping on the couch or tantruming for the video. In fact, by Mom learning how to handle Lucy's tantrums in this situation, she may be able to apply this new skill—and new way of looking at Lucy's behaviors—in other problem areas.

Why Are We Talking About ABA?

To date, ours remains one of the few books on AS to recommend ABA. Why is that? If you have read other books, attended conferences, or spent time on the Web, you may have noticed a clear anti-ABA bias even among some of the most prominent AS authorities. After spending a year and a half training and teaching in an ABA school, Patty believes that most anti-ABA bias is at best out of date, and at worst uninformed. Anyone who you hear describe ABA as "a system of rewards and punishments" simply doesn't understand ABA or the principles of behavior on which it is based. After hearing from countless parents whose children's choices and potential are limited by deficits in the types of skills ABA is so effective in teaching, we feel strongly that parents should at least understand what ABA is about and consider it if their child's needs warrant it.

A few years ago, few parents of children with AS ever heard the terms *ABA* or *applied verbal behavior* (AVB, discussed in the next section). One reason for that was that most children with AS were diagnosed during their school years. Now that pediatricians, teachers, and other professionals are more aware of the early signs of all forms of PDDs, even children with AS are being diagnosed earlier. If your child is identified and classified prior to age three (when he might receive early intervention services) or from age three through kindergarten (when he might receive preschool services), the dominant therapy available will probably be ABA or AVB, in addition to speech therapy, occupational therapy, and physical therapy, if appropriate.

According to Dr. Bobby Newman, a psychologist, Board Certified Behavior Analyst, and director of training for the Association for Metroarea Autistic Children, Inc., in New York City, "ABA assumes that behavior is determined, and that there are laws of behavior that we can study. Once we understand the laws of behavior, we can make certain predictions about what kinds of behavior will occur in certain circumstances. If we can manipulate some of the variables, then we may be able to bring about some behavioral change."

ABA systematically identifies target behaviors and skills and then teaches them by breaking each skill down into small steps that are mastered individually and by reinforcing desirable skills and behaviors through rewards (bits of food, tickles, hugs, enthusiastic praise) that are known to be motivating for that particular child (these are called *reinforcers*). At the same time ABA ignores undesirable behaviors or corrects them in a neutral manner that ignores the behavior without ignoring the student (although to the untrained eye, it may appear that the therapist is doing exactly that).[7] Children with severe autism may receive up to forty hours a week of intensive one-on-one therapy, but a less rigorous schedule would be appropriate for less pervasive behaviors. Regardless of what behavior or skill ABA is used to address, for the method to succeed, parents and others in the child's life must also respond to the child's behaviors using the same repertoire of responses and reinforcement.

When It May Be Appropriate

Theoretically, ABA can be used to address problematic behaviors, including perseverative behaviors, stigmatizing behaviors, and some types of tantrums and outbursts. Although there is a general misconception that ABA is only for younger children with AS or children who have other forms of PDDs, an experienced therapist can work with persons of any age and at any level of functioning. ABA's approach to analyzing behavior based on observation and collected data can be useful if your child is exhibiting behaviors that "make no sense" or seem to "come out of nowhere." Needless to say, before putting any ABA program into effect, you, the ABA therapist, and any other professionals working with your child should be sure to rule out other possible causes of problem behaviors (such as comorbid disorders, neurological problems, sensory issues, and so on).

How It Works

ABA is based on the premise that any human behavior can be analyzed and understood according to the principles of behaviorism. This relationship is often expressed in terms of ABC: *antecedent* (what occurs before the behavior), the *behavior* itself, and the *consequences* (by which we mean the response the behavior elicits from others, not a punishment). A crucial part of an effective ABA approach to any behavior is determining the function of the behavior; in other words, why does Janie panic whenever she hears the family car start? What purpose does that panic and the reaction it prompts serve for her? What is it about the response to her panic that reinforces the behavior and increases the likelihood that it will recur and/or increase? What alternative consequence will decrease the likelihood that Janie will panic? And so on.

Another important aspect of ABA is the understanding of reinforcers. Essentially, any behavior that is reinforced will be more likely to recur and become more prevalent than one that is not reinforced. It is important to understand that in ABA terms a reinforcer is not necessarily what most of us would consider a "reward" or a "punishment." Rather, a reinforcer is a consequence of an individual's behavior that increases the likelihood that that behavior will recur. For one child, an effective reinforcer might be a tiny bite of a favorite food; for another, it might be the chance to look at a book about trains for a few moments, or a high-five, or a big smile and behavior-specific praise ("Great reading that passage," "Nice folding your pants"). Once the reinforcer is identified, the therapist would then determine how and when that reinforcer would be used (every time, as is often the case when a learner is acquiring a new skill, or intermittently, as it might be once the learner has mastered a skill and we are trying to thin or fade the reinforcement). Ideally, reinforcers are thinned as the skill is mastered and then removed once the learner demonstrates the skill across different environments and situations (this is called *generalization*). For example, to encourage a child to turn and look at you when his name is called, you might reinforce him every time. As the response becomes more consistent and independent, you will slowly fade the reinforcement.

To give a basic idea of how ABA might work for a child with AS, let's look at a grossly oversimplified example with a very simple solution. (Bear in mind that the factors determining behavior can be extremely complex.) If Timmy kicks his desk every morning "for no apparent reason," an ABA therapist would study the situation to determine what function Timmy's kicking was truly serving. Since the consequence of his kicking to date has been removal from the classroom, and every time Timmy kicks he is removed from the classroom, then the removal is viewed as a possible reinforcer. We also cannot ignore the fact that even though—to the teacher's way of thinking—this removal constitutes a "punishment" and should serve as a disincentive that discourages the kicking, it does not. How do we know that it does not? Because Timmy is still kicking.

An ABA therapist would study the situation and try manipulating variables that might be serving as antecedents to help answer the question "What is prompting Timmy's kicking?" This may take some trial and error: Is it the noise of the PA system from the morning announcements? The packet of worksheets that are placed on his desk? A general need to escape the classroom? The therapist will test each hypothesis by analyzing every aspect of the behavior. If one day Timmy's teacher does not place a packet of worksheets on his desk and he does not kick, then it would be reasonable to work out a plan based on the premise that Timmy is kicking to avoid schoolwork. Timmy may not be thinking of it in exactly those terms, and he may never have "planned" to get out of doing his work by kicking, but once he kicked and was removed from the classroom, he accidentally happened upon a behavior that produced a consequence that achieved what he considers a desirable outcome. Like Lucy, he's hit on what is to *him* an effective means to a desirable end.

The next step is to look at the consequence of Timmy's kicking—removal from the classroom and from the work—as the reinforcer that is driving this inappropriate behavior. In this case, the therapist might advise one of several possible alternate consequences. The teacher could ignore the kicking (which may be difficult) or have Timmy removed from the classroom to a place where he would still have to complete his work. In addition, the therapist might introduce other reinforcers—such as an immediate reward for doing the work in the alternate setting, then for doing the work at his desk, and then for doing the work at his desk without kicking—to increase the likelihood that the acceptable behavior would occur again. The ultimate goal would be to fade the reinforcer (a sometimes complicated matter) as Timmy gained the ability to control his kicking himself. The important thing to remember, however, is that the teacher and everyone working with Timmy would be vigilant in ensuring that the inappropriate behavior not be reinforced by their responses—and, equally important, that they provide prompt verbal praise and other known reinforcers for the desired behavior. "Catch them being good" is a good motto to bear in mind. In the beginning, it might be advisable to praise Timmy as often as every few moments for staying in his seat and doing his work.

What We Know About ABA
and Asperger Syndrome

The potential role of ABA in AS is still sketchy. The bulk of research done on ABA and autism spectrum disorders focuses on individual case studies of individuals whose diagnoses are more indicative of autistic disorder or PDD-NOS. You should also be aware that chances are good that most ABA therapists have spent most, if not all, of their time working with such children. It is impossible to generalize about how any particular ABA teacher views certain ASD-related behaviors. However, it is generally true that among ABA therapists whose experience is with children on other parts of the spectrum, there may be much less tolerance for behaviors such as stereotypical behaviors, noncontextual verbalizations, abnormal eye gaze, and unstructured time than there is in the AS community. Nonetheless, we have heard from parents who credit ABA therapy (though used in a program less intensive than forty hours a week) with impressive gains in diminishing their children's problem behaviors and teaching new, appropriate skills. Although you may read experts' warnings that ABA is not a quick fix for teaching and reinforcing appropriate behaviors, that is precisely how some parents of children with AS have used it, with positive results.

It is important not to confuse ABA the philosophy with certain ABA techniques that have come to define it. Discrete trial teaching is just one technique, a highly structured sequence of exchanges between a teacher and a student consisting of a teacher-directed antecedent, or stimulus, the learner's behavior or response, and the consequence. For a student learning simple motor imitation, a discrete trial might look like this: the teacher establishing a readiness response (saying the student's name, "Get ready," "Let's start," establishing eye contact, or any other exchange that the student recognizes as a signal that it's time to attend and that the teacher knows indicates that the student is paying attention), then saying, "Clap hands" (antecedent, stimulus), the student clapping his hands (behavior, response), and the teacher then reinforcing with praise, smiles, a piece of a preferred food, or access to a favored activity (consequence). If the student erred or did not clap his hands, the teacher would correct the error in one of several possible ways, depending on the student's abilities, past performance, and other factors. She might model clapping hands, clap the student's hand in a hand-over-hand manner, and so on. If the student is learning to clap hands, she might teach errorlessly and, for instance, clap his hands hand-over-hand right after saying "Clap hands," then offer reinforcement and praise. Discrete trial teaching often occurs in massed trials. That means that this student would be asked to "clap hands" in five, ten, fifteen regularly scheduled trials (for example, once every school day or session day). More complicated responses, such as setting a table or completing a sheet of math problems, might call for fewer trials.

There are ABA therapists who insist on using discrete trials with children. Because of more severe deficits in language skills and social understanding, it might be appropriate to teach a child with a different spectrum diagnosis to respond "Fine" every time someone asks, "How are you?" And this could be done using discrete trials with a teacher and then generalized through practice with other people. However, a child with AS needs to learn a full repertoire of responses to the question "How are you?" and have some understanding of when each response is appropriate. There is little evidence that such understanding can be taught using discrete trials. On the other hand, a clearly defined response, discrete trial teaching methods (including at first errorless teaching and graduated guidance), and massed trials may be just what some children with AS need to learn to cut with scissors, fold clothes, or dress independently. ABA can also be very effective in dealing with toileting issues.

Further, some children with AS, because of their advanced cognitive abilities or comorbid conditions, may find the repetition and some therapists' neutral vocal and emotional tone confusing, even distressing. Fortunately, this is not the demeanor of a good ABA therapist, who is enthusiastic and engaging. Good ABA therapists pride themselves on creating relationships with their students that are reinforcing. There is also a danger in seeking to extinguish behaviors that may have strong neurological bases (for example, responses that result from an anxiety disorder, or tics from Tourette's syndrome), although an accomplished ABA therapist may be able to teach alternate, more appropriate responses (for example, teaching a child to replace a socially stigmatizing tic or stereotypy with squeezing a Koosh ball imperceptibly in his pocket).

ABA is distinguished by the scrupulously detailed written records therapists keep to track and quantify the frequency, duration, and intensity of specific behaviors and the detailed teaching procedures used. Careful attention is paid to the systematic use and fading of prompts. The direction of the therapy is determined by the data collected, not by a teacher's or a parent's impressions or "feelings" about how a child is doing. If the teacher determines that mastery for cutting a straight line is 80 percent (eight of ten trials, or four of five, or sixteen of twenty) accuracy over three (or four or five) days, and accuracy is defined as the line being cut straight within one-eighth inch (or one-sixteenth inch or no margin) on either side, Sidney will not move on to cutting an L until he has met that criterion. This reduces the chances that Sidney will start working on cutting Ls without the required skills. Such systematic teaching is geared toward creating conditions under which the student can most quickly and accurately learn the correct responses and skills.

For these reasons, and because of the many studies published on programs using ABA, some professionals and educators consider it "more scientific" than other common interventions. As a result, a growing number of health and education officials are identifying ABA as the "most effective" intervention for children with all forms of PDDs. This is prompting a rush to get educators and other therapists trained in ABA through programs that are incomplete and insufficient. Mastering ABA requires years of training. No one can be considered an ABA therapist, expert, or consultant on the basis of taking a single course or seminar, reading a few books, or working under the occasional supervision of an ABA expert. Improperly applied, ABA can reinforce undesirable, even dangerous behaviors and exacerbate underlying comorbid psychiatric or emotional disorders. We caution parents to refuse to submit their child to any ABA program or treatment that does not include the direct hands-on involvement of at least one certified ABA therapist who has experience with AS. Demand to see credentials. Ideally, if your child has complicating issues, the ABA therapist should also be a licensed psychologist. (See "Recommended Resources" on page 188 to find certified ABA therapists.)

Before you consider ABA therapy for your child, consult with other professionals who work with him. Ask them about their experience with ABA (though you may find harsh criticism of the method; not all professionals truly understand ABA) and whether they know of any other children with AS who have benefited from it. If they do, ask specifically what types of behavior it addressed and, alternately, any behaviors for which it proved ineffective. Don't be shy about asking for references, from both former supervisors and employers and clients.

Generally speaking, the professional consensus is that children with AS do not need ABA therapy as urgently as they need social skills training. However, depending on your child's behaviors, it may be wise not to view this strictly as an either/or question. "No matter what the problem is," psychologist Bobby Newman says, "my basic question is, 'Okay, the student is functioning in this particular setting. Is he functioning as well as he could? If not, what do we need to teach him to do to help him function better? And if he is functioning adequately in that setting, what does he need to learn or what behavior does he need to eliminate in order to move to the next less restrictive setting?' I believe ABA gives choices. If I don't have a skill, I don't have a choice. If I can't leave the house without having the television set on a certain channel without feeling anxious, I have no choice. I have no freedom. But if I have the skill to be able to leave the house without the television on that channel, now I have a choice."

Where to Find ABA Therapy

Your first challenge will be to find a certified ABA therapist in your area, preferably one with AS experience. A good place to start is the Behavior Analyst Certification Board's Web site, which lists certified therapists (see page 188). Your school district's special education administrators, teachers, or a local AS- or ASD-related support group may be able to put you in touch with ABA-trained therapists in your area. You might also want to contact local special education schools or programs, including those that provide early intervention and preschool services. Some organizations, universities, hospitals, and adult education programs offer training in ABA for parents.

Issues to Consider

Of all ASD therapies, ABA is probably the most controversial and the least understood. Read all that you can about it and contact, through support groups or the Internet, parents of children with AS who have tried it. Be prepared: Parents either love it or hate it. Try to pay attention to what types of behaviors were being addressed, the experience and background of the therapist, and other factors about the child (such as comorbid diagnoses) that may have complicated the outcome.

Due to the shortage of qualified ABA therapists, your child's therapy may be provided by a therapist working as an independent contractor, or freelancer, in your home. If possible, try to find an ABA therapist through a licensed agency that provides early intervention or preschool services or through a parent support network or group whose members may each know several therapists. Your school district's special education office should be able to help you with this. You should know that national certification of ABA therapists through the nonprofit Behavior Analyst Certification Board began only in 2000. As a result of the lack of certification until now and the shortage of qualified therapists, there is nothing to prevent anyone, regardless of training, from presenting himself as a qualified therapist. In addition, even an eminently qualified ABA therapist may have had limited direct experience with children with AS. Don't be afraid to ask. What might be appropriate, standard practice for a child with a different ASD may be not only inappropriate but harmful to a child with AS. Bear in mind that a freelance therapist working in your home who is not hired through a licensed agency or under the direct supervision of your school district is, by definition, working without the supervision or input of more experienced superiors.

Depending on your child and the behaviors you want to address, ABA therapy can be stressful. Often inherent in the process is a phenomenon known as the "extinction burst," essentially an increase in the intensity, frequency, and severity of the target behavior that precedes its extinction. If, for example, your child is having difficulty at school, you may choose to postpone ABA until summer.

If you do go forward with ABA therapy, be sure that everyone who works with your child is aware of the behavior you are addressing and the appropriate ABA response. Consistency of response in every setting is key to the therapy's success. So, for instance, if Nancy's therapist has determined that the appropriate response to her snapping her fingers as she speaks is a particular gestural cue or a touch on the shoulder, everyone—parents, teachers, grandparents, baby-sitters—should be doing it, every time the behavior occurs.

Recommended Resources

BOOKS

Bobby Newman, *When Everybody Cares: Case Studies of ABA with People with Autism* (New York: Dove and Orca, 1999) and *Graduated Applied Behavior Analysis* (New York: Dove and Orca, 2002).

WEB SITES

Behavior Analyst Certification Board
Metro Building—Suite 102
Tallahassee, FL 32308-3796
www.bacb.com
This Web site includes a current listing of nationally certified ABA therapists.

www.christinaburkaba.com/
Christina Burk, M.A., is a behavior analyst. Her Web site is a treasure trove for parents who have questions about ABA, VB (see next section), and related issues.

VERBAL BEHAVIOR

You might hear someone refer to verbal behavior (VB), or verbal behavior analysis (VBA), or applied verbal behavior (AVB) as a "new" therapy or something "different from" ABA. Some refer to it as NET (for Natural Environment Training, a component of VB that focuses on working with the child in his natural environment and using his interests and activities to shape the teaching) or "the Carbone method."[8] Technically, VB should not be separated from ABA, since it is a teaching method that uses the principles of ABA, and, most important, the theory behind it was articulated by B. F. Skinner, the father of ABA. Skinner's 1957 landmark work, *Verbal Behavior,* set forth the argument that verbal behavior—what we say and why—is really no different from any other kind of observable behavior. Skinner contended that language is learned through a series of interactions in which behavior is either reinforced or punished, and that we can analyze different types of language in terms of their function.

Skinner and other behaviorists focused only on observable, external behavior; what a person said (or signed or wrote). Skinner was not interested in how internal mental states—memory, imagination, consciousness, and so on—might influence what someone said.[9]

What It Is

Verbal behavior uses the principles of ABA to promote expressive language; in other words, to encourage children to speak, by manipulating the environment to set up natural antecedents that will promote language by establishing associations between objects, actions, and anything else we have a word for with the actual object, action, quality, and so on. VB has its own jargon, invented by Skinner as well. A request is *mand,* a noun is a *tact.* In VB, then, "ice cream" could be both a mand (when it is requested) and a tact (when the child correctly identifies a photograph of ice cream). In VB, learners are said to be *manding, tacting,* and so on.[10]

When It May Be Appropriate

For a child with Asperger Syndrome who, according to *DSM-IV-TR* criteria, does not have an expressive speech delay, there may be a place for VB. Though for learners on other points on the spectrum, it is used to elicit basic language and establish imitation skills (usually not issues for children with AS), it can also be effective for teaching more complex and higher-level forms of language such as answering "Wh" questions and fill-ins, what AVB terms the *intraverbal.* Intraverbal exchanges do not depend on imitation of what someone else has said but may require prompting or modeling to elicit a response. The reinforcers are natural and social. Intraverbals require the child to attend and respond to another person's language, a crucial skill.

VB's emphasis on teaching to mastery, fluency, and spontaneity may be a welcome alternative to less structured approaches or those that do not adequately recognize or reinforce learner initiative.

How It Works

VB in action can look quite different from ABA, especially its discrete trials. For example, in teaching manding in VB, the teacher would follow the child's lead, determine something the child would want, set up a situation in which it would be visible but not readily available (say, a juice box on a shelf the child could not reach or a cookie in the teacher's hand), then use very specific techniques to elicit the word *juice* or *cookie* (or approximations, and, in the case of children who are nonverbal, perhaps signing). The reinforcer here would be the actual object the child requests, as opposed to what sometimes occurs in ABA discrete trials, which is the presentation of a cookie for the child saying something totally unrelated, like *cat*. VB also emphasizes allotting working in the natural environment (the NET), where the teacher would appear to be following the child's lead and seizing upon any and every opportunity to reinforce verbal behavior. For example, if a child were to walk toward the bubble wand on a table, the teacher would hold it up and repeat the word *bubble* three times, each time moving the bubble wand closer to the child. If the child makes a vocal approximation or says the word *bubble,* he receives the wand immediately. Proponents of VB also argue that because language is taught in ways that make it always functional, it helps to promote more natural prosody (the tone, volume, and rhythm and other "nonword" qualities of speech) and learner initiative.

What We Know About VB and Asperger Syndrome

We know very little at this point, but as more teachers, speech pathologists, and other therapists are trained in it and as more children with AS are diagnosed younger, research will certainly emerge. For now, however, you should make your decision based on your child's needs and discussions with potential therapists. If your child receives early intervention or preschool services, and the only form of therapy available is ABA, you should consider requesting that language objectives be addressed using VB rather than discrete trial ABA. For further information, such as where to find VB, questions to ask, and what parents can do to help, see above regarding ABA.

Recommended Resources
See above regarding ABA; and
Carbone Clinic
www.Carboneclinic.com

To see a video of Dr. Carbone discussing VB, go to the Web site of
POAC of New Jersey:
www.poac.net/default.aspx (scroll down left navigation bar)

AUDITORY INTEGRATION TRAINING (AIT)

Auditory integration training is one of the more controversial interventions here. Unfortunately, research on AIT is neither plentiful
nor definitive, and the procedure does not produce the desired outcome for everyone. In fact, the American Academy of Pediatrics has
adopted a position recommending against the use of AIT. The
American Speech-Language-Hearing Association (ASHA), the largest "professional, scientific, and credentialing" organization for
speech-language pathologists and other speech, language, and hearing professionals, has come out against AIT, too. Although there are
several highly complex theories behind AIT, it is unclear precisely
how it changes behavior.

Most recently, it's cropped up in the media in association with
ASDs through coverage of the child savant jazz pianist and composer
Matt Savage. Matt, who was diagnosed with PDD and hyperlexia at
age three, could not tolerate such everyday sounds as windshield
wipers. After Bérard AIT, his parents claim, Matt began showing an
interest in the piano and began writing his own songs. He began
recording with the Matt Savage Trio at age seven; by twelve, he had
released five acclaimed albums.

What It Is

There are several forms of AIT. The two that are most associated
with ASDs were developed independently by two French doctors.
More than forty years ago Dr. Alfred Tomatis developed his audio-
psycho-phonology approach using predominantly high-frequency
sounds as well as the voices of the patient and his mother, songs, and
stories. The therapy involves about one hundred hours of listening.
Critics of Tomatis say that his claim that problems in hearing and auditory processing may be rooted in emotional problems and experiences (thus the use of the mother's voice in the therapy) is outdated.
Among those critics is Dr. Guy Bérard, who developed his method

for AIT in the 1960s. Bérard's approach is less psychologically based than Tomatis's. Based on the results of extensive audiological tests, the therapist programs a special sound amplifier to modify music from regular CDs (so a patient might be listening to Hank Williams or Madonna) by eliminating high and low frequencies. It is important to stress that patients are not just "listening to music," but listening to music that has been sonically altered according to the individual sensitivities revealed through prior testing. Bérard's AIT usually involves two half-hour sessions, spaced a minimum of three hours apart, every day over the course of ten days. Both Bérard's and Tomatis's AIT can be administered only by a trained professional, usually an audiologist.

In addition, there are a number of other listening programs— among the better known are Earobics, Train Time, and Fast For-Word—the makers of which claim to address a wide range of auditory and learning problems. Programs such as Earobics and Train Time involve a onetime cost (for the purchase of the CD-ROM) and are designed for use in the classroom and the home. Fast For-Word sessions may take place in a clinician's office or be done at home using an Internet hookup so that your child's progress can be monitored by Scientific Learning Corporation, the company that makes the program. Fast ForWord is considerably more expensive (approximately $1,000 for the at-home program, which is monitored by a trained professional, as opposed to $50 to $200 and more for an unmonitored program such as Earobics).

When It May Be Appropriate

Children who are diagnosed with central auditory processing disorder (CAPD) (also referred to as auditory processing disorder, central auditory disorder, auditory perceptual problems, or central auditory dysfunction) have extreme responses—pain, anxiety, panic—to everyday sounds and noises; have hyperacute hearing; have processing difficulties; and have difficulty attending and focusing or other behaviors that suggest ADHD/ADD or other learning disabilities. Preliminary research suggests that abnormalities in hearing and in processing are extremely common among persons with PDDs. (See pages 52 and 81 for a fuller description of AS-related hearing problems.)

How It Works

Essentially, every AIT program attempts to address some form of auditory processing disorder. (For more information, see "Central Auditory Processing Disorder," page 81.) There are highly technical explanations of CAPD, but for most parents, it is enough to think of a child with CAPD as a child who can hear normally but whose mind cannot sort or make sense of what he hears. Normal hearing does not equal normal listening. In other words, a child with profound CAPD issues may well pass a typical hearing test with flying colors. The problem, then, is not what is heard but how it is heard and how the brain responds. As one handout on the topic available online put it, "The child can hear, but listening is the problem. Think of the problem you would have if you suddenly found yourself in England at the time of Shakespeare. The speech is English, but in a strange, accented style with different constructions and meaning."[11] The goal of AIT is to help people with AS understand what they hear.

Some therapists view CAPD as another form of sensory integration disorder, and that seems to make sense, considering how many of our abilities and responses are shaped not only by what we hear (the sounds themselves) but how we hear them and how our brain processes them. Our hearing affects not only how we perceive and understand the sounds we hear but our abilities to:

- Focus and attend
- Initiate appropriate, purposeful activity
- Modulate sensory stimulation
- Accurately perceive balance and movement
- Cope with gravitational insecurity
- Develop appropriate speech and language skills
- Develop socially and emotionally
- Master praxis (the ability to plan, organize, and carry out voluntary actions) and sequencing (the ability to recognize patterns and to organize thoughts and objects in a logical order)
- Develop eye control

Diagnosing CAPD is a challenge, because hearing is so subjective. Persons with CAPD have nothing against which to compare their "distorted" hearing. A child with CAPD, for example, cannot possibly know that the sound of water running in a sink should not be physically painful to hear. He does not know that the sound of other students walking quietly outside the closed classroom door should not be as loud as the voice of the teacher speaking directly to him. Yet that's the way some persons with CAPD hear the world. It's not surprising, then, that they may respond with confusion, anxiety, and what appears to be an inability to pay attention. Children who find what they hear at times physically painful or unusually frightening may become nervous, anxious, avoidant, whiny, or physically aggressive when subjected to sounds they are sensitive to. Tellingly, Dr. Bérard's book on his method is entitled *Hearing Equals Behavior.* The responses of older children and adults who successfully underwent AIT provide a glimpse into what some younger children may be experiencing. One child announced after a single AIT session, "Mom, the world sounds so peaceful now." Another, on the last day of a ten-day treatment, surprised his parents by exclaiming, "I can finally hear what you are saying!"

What We Know About AIT and Asperger Syndrome

As yet there are few hard statistics on the prevalence of CAPD among persons with AS. However, autism expert Dr. Bernard Rimland has reported that sound sensitivity is an issue for perhaps 40 percent of people with autism. Our OASIS Survey on Hearing and Noise found that while 10 percent of the respondents' children were officially diagnosed as having CAPD, from 50 percent to 75 percent reported their children having difficulties that are indicative of the disorder.

Where to Find It

As awareness of CAPD grows, more professionals who work with our children are recognizing it. However, only an audiologist should be diagnosing CAPD (although speech pathologists and other therapists may recognize signs and suggest evaluation by an audiologist). Many CAPD- and ASD-related Web sites post lists of practitioners and organizations that provide AIT. You can also locate a practitioner through the "Recommended Resources" listed on page 197.

Questions to Ask

Before you begin, do your research and determine which (if any) method of AIT may be appropriate for your child.

- Ask the practitioner about his background, his experience with the methods he offers, and his experience with children like your own. How many children has he treated? Roughly what percentage showed significant improvement?
- Provide the practitioner with any evaluations and reports you have on your child (speech and language, neurological, psychological, occupational therapy, etc.). Be sure you have thoroughly discussed your child's particular challenges before the training begins and that the practitioner has a good idea about your child's basic temperament, sensitivities, and usual behaviors.
- Your practitioner should know about any medication your child is taking (including over-the-counter and "natural" alternative products and supplements).
- If at all possible, try to speak with parents who have worked with the practitioner.
- If the practitioner is not an audiologist, find out if there is an audiologist with experience in the method of AIT you will be using available to do the pre-training diagnostic testing and the post-training follow-up evaluations.
- Ask about the schedule for pre- and post-training examinations and evaluations. When will they occur? Are they included in the cost of the training, or will they be charged as separate visits?
- Be sure you have a clear idea about the schedule of treatment.
- Ask specifically about what happens if, for instance, your child cannot complete the training due to illness, family emergency, adverse reaction, and so on.
- Ask the practitioner what time of day he would prefer to see your child during the training. Generally, most children are best early in the day, before school.
- Find out about what to expect during the actual training sessions.

Ask to visit the room where the training will occur with your child. Will you be allowed to stay with your child? Can your child have drinks or snacks in the room during the training? If your child can have snacks, try to avoid overly sweetened treats or foods and drinks that contain caffeine.

• Ask about possible changes in behavior during and after the training. Agitation, hyperactivity, mood swings, aggression, nausea, and changes in eating and sleeping patterns have all been reported during training. While most are temporary, lasting only a day or a few days, some may persist for two weeks or more.

• Inquire about the cost. Most insurance companies will not cover AIT. Depending on your coverage, it may be possible to have the diagnostic testing and evaluations paid for. Costs vary, depending on the method used and the practitioner, but may range as high as $1,000 or more for a series of training sessions or less than $50 for the onetime purchase of a program such as Earobics.

• Once your child has been evaluated and/or treated, ask the practitioner or audiologist to explain the test results to you in plain English. Ask for specific information on what you can do at home and what teachers can do in school to help your child. If you believe that hearing issues are causing problems in school, also ask that the practitioner prepare a written report for your child's school that includes specific suggestions for helping him in the classroom (for example, being seated near the teacher's desk, or being excused from loud, noisy activities or places, such as school pep rallies).

What Parents Can Do to Help

If your child has been diagnosed with CAPD, you can do many things to make his environment, at home and in school, more comfortable. Be patient, understanding, and accommodating. To the extent possible, avoid noises and sounds that provoke panic responses. Try to be more conscientious about the "noise environment" wherever your child is, but don't be afraid to test your child's ability to cope with troublesome sounds whenever you can do so safely and you can leave the situation immediately if there is a problem. Do all that you can to "clear the field," so to speak. To expect your child to understand you as you talk over the stereo, radio, television, or another conversation is asking for frustration. At home, be sure you have your child's attention before you start speaking. Use a code word or a gesture, such as a light tap on the shoulder or pointing to your ear to indicate that it's time to listen. Speak clearly and slowly, using shorter sentences, and give one- or two-step (as opposed to five- and six-step) directions or explanations. Gradually work on building up the number of steps your child can follow. Check with your child to see if she heard and/or understood what you said, and teach her to recognize when she may have missed or misunderstood something and how to ask the speaker to repeat or clarify what was said.

Work closely with your child's teacher to ensure that her hearing difficulties are recognized and accommodated. Keep in mind that many classrooms are, acoustically speaking, not the most conducive environments for learning. Your child might require seating closer to his teacher or away from other auditory distractions (the air conditioner, the open doorway to the hall, the class computer and printer station). Some students have benefited from using a system whereby the teacher speaks into a small wearable microphone and the sound is conveyed to a headset the student wears. You can learn more about such devices from your child's audiologist or speech pathologist.

Notes and Comments

Despite reports that children who listened to regular, untreated music through regular equipment and headphones showed similar improvements to children who underwent AIT, only an audiologist who specializes in AIT can determine what may be effective for your child. And only an audiologist can conduct the type of assessment needed to determine what improvement may occur.

Recommended Resources
The Georgiana Institute
www.georgianainstitute.org
Site includes lists of AIT practitioners organized by country and
    state.

The Society for Auditory Intervention Techniques (SAIT)
www.up-to-date.com/saitwebsite/table.html
This Web site contains many research articles on AIT.

Dr. Guy Bérard
www.drguyberard.com

Scientific Learning Corporation (maker of Fast ForWord and other
    programs)
www.scientificlearning.com

Cognitive Concepts (makers of Earobics, which offers different pro-
    grams for children, adolescents, and adults)
www.earobics.com

SOCIAL STORIES AND COMIC STRIP CONVERSATIONS

Social Stories and Comic Strip Conversations are two different but related approaches to helping people with AS and other PDDs develop a
clearer understanding about a wide range of social information.
Though each uses a different technique, and one may be more effective in a given situation, they both do essentially the same thing: make
explicit—through words, drawings, or both—the kind of information
about social behavior, routines, goals, and academic skills that people
with AS have difficulty picking up. Both methods are based on the
premise that inappropriate or undesirable behavior arises from a lack
of understanding of what's appropriate or desirable in a given situation. Social Stories may be applied to a wider range of situations;
Comic Strip Conversations, on the other hand, are graphic illustrations
of conversations—past, present, or future—and "systematically identify
what people say and do, and emphasize *what people may be thinking.*"[12]
Carol Gray, an educator and expert on autism who created both Social
Stories and Comic Strip Conversations specifically to address the types
of problems children with ASDs face, says that there are no firm
"rules" regarding which method is best suited to a given situation, but
she has made some general observations about each.

Social Stories tend to be more accessible to younger children,
who can read the stories themselves or have them read to them.
Writing a Social Story does require that its author (you or another
adult) fully understand the issues from the perspective of the child.
Writing a Comic Strip Conversation, in contrast, demands a fact-

finding effort on your part. Unlike a Social Story, a Comic Strip Conversation is a collaborative effort between you and the child (or you and several children). Part of the process involves asking questions and "drawing" the conversation to reflect the child's answers.

The beauty of both methods is that anyone can learn how to create them, or work with the child to create them. As long as you have paper and pencil handy, they can be created anywhere; they are portable; they can be referred to as many times as necessary. Notebooks containing the Social Stories and Comic Strip Conversations about skills, fears, and issues that a child is working on or has mastered offer a great opportunity for him to see concrete evidence of his progress.

What We Know About Social Stories and Comic Strip Conversations and AS

Both Social Stories and Comic Strip Conversations have been in use since the early 1990s. They have gained wide acceptance from authorities on AS and ASDs, who view them as an effective way of overcoming social difficulties resulting from problems with theory of mind and social understanding. Because they were created by an educator and designed to work with students in the school environment, they are practical as well.

SOCIAL STORIES

What They Are

A Social Story is a brief (100- to 500-word) narrative that describes a situation (who, what, where, why, when), explains the feelings and/or thoughts of everyone involved (including the child for whom the story is written), and gives some direction regarding appropriate response. Although a Social Story may seem "simple," it's important to remember that it must reflect the child's perspective, and that may require some detective work. If a child is nervous about going to a movie theater, and you write a Social Story based on your assumption that the issue is the hubbub around the snack bar, it won't work if the real problem is the child's fear of the restroom's self-flushing toilets.

Nor can you use a Social Story to prescribe or dictate desired behavior without offering an adequate description of the situation or of the feelings, thoughts, or actions of others. It may help to remember that the primary purpose of a Social Story is not to dictate appropriate behaviors and responses but to increase a child's awareness and understanding. Ideally, this understanding will make it easier for the child to demonstrate the desired behavior. After writing and reviewing thousands of Social Stories, Carol Gray developed the "Social Story Ratio," which is the key to a Story's effectiveness. In her formula, for every directive sentence ("do this" or "say that"), the story must include two to five sentences that are descriptive and/or offer perspective on why someone might do, say, or think something.

Let's use an example from the "Social Story Kit"—a clear, concise guide to writing Social Stories that appears in all Social Story collections (see "Recommended Resources," page 205). For illustrative purposes, we have indicated the type of sentence that follows in italics. In a real Social Story, the text in regular type would run as a full paragraph without the descriptive terms at the left.

Descriptive: Sometimes a person says, "I changed my mind."
Perspective: This means they had one idea, but now they have a new idea.
Descriptive: There are many situations where a person may say, "I changed my mind."
Perspective: It is safe for someone to change their mind or want to do something else. Sometimes the new idea or the new thing they want to do is better than the old one.
Descriptive: I will work on staying calm when someone changes their mind.
Descriptive: It is important to try to stay calm.
Descriptive: This keeps everyone safe.[13]

Word choice is also important. Obviously, the Story must be written at the child's level of understanding. In addition, the writer must avoid terms and expressions that may be interpreted too literally. Words such as *always, never,* and *every* may cause confusion or distress. For example, you would not write "Every day I ride my bicycle to school," even though most people would understand that implicit in that statement are such mutually understood exceptions as days when there is no school, days with inclement weather, days when the child might be home from school ill. In a Social Story you would write "Sometimes I ride my bicycle to school." It is wise to exercise extra caution in phrasing the directive sentences in such a way that they don't create an atmosphere of unrealistic expectations and inadvertently set the stage for failure. "I can," "I will," "I should," or "I must" statements have no place in a Social Story. Not only may a child not be able to comply with the directive, he may be hindered from doing so by circumstances entirely beyond his control. Instead, begin directive sentences with: "I will try to . . ." "I will work on . . ." "I may [do something] . . ." "I can try to [do something] . . ." and so on. Be sure directive sentences are positive and focus on the appropriate, desired response or behavior, not on the problem behavior the Social Story is designed to address. Remember that for many of our children, simply having the understanding necessary to make the effort is a victory unto itself.

When They May Be Appropriate

You can use a Social Story to help a child with AS:

- Learn a routine, such as how to get dressed or how to set the table
- Prepare for an event or situation that is either unfamiliar or difficult, such as attending a birthday party or the first day of school
- Foster understanding of behaviors and identify appropriate responses, such as what to do when one feels angry or afraid generally or in specific situations
- Recognize social cues and respond appropriately, such as "Why and How I Show People I Love Them"
- Learn how to achieve a goal using step-by-step instructions, such as "Going to McDonald's"
- Understand how to identify fictional, inappropriate interactions and events in movies, videos, video games, and other forms of fiction and media
- Learn how to apply knowledge, such as how to make change or tell time, to practical situations.

Notes and Comments

Although the Social Story technique is easily learned, there are specific guidelines crucial to its successful application. These are found only in the Social Story books and video.

COMIC STRIP CONVERSATIONS

What They Are

A Comic Strip Conversation is exactly what it sounds like: a hand-drawn comic strip (or a single panel) that illustrates social communication. A parent or teacher may draw the conversation, but it is best approached as a joint project in which the child is an active partner. It can be used to help a person with AS understand an exchange or event that occurred in the past or to help that person prepare for a future interaction. For example, you might use a Comic Strip Conversation to explain to a child with AS why his sister cried when he told her that her games were all "stupid," or how to greet a friend.

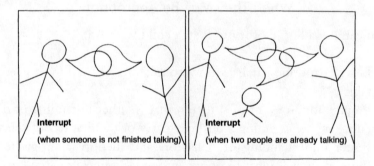

Interrupt:
When my words bump into words from other people.

In Carol Gray's Comic Strip Conversations, different types of thought and word bubbles are used to illustrate different types of verbal exchanges. In this one, the figures' interrupting one another is shown by overlapping word bubbles that appear to literally "step on" what another person is saying. (From *Comic Strip Conversations: Colorful, Illustrated Interactions with Students with Autism and Related Disorders,* Carol Gray [Arlington, TX: Future Horizons, 1993]. Reproduced by permission of Future Horizons.)

You don't need to be an artist to draw Comic Book Conversations; stick figures will do. The technique is fully explained in Carol Gray's short book, *Comic Strip Conversations: Colorful, Illustrated Interactions with Students with Autism and Related Disorders*. Comic Book Conversations use the same visual vocabulary as comic books: text bubbles with tails that point to the speaker for spoken words, cloudlike bubbles for thoughts. Overlapping text bubbles signify what it "looks like" when someone interrupts; for instance, large letters spell out words spoken loudly and smaller letters indicate words spoken softly. Different emotions may be indicated by colors. Carol Gray has developed a "color vocabulary," but you can change these to suit your child's preference. Just remember to use the colors consistently (for example, blue will always mean happiness; red, anger; and so on).

When They May Be Appropriate

Comic Book Conversations usually illustrate communication and social interaction. They've been shown to be effective in helping some people with AS better understand the thoughts, emotions, and words of both themselves and others.

How They Work

The comic strip format helps a child with AS because it "freezes" the action (which makes postevent analysis possible) and because it offers insight into the thoughts and feelings of others. A Comic Strip Conversation takes the many levels of social communication—emotion, facial expression, tone of voice, speech—and breaks them down into discrete components. Once drawn, a child can revisit or become familiar with a situation at his own pace without the distraction and stress of actually being in the situation. For example, using both a text bubble and a thought bubble, you can effectively illustrate another person saying "You can't catch me!" while thinking "I really want Sean to follow me because he is my friend and I like playing with him." This level of understanding is often simply not accessible to a child with AS. For Sean, who interprets "You can't catch me" as an insult or a taunt, a vivid, visual representation of the "thought behind the words" may be the difference between being able to play comfortably among peers and not.

A Comic Strip Conversation as social autopsy.

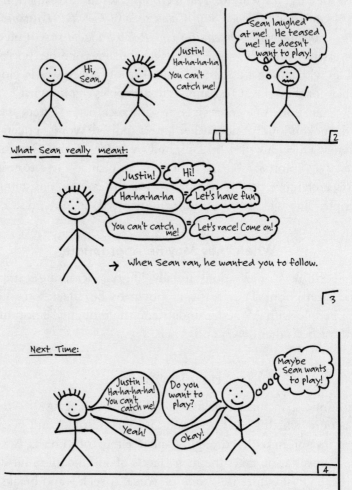

This Comic Strip Conversation is based on a true story. Justin became upset when he "read" Sean's playful invitation to join him according to the literal meaning of Sean's words and a noncontextual interpretation of Sean's actions. Justin interpreted Sean's playful "Ha-ha-ha-ha" as "He was laughing at me" and Sean's "You can't catch me" as a boast or insult rather than an invitation. When Sean turned to run (expecting Justin to follow), Justin saw that as a sign that Sean did not want to play with him. The Comic Strip Conversation in panel 3 is designed to give Justin some insight into what Sean really meant and expected. Panel 4 demonstrates how to ask for clarification when someone's meaning is not clear.

What Parents Can Do to Help

If you do decide to try Social Stories and Comic Strip Conversations, consult one of Carol Gray's books or work with someone who knows the technique and follow Gray's guidelines completely. Even if you don't write a Social Story or sketch out a Comic Strip Conversation for every problematic situation, it is well worth the time and effort to familiarize yourself with the approach. Simply thinking through a situation and breaking down the ideas as you would to write a Social Story can help you learn a simpler, clearer way of communicating orally with your child.

Recommended Resources

Carol Gray, *Comic Strip Conversations: Colorful Illustrated Interactions with Students with Autism and Related Disorders* (Arlington, TX: Future Horizons, 1994).

———, "Social Stories 10.0: The New Defining Criteria and Guidelines," in *Jennison Autism Journal,* vol. 15, number 4, pp. 2–21. The latest word from Carol Gray. Note that the journal is now known as *Autism Spectrum Quarterly* and available from www.ASQuarterly.com or www.thegraycenter.org. This is Gray's most recent revision of the Social Stories guidelines.

———, *Taming the Recess Jungle* (Arlington, TX: Future Horizons, 1993).

OCCUPATIONAL THERAPY (OT)

What It Is

Occupational therapy is a health care specialty concerned with developing, strengthening, and restoring the patient's ability to perform the tasks of daily living. It emerged as a specialized field in the wake of World War I, which left millions of survivors who were physically and/or neurologically disabled. Disabled persons who were taught to regain some degree of ability with OT had quicker and more satisfactory outcomes than those who remained inactive. The term *occupation* refers not simply to paid work but to any goal one wishes to achieve.

OT recognizes and addresses nervous system (brain- and nerve-related) dysfunction that may give rise to challenges in all areas of life—intellectual, personal, social, psychological, emotional, and vocational. Occupational therapists treat patients whose problems arise from a wide range of causes: physical injury, birth defect, aging, psychological disability, illness, and developmental disability.

When It May Be Appropriate

For children with AS, OT may address many different types of nervous system dysfunction. Because many children with AS have two or more of these problems, OT can make a positive difference in several different areas, including problems with handwriting, learning, fine- and gross-motor skills, motor planning (dyspraxia), and general clumsiness.

Another area in which OT can be helpful is sensory integration disorder (SID), also known as sensory integration dysfunction, the inability of the brain to effectively and efficiently process sensory stimuli. Experts estimate that between 12 percent and 30 percent of all children have some degree of sensory integration disorder. Of those receiving OT for SID, about 80 percent are boys. Although there are no hard statistics regarding the prevalence of SID among children with AS, Dr. Hans Asperger noted unusual sensitivities to sensory stimuli, including sound, in his original 1944 paper.

It is not unusual for a child with AS to have problems in both areas and to receive OT for both. In many cases, the causes and the corrective therapy overlap. In fact, determining which disorder gave rise to which disability often comes down to a chicken-and-egg question. Is Aaron averse to handwriting because he lacks fine-motor and motor-planning skills? Or is it because he has always shown general tactile defensiveness when anything touches his hands? Or did his development of fine-motor and motor-planning skills get "stopped" because his tactile defensiveness made him less likely to crawl and explore?

Occupational therapy should be considered for any child who:

• Has deficits in or seems to be behind his peers in mastering such skills as feeding, dressing, and grooming himself; bouncing, catching, and throwing balls; writing, drawing, coloring, painting, working with clay or Play-Doh; or jumping, hopping, running, skipping, and climbing.

- Seems unusually sensitive to touch, sound, smells, or visual stimuli. For example, a child who goes to great lengths to avoid being touched or hugged, covers her ears and becomes distressed at certain sounds, reacts violently to particular scents, or appears to become disoriented or distracted during tasks that require tracking a moving object or copying material from a blackboard.
- Is unusually averse to certain places, situations, or experiences. For example, a child who tantrums upon entering a department store for "no apparent reason" or who is unusually whiny and "picky" about the clothes he wears.
- Is unusually active or inactive for his age.
- Seems clumsy or uncomfortable even when performing simple tasks such as walking, opening a jar, or following simple directions such as "Put your left hand on top of your head."
- Gives the impression of "not knowing what to do with himself" by being unable to sit or stand still; or assumes unusual postures while sitting, standing, or walking.
- Generally appears, to borrow a title from an informative book on the topic, "out of sync."

A complete list of the symptoms and behaviors that may suggest SID could include over a hundred items, some of which are polar opposites. So, for example, a child who is averse to spinning and a child who craves it, a child who seems to hear "too well" and a child who seems to hear poorly, a child who seems to smell and react to everything and a child who seems to have no sense of smell, a child who grasps objects too tightly and a child who grasps objects too loosely may all have SID. A child with SID may enjoy or avoid messy activities such as finger painting; he may seek out deep-pressure types of touch like hugs or become distressed at merely being brushed up against; he may have a stiff, rigid posture or appear overly relaxed, loose, even "floppy." We include these examples because SID is an area that few pediatricians, educators, and other professionals know much about. Sometimes parents may hear that a child who overreacts to pain may have SID and conclude, erroneously, that their own child, who underreacts to pain, does not. In fact, it is possible that both children would have SID.

How It Works

We know that from the first moments of life, children learn through their senses. Typical neurological development is the result of a complex and constant exchange of sensory information. Just as a child must sit before crawling, crawl before standing, and stand before walking, healthy neurological development depends on mastery of a specific sequence of tasks. Learning a discrete skill, such as writing, is actually the result of having learned and mastered countless other skills over a lifetime.

Key to that is the brain's ability to accurately process sensory information and to organize it in such a way that a child is capable of responding appropriately and comfortably to his environment. Proper sensory integration is a major component of neurological development. It sets the stage for emotional security, behavioral self-regulation, and learning. When dysfunction occurs in one area, it produces a ripple effect through the entire learning chain. So, for example, a child with tactile sensitivity may avoid touching objects and exploring her environment. As a result, she will not spontaneously seek out other experiences and activities that foster further sensory integration. A child who avoids exploring her environment is starving her brain of the sensory stimulation necessary to healthy development.

Location and Functions of the Sensory Systems

SYSTEM	LOCATION	FUNCTION
Tactile (touch)	**Skin**—density of cell distribution varies throughout the body. Areas of greatest density include mouth, hands, and genitals.	Provides information about the environment and object qualities (touch, pressure, texture, hard, soft, sharp, dull, heat, cold, pain).
Vestibular (balance)	**Inner ear**—stimulated by head movements and input from other senses, especially visual.	Provides information about where our body is in space, and whether we or our surroundings are moving. Tells about speed and direction of movement.

Proprio-ception (body awareness)	**Muscles and joints**— activated by muscle contractions and movement.	Provides information about where a certain body part is and how it is moving.
Visual (sight)	**Retina of the eye**— stimulated by light.	Provides information about objects and persons. Helps us define boundaries as we move through time and space.
Auditory (hearing)	**Inner ear**—stimulated by air/sound waves.	Provides information about sounds in the environment (loud, soft, high, low, near, far).
Gustatory (taste)	**Chemical receptors in the tongue**— closely entwined with the olfactory (smell) system.	Provides information about different types of taste (sweet, sour, bitter, salty, spicy).
Olfactory (smell)	**Chemical receptors in the nasal structure**—closely associated with the gustatory system.	Provides information about different types of smell (musty, acrid, putrid, flowery, pungent).

(From *Asperger Syndrome and Sensory Issues: Practical Solutions for Making Sense of the World,* Brenda Smith Myles, Katherine Tapscott Cook, Nancy E. Miller, Lousann Rinner, Lisa A. Robbins [Shawnee Mission, KS: Autism Asperger Publishing, 2000]. Reproduced by permission of the Autism Asperger Publishing Company.)

Sensory integration therapy (SIT) addresses sensory dysfunction through activities that both stimulate the various senses and require that a child organize those stimuli to respond appropriately. Neurologically typical children do this naturally; as they play, they receive the sensory stimulation and refine the appropriate responses that compel them to try other activities and seek out other sensory experiences. Children who receive SIT usually find that it's fun. Bouncing a ball, swinging in a tirelike swing, and doing "wheelbarrow walking" are just a few of hundreds of standard but very playlike SIT techniques. OT may also involve working with puzzles, games, and objects that are manipulated (like stringing beads or digging small "buried" objects out of a ball of putty or clay). Some parents are surprised to discover that SIT does not "teach" the skill of holding a pencil properly by having the child practice holding a pencil, for example. Instead, OT uses different techniques to increase the child's mature sensory integration of those senses and the neurological response crucial to the process of holding a pencil to write.

The theory that explains SID and the methods used to treat it were first developed in the 1960s by Dr. A. Jean Ayres, an occupational therapist and educational psychologist. Initially rejected by the occupational therapy community, Dr. Ayres's assertion that sensory integration is key to the development of the mind, the brain, and the body has found broader acceptance in recent years. *Sensory integration,* a term she coined in the late 1960s, refers to the brain's ability to organize sensory input, or information, received not only through the five "far" senses (taste, touch, sight, smell, and hearing) but also through the so-called near senses. These are the tactile sense, or what is felt through the skin (touch, temperature, movement); the proprioceptive sense, or what is felt through the position and movement of the muscles and joints (essentially where our bodies are in space, where we are in relation to gravity); and the vestibular sense, which is what our inner ear conveys to our brain about balance, body position, gravity, and movement. Dr. Ayres also believed—and the success of OT for SID seems to bear it out—that therapy can essentially "retrain" the brain to integrate sensory input normally.

The impact of any dysfunction in the far senses is easy for most of us to comprehend. However, the role of the near senses is somewhat more abstract and difficult to conceptualize. Some examples of dysfunction in the near senses may help illustrate the point. Examples of tactile dysfunction would include being repulsed, extremely distracted, or uncomfortable, even nauseated, by the feel of a particular fabric against the skin, the texture of glue or finger paint, or a pat on the back.

One form of vestibular dysfunction many airline passengers know well is that feeling of being slightly off balance as a result of pressure in the inner ear. For children who live with vestibular dysfunction, the feelings may be constant and more extreme. As mentioned earlier, one child may crave intense spinning, and another may panic at even turning around to walk in a different direction. Observing a child with vestibular dysfunction may give the impression that his left hand doesn't know what his right hand is doing, and that would not be far off the mark. These children will not automatically use their hands or bodies to "help" them execute tasks. For instance, there will be no coordination between the hand that wields the scissors or the pencil and the hand that moves or steadies, as the case may be, the paper. Children with vestibular dysfunction may also experience gravitational insecurity, which manifests in a fear of jumping, swinging, hopping, or any other activity that takes their feet off the ground.

For most people, proprioceptive dysfunction is perhaps the most difficult form of SID to conceptualize. If your brain processes and organizes proprioceptive information, you are receiving sufficient sensory feedback from everything you do to keep your mind alert. You don't need to stop and consciously think about (or look to see) where your hands or your feet are, for example. You position your body without consciously thinking, and you move through space without consciously noticing the distance between your arm and the wall, or your foot and the steps you're climbing. Your brain instantaneously "calculates" the correct angle, speed, and muscle force needed for every movement. As a result, you don't bump into objects or accidentally crush an egg when you pick it up.

Vestibular dysfunction disrupts the automatic processing of information regarding the position of the head in relation to gravity and movement. Remember that foggy, out-of-sync, off-kilter sensation you have when your ears have not yet "popped" after a flight? Dr. Ayres viewed the vestibular system as the "unifying" system and believed that problems there led to "inconsistent and inaccurate" processing of sensory input through other senses. The vestibular sense signals the brain to relax or contract muscles throughout the body to adjust for movements as seemingly minute as sitting in a chair or as obvious as running. It makes it possible for us to hold our heads upright, coordinate the actions of both sides of the body, and to maintain our balance during activities as simple as walking up a flight of steps. Deficiencies in this system may manifest in a range of problems with motor planning, auditory-language processing, visual-spatial processing, muscle tone, balance, movement, and bilateral coordination. Vestibular problems may explain why one child seems to constantly "melt" into his chair or lean his upper body against his desk. A child who has not established a dominant hand by kindergarten or who has trouble putting together simple puzzles may have vestibular problems.

What We Know About Occupational Therapy and AS

While educators, doctors, and other professionals who deal with PDDs usually understand the role of OT, you may encounter professionals who are not as well informed. This is particularly true with sensory integration disorder, which is not widely known outside the disability community. Though there are standard instruments for diagnosing deficiencies in individuals, it is difficult to measure some of the results of OT objectively; for example, increased gravitational security or decreased sensitivity to a particular stimulus. A large percentage of parents whose children receive OT note improvement in one or more areas.

Where to Find It

Occupational therapists can be found in private practice and/or working in schools, hospitals, therapy centers, and doctors' offices. Occupational therapy is considered a related service under IDEA.

What Parents Can Do to Help

Whenever your child is evaluated, be sure that he's tested by an occupational therapist for possible deficits in skills or sensory integration disorder.

Sensory integration dysfunction is one of those "invisible" challenges that people untouched by it find difficult to conceptualize. You may find yourself explaining it many times, to family members, teachers, baby-sitters, even strangers. First, recognize that sensory integration disorder presents a potentially serious problem that is much greater than the sum of all its parts. It's discouraging to hear a parent say, "So my four-year-old daughter doesn't like to swing or color? What's the big deal?" The "big deal" is that the four-year-old who doesn't swing or color could become the second-grader who is still struggling mightily with printing letters, cutting shapes with scissors, and participating in age-appropriate playground activities.

Sensory integration disorder is not a problem that simply goes away by itself. Over time, some children become less sensitive or less averse to certain sensory experiences, but it would be inaccurate to say that these problems can be outgrown. An occupational therapist who is trained in sensory integration techniques will probably offer guidance on ways to help your child cope with SID and perhaps help reduce some sensory sensitivity. Opportunities to enhance your child's level of sensory integration abound. In her excellent book *The Out-of-Sync Child* (see "Recommended Resources," page 214), Carol Stock Kranowitz makes a compelling case for what she calls "a balanced sensory diet," something typical children actively seek but that children with SID lack. A well-rounded sensory diet will be specifically tailored to meet the needs of your child and will combine activities with different goals: organizing, calming, and alerting. Your occupational therapist can give you techniques and activities to do at home.

Second, remember that sensory sensitivities are real and may even be terrifying for your child. Telling your child to just "ignore" how uncomfortable his shirt feels is not only ineffective but communicates to your child that you don't appreciate the difficulties he faces. Parents sometimes find themselves prodding a child into an activity he is averse to in the mistaken hope that if he only goes down the slide enough times or only chews meat enough times, "he'll get used to it." In fact, what you'll get is a child who will continually feel insecure, anxious, and afraid. If simple exposure were the answer to sensory integration problems, they would not exist in the first place. At the same time, do not rule out different therapeutic approaches (behavioral and cognitive behavioral) to desensitize children to certain uncomfortable stimuli. It may not be worth the discomfort and effort to teach Sally to tolerate the feel of chalk; however, when you consider the implications for safety (not to mention hygiene) of an oversensitivity to water on one's face, additional intervention may be in order.

Questions to Ask

- What problems does my child have? And can you please explain them to me in plain English?
- How do these problems affect my child in terms of daily activities?
- How do the activities you'll be doing with him as part of therapy help him? What are the goals of this therapy?

- What can I do at home and what can his teacher do in the classroom to help address these issues?
- What are some specific activities that will have therapeutic value for my child?
- What are the elements of a good "sensory diet" for my child? How often should we have him engage in these activities?
- Are there any activities he should avoid for now?
- Are there any other types of evaluations or professionals you believe we should consider? If so, why?

Recommended Resources

Anne G. Fisher, Elizabeth A. Murray, and Anita C. Bundy, *Sensory Integration: Theory and Practice* (Philadelphia: F. A. Davis Company, 1991). Although written for occupational therapists, this highly technical book includes many useful tips and illustrations.

The New York State Occupational Therapy Association, "Occupational Therapy for Learning Disabilities," an excellent two-page paper of interest to any parent whose child's OT issues affect learning. Available at http://www.nysota.org/mentalretardation.

Brenda Smith Myles, Katherine Tapscott Cook, Nancy E. Miller, Louann Rinner, and Lisa A. Robbins, *Asperger Syndrome and Sensory Issues: Practical Solutions for Making Sense of the World* (Shawnee Mission, KS: Autism Asperger Publishing, 2000). The beauty of this slim, information-packed book is how clearly it explains a complex, often confusing subject.

Carol Stock Kranowitz, *The Out-of-Sync Child: Recognizing and Coping with Sensory Integration Dysfunction* (New York: Perigee, 1998) and *The Out-Of-Sync Child Has Fun: Activities for Kids with Sensory Integration Dysfunction* (New York: Perigee, 2003).

SPEECH AND LANGUAGE THERAPY

What It Is

The term *speech and language therapy* encompasses a wide range of therapeutic practices involving patients of all age groups and addressing problems that range from difficulty swallowing to regaining the ability to speak and understand following trauma or illness. When working with children with AS, speech and language pathologists or teachers may engage in many different exercises to address different aspects of the deficit. However, the ultimate goal is to help children with AS develop, through explicit teaching, the social communication skills they cannot learn through "social osmosis," as most other people do.

When It May Be Appropriate

Because AS so profoundly affects the social use of language, most children with AS will need some form of speech and language therapy. Though you will probably hear the two types of therapy referred to simply as "speech," there are differences between speech therapy and language therapy. Speech therapy usually addresses issues of basic speech, namely correct articulation. Language therapy deals with problems in understanding (receptive) or expressing (expressive) words, both verbal and nonverbal. Children with AS usually experience difficulty in the areas of semantics (the use of words to express literal meaning), pragmatics (the social use of language), presupposition (the ability to recognize and tailor one's communication to a conversational partner's understanding, beliefs, and relationship to the speaker), and social discourse (essentially, the ability to initiate, maintain, and end a conversation in a socially appropriate manner).

There is some confusion in this area, because one of the diagnostic criteria that distinguishes Asperger Syndrome from other pervasive developmental disorders is the absence of speech delay before age three. Some have interpreted this to mean that children with AS have "normal" speech development. In view of the many language problems children with AS often have, some authorities have begun to question whether that early speech development should not be more accurately characterized as "normal appearing." As Dr. Diane Twachtman-Cullen notes in her book on students with ASDs *How to Be a Para Pro:*

At the more able end of the autism spectrum continuum . . . one finds individuals who often *appear* to understand and use language at a rather high level. In fact, individuals with Asperger syndrome are thought by many to have *normal* language. This, however, is not the case. Thus, it is important to note that even though students with AS may appear to have *superficially* normal language expression (in terms of grammar and syntax), and even though they may evidence advanced vocabulary usage, they nevertheless manifest difficulty in *social communication*—that is, in the *comprehension and use of language for the purposes of receiving and sending messages.*[14]

We learn what we are taught and express what we know through language. It is possible for a child who has kept pace academically through the early elementary grades to encounter difficulty later when schoolwork requires greater independence and understanding of abstract concepts. Also bear in mind that difficulties with language may also manifest as problems in mathematics and social skills. Your local school district may resist even evaluating a child with AS for speech and language problems because he may be extremely talkative and have an impressive vocabulary. You should know that IDEA specifies that one goal of evaluation is to identify *all* of the *possible* deficits a child may have and to test specifically for those known to be related to a specific disorder. The prevalence of speech and language disorders among persons with AS is well established; indeed, some consider speech and language therapy the most important intervention.

Your child should be evaluated for speech and language therapy if he or she:

- Misinterprets or misunderstands the words and actions of others
- Has difficulty understanding nonverbal aspects of communication (facial expression, gestures, body language, tone of voice)
- Often interprets oral and written language literally
- Has difficulty using and maintaining appropriate speech volume and intonation (for example, has a "flat" tone)
- Has difficulty initiating, maintaining, repairing, and ending a conversation in a socially appropriate way
- Fails to appreciate the listener's level of interest in and/or understanding of a topic, so that he or she provides too little or too much information
- Has difficulty understanding or talking about abstract concepts, such as time ("yesterday," "next week"), states of mind, and ideas, particularly those of other people
- Seems to take an unusually long time to respond to questions and statements from others; may seem not to be hearing

- Often seems to miss the larger message or the theme of conversation, stories, books, movies, television programs, and other forms of storytelling.

How It Works

There are so many different techniques and methods a speech and language therapist might employ, it is impossible to cover them all. Creative speech and language pathologists tailor their approach to address the needs of the individual. Sessions may include elements of social skills training, auditory integration training, occupational therapy, and play. To encourage more appropriate communication, role-playing, videotaping the child, and group sessions may be used. (Because there is this overlap between speech and language therapy and social skills training, please read the section on Social Skills Training that follows.)

What We Know About Speech and Language Therapy and AS

When designed for a child with AS and carried out correctly, speech and language therapy can help children improve their social communication skills as well as their ability to listen, attend, ask and respond to questions, and comprehend written and spoken language. Because atypical speech and language development is the core defining deficit in all autism spectrum disorders, speech-language pathologists usually have some training and/or experience in this area, if not with AS specifically. There is a large and growing body of literature on speech and language therapy and AS and related language-based disorders, such as semantic-pragmatic language disorder (SPD) and nonverbal learning disability (NLD or NVLD).

Where to Find It

Speech and language therapy is considered a related service under IDEA, and most public and private schools have speech-language pathologists on staff. Speech-language pathologists also practice in a wide range of medical and educational settings; some are in private practice.

Questions to Ask

- What is your experience with children with ASDs and AS specifically?
- Would you please explain the deficits you'll be addressing and give me everyday examples of how each deficit affects my child, both at home and at school?
- What can we do at home and what can his teachers do in school to support the work you'll be doing with him?
- From what you have observed working with my child, would you recommend further evaluations for other, related conditions, such as central auditory processing disorder, sensory integration disorders, or reading or other learning disability? Would you recommend occupational therapy?

What Parents Can Do to Help

Ask your child's speech pathologist for any "homework" that might be appropriate. He or she may recommend computer programs, videos, books, or techniques for home.

Recommended Resources

Sabrina Freeman and Lorelei Dake, *Teach Me Language: A Language Manual for Children with Autism, Asperger Syndrome, and Related Developmental Disorders* (Langley, B.C., Canada: SKF Books, 1997) and *The Companion Exercise Forms for Teach Me Language* (Langley, B.C., Canada: SKF Books, 1997).

Michelle Garcia Winner, *Inside Out: What Makes a Person with Social-Cognitive Deficits Tick?* (San Jose, CA: self-published, 2000), online at www.socialthinking.com.

SOCIAL SKILLS TRAINING

What It Is

Just about everyone agrees that children with AS need social skills training. Some contend that it is the single most important intervention. Unfortunately for parents, not everyone agrees on what that training should include or how to teach it. Ideally, social skills training breaks down and teaches specific social skills—taking turns, conversation, sharing, joining a group, working with others toward a common goal, understanding facial expressions, tone of voice, and so on—and it provides a "safe" place in which to practice them. There are countless ways to teach such things, but not all are equally effective for children with AS or for any particular child with AS. A talented group leader or therapist should make the group sessions fun, too. Remember, it is not enough for your child to learn how to greet a new acquaintance appropriately. He also needs to acquire that skill in an environment that is positive and reinforcing and will leave him with the impression that other individuals may be worth the time and the trouble to get to know.

Ideally, a social skills group contains four to six children. It is large enough to give each child a number of other group members to "practice on" but small enough to allow for critical individual attention. The group should be led by someone with a background in child development or psychology (social worker, psychologist, psychiatrist, therapist), and extensive experience with Asperger Syndrome is preferred. Social skills therapy is also used for children who have emotional and behavioral issues, as well as those with other specific disorders (ADHD, etc.). It is important that a child with AS be placed in an AS or HFA group. Some groups include only children with AS, while others also bring in "coached" neurotypical children to model appropriate peer behavior. In one social skills group we know, the children rehearsed and then ordered their own desserts at an ice-cream shop, role-played appropriate responses to teasing and bullying, practiced making telephone calls to each other, and worked together as a group on a play, which was videotaped and shown later to parents at a "premiere."

The idea of social skills training is neither new nor exclusive to spectrum disorders. It has been a key component in the education of individuals with a wide range of issues, diagnoses, and challenges. One of the most popular general social skills curricula is Skill-Streaming, which is designed to help students of all ages (books and videos are targeted at specific age groups) who, according to its home page, "display aggression, immaturity, withdrawal, or other problem behaviors. It is designed to help youngsters develop competence in dealing with interpersonal conflicts, learn to use self-control, and contribute to a positive classroom atmosphere." Although not specifically designed for use with students with spectrum disorders, it is one of the most widely used programs in schools, and we know of several children with AS who have used it with success when therapists made necessary modifications based on individual skills and needs.

There is such a need for good social skills programs and no real means of regulating them that virtually anyone can hang a shingle and offer a program. The problem with this is obvious. We recently heard about a so-called social skills program where the leader (a special education teacher) had the group of elementary school children whose diagnoses ranged across the spectrum sit in a circle and answer the question "How do you feel about being here today?" The techniques and objectives of a social skills program developed for, say, children who have ADHD, whose parents have recently divorced, who are dealing with grief, or who have problems with garden-variety shyness probably will not be very effective for a child with AS. All types of professionals can and do offer social skills training: psychiatrists, psychologists, social workers, school counselors and school psychologists, teachers, and others. There is no accrediting body for social skills training in the realm of ASDs. Perhaps the most important "credential" for working with children who have AS is probably experience working with children with AS.

When It May Be Appropriate

Most children with AS can benefit from some form of structured instruction and practice in social skills. According to special education authority Richard Lavoie, "Social skill development is one of the greatest challenges that parents of special needs children face. The social competence of a child will determine his self-esteem, friendships, and adjustment to school life. Most important, social competence will determine his ultimate success and adjustment in the adult world."[15]

While Lavoie was speaking of children with special needs generally, the need to acquire, practice, and master social skills is even more urgent for the child with AS, whose disability is often invisible and whose words and actions may easily be misinterpreted by others. Contrary to the impression they may sometimes give, children with AS are interested in their peers and many of them long for companionship. The problem is that in social situations, a child with AS does not know "automatically" how to behave in a manner that is conducive to creating and sustaining relationships with others. Few would disagree that friendship is an important part of life, a source of satisfaction and joy. Most of us find it impossible to imagine our lives without friends.

How It Works

Social skills training makes it possible for the child with AS to do what AS prevents him from doing automatically, naturally, and fluently for himself: observing, processing, and imitating appropriate social behavior naturally. Social skills training takes a social activity—say, for example, answering the telephone or initiating a conversation with a classmate—and, in Dr. Tony Attwood's words, "freezes the action," breaks down the steps of the activity, and clearly explains the applicable social "rules." The crucial element of social skills training in a group is the "sheltered" practice with peers, something that one-on-one therapy with an adult cannot provide.

What We Know About Social Skills Training and AS

There have been few studies on the efficacy of social skills training, which isn't surprising, considering how difficult it is to objectively measure progress. Nonetheless, most experts agree that social skills training is one intervention every child with AS should have, in one form or another.

Using Computer and Video Technology

One of the most exciting tools for social skills training comes from Dr. Simon Baron-Cohen and colleagues at Oxford University. His *Mind Reading: An Interactive Guide to Emotions* is a CD-ROM or DVD computer program that presents 412 distinct human emotions, grouped into twenty-four different categories, each with facial expression, tone of voice, and inclusion in a brief, simple story. The design of the program is clean and bright; it is easy to navigate and fun to use. Unlike earlier attempts at "emotion teaching" computer programs, which used drawings or amateurish video clips, this one is sleekly professional. The faces are those of professional actors—both American and British, which offers a wide range of different accents—including Daniel Radcliffe, aka Harry Potter.

In the Emotions Library section, each of the 412 emotions is accompanied by several video clips, each showing different types of people (male, female, young, old, of different ethnic backgrounds) and audio clips, in which an actor speaks using that emotion. The Learning Centre contains lessons and quizzes specifically tailored to meet the needs of persons with ASDs. You can test drive and order this program at its easy-to-use Web site: www.human-emotions.com.

Where to Find It

Ask your child's doctors, therapists, and teachers for recommendations. Social skills groups are run by private practitioners, hospitals, universities, and nonprofit organizations, including religious institutions. If you choose a group that is run by a licensed physician or therapist, some or all of the cost may be covered by health insurance.

Questions to Ask

- How long has this group been meeting?
- Who is the group leader? What is his/her experience working with children with AS?
- What do you consider the primary goals of the group? What specific skills will you be working on? Can you give me some idea of the activities you'll be doing to help teach those skills?
- Tell me about the actual meetings: When do they meet? How often? How long are the sessions? What is the cost? Do you break for summer or continue having sessions?
- How many children are in each group?
- What types of diagnoses do the other children have? What are their ages?
- What are some things we can do at home and his teacher can do at school to reinforce what he learns here at group?
- What are the rules of behavior for the group?

• Is it possible for me to observe a group in session? If not, are there other parents I can call to ask about their experience with the group?

More Thoughts on Social Skills

Formal social skills training is important, even crucial, for children with AS. For social skills training to be effective, however, parents, teachers, and others who work with our children need to take advantage of every possible moment to teach, reinforce, and expand it every single day. If learning to use the telephone is a current objective, let your child make that routine call you make to your spouse to remind him or her to pick up milk on the way home. If your child is learning to ask for assistance, send him to the neighbor's house to borrow a cup of sugar or a blank CD (after you call and set it up first). In school, ask your child's teacher to send him on a daily errand to another classroom or the principal's office. We talk more about this in the chapters that make up Part Three.

Recommended Resources

Jed Baker, *Social Skills Training for Children with Asperger Syndrome, High-Functioning Autism, and Related Social Communication Disorders: A Manual for Practitioners* (Shawnee Mission, KS: Autism Asperger Publishing Company, 2002).

Steven E. Gutstein, *Autism/Aspergers: Solving the Relationship Puzzle* (Arlington, TX: Future Horizons, 2000); and, with Rachelle K. Sheely, *Relationship Development Intervention with Young Children: Social and Emotional Development Activities for Asperger Syndrome, Autism, PDD and NLD* (Philadelphia: Jessica Kingsley, 2002).

Patricia Howlin, Simon Baron-Cohen, and Julie Hadwin, *Teaching Children with Autism to Mind-Read: A Practical Guide* (Chichester, England: John Wiley & Sons, 1999).

Jeanette McAfee, *Navigating the Social World: A Curriculum for Individuals with Asperger's Syndrome, High Functioning Autism and Related Disorders* (Arlington, TX: Future Horizons, 2002).

SkillStreaming: For more information on books and videos by the developers of SkillStreaming, Dr. Arnold P. Goldstein and Dr. Ellen McGinnis, go to www.skillstreaming.com/.

PSYCHOTHERAPY

When we say "psychotherapy," we mean individual, one-on-one cognitive behavior "talk therapy" that is designed to help change, modify, and/or replace dysfunctional behaviors and inaccurate perceptions and self-perceptions. Freudian-style psychoanalysis, psychodynamic therapy, family therapy, group therapy, and most other psychotherapeutic approaches are not recommended for children with AS. Also inappropriate are:

- Any therapeutic philosophy that is confrontational, aggressive, or holds the patient entirely responsible for all of his feelings and actions
- Any therapeutic approach that considers AS and related disorders to be the product of poor or incomplete maternal bonding, early emotional trauma, the "choice" of the person with AS, and so on
- Any therapeutic approach that views AS as anything other than a neurological anomaly or disorder
- Any therapeutic approach that dismisses or fails to accept as valid professional diagnoses of other, comorbid conditions (ADHD, OCD, Tourette's syndrome, anxiety disorder, depression, etc.)

When It May Be Appropriate

It is important to understand what cognitive behavior therapy can do and what it cannot do for the child with AS. Its purpose is not to "treat" the Asperger Syndrome itself, but to help the child deal with the specific emotional difficulties that result from having AS or the neurological anomaly that gives rise to AS. A psychotherapist who understands AS can also teach social skills, self-monitoring, relaxation, stress management, and a repertoire of appropriate behaviors. Because persons with AS are at high risk for depression, anxiety, and suicide, especially consider psychotherapy for your child if he meets any of the criteria for depression (see page 71) or anxiety (see page 69).

These criteria are the typical symptoms of anxiety and depression; however, persons with AS may exhibit other behaviors instead of or in addition to those listed. A person with AS may begin devoting more (or less) time to or talking more (or less) about his special interest. He may have more emotional outbursts and tantrums or seem more emotionally sensitive than usual. Another possibility is that you may not notice new symptoms, but behaviors that are common to your child may change in frequency, intensity, or duration. Or you may see new behaviors that are not usually associated with depression and anxiety but that are known to arise in persons with autism spectrum disorders. Some of these might include echolalia, repetitive motor movements, rocking, spinning, or desire for light touch or deep pressure.

What It Is and How It Works

Cognitive behavior therapy is a type of psychotherapy widely used as the primary or adjunctive treatment for many disorders. It is based on the premise that emotional disorders arise from dysfunctional or distorted thinking. Cognitive behavior therapy teaches patients to recognize and monitor their emotions, evaluate the validity of their perceptions about persons and situations, and develop appropriate, functional responses. This can be accomplished through talking with a therapist, role-playing, games, and other therapeutic activities.

Given the challenges persons with AS face in understanding not only other people's thoughts, feelings, and intentions but their own, typical cognitive behavior therapy has proved somewhat limited in helping effect change. The main stumbling block is that persons with AS may lack the basic level of self-awareness, social understanding, theory of mind, and linguistic ability (particularly when discussing such abstract concepts as emotions, thoughts, feelings, and intentions) necessary for effective cognitive behavior therapy. Parents whose children have undergone some form of cognitive behavior therapy prior to their Asperger diagnosis often report that it was ineffective, confusing, or stressful.

What We Know About Cognitive Behavior Therapy and AS

In the hands of a therapist who is familiar with AS and willing to work with your child, cognitive behavior therapy can be very effective. However, it is crucial that you and your child's therapist understand the need to tailor the therapy with an eye to explicitly teaching the basic social, emotional, and linguistic skills most of us assume we never actually actively "learned." You might want to consider cognitive behavior therapy for your child if you lack access to a good social skills group.

Where to Find It

Psychotherapists work in a wide range of settings: in private practice; through public and private agencies; in schools; and in hospitals, clinics, and other health care settings.

Questions to Ask

- What is your experience working with children with AS?
- What do you feel are my child's specific problems and how do you think they should be addressed?
- What activities will you be using in therapy?
- What specific skills will my child be learning in the course of therapy?
- What can we do at home and what can his teachers do at school to reinforce and support what you'll be doing?
- Are you knowledgeable about and taking into account my child's other, comorbid conditions?
- What other therapies and/or interventions would you recommend that we explore, and why?

Recommended Resources

Tony Attwood, "Modifications to Cognitive Behavior Therapy to Accommodate the Cognitive Profile of People with Asperger's Syndrome," August 1999, online at www.tonyattwood.com/paper2.htm. Required reading for any parent or mental health professional working with a child who has Asperger Syndrome.

SPECIAL DIETS: CASEIN- AND GLUTEN-FREE

The use of special diets that eliminate casein (found in dairy products) and gluten (found in wheat, other grains, and processed foods) has long been an area of interest in the autism community. The theory behind these diets is complex but boils down to the idea that when inadequately digested, the protein molecules found in casein and gluten result in amino acid chains (called *peptides*) that adversely affect neurological function. There is no doubt that among some individuals on the autism spectrum, gastrointestinal and digestive problems do occur, including celiac disease (intestinal damage caused by malabsorption of certain nutrients) and dermatitis herpetiformes (a skin rash that is often accompanied by tissue damage in the intestine). It is important to understand that these are not food allergies in the usual sense. Even if your child's test for allergies for milk or wheat comes back negative, it does not necessarily mean that he might not benefit from the elimination of casein or gluten.

The interest in these diets has been spurred by the anecdotal accounts of parents and professionals who have seen marked success with them. Only recently, however, have research studies on the diets and their effectiveness in ameliorating or eliminating autism-related symptoms and behaviors been conducted.

We have heard from parents whose children's AS symptoms were considerably reduced through a wheat- and milk-free diet, but these approaches seem to have a higher rate of success in children with autistic disorder than those with AS. Despite all the attention such diets receive in other ASD communities, we have found little interest in them at OASIS. When we polled OASIS members on the topics they would like to see covered in this book and on their experiences with such diets, the response was weak at best. The few who did report having tried the diets were disappointed and saw little or no change.

On the positive side, it can be argued that a dietary change is a lot less intrusive than some other therapies and carries less risk of side effects than just about anything else. Such dietary restrictions may be very difficult to adjust to, and the cost of special foods and lack of convenience are considerations, but families who have found them helpful say they learn to cope and it is well worth the effort.

Recommended Resources
GFCF Diet
www.gfcfdiet.com/

OTHER THERAPIES AND INTERVENTIONS

At last count, there were dozens of other proposed therapies and interventions purported to be of potential benefit to some persons with AS. Unfortunately for parents charged with making the decisions, the amount of hard science on most of them is sketchy or premature at best. Due to the wide variations from one person with AS to another in terms of symptoms and, we may learn, causes of symptoms, there is no one-size-fits-all therapy to be found here, either. And, at the risk of editorializing, we must say that we have found the most vehement advocates to be those who believe that simply because a course of cranial sacral manipulation worked wonders for their child or for the children they treated, everyone should be trying it. You will find that often the most vociferous and intolerant advocates for a particular approach are either parents for whose child it has worked or the practitioners who provide it. And though either may be honest and truthful, they are not often, scientifically speaking, objective. One of the mysteries of autism generally and AS in particular is how many dozens, if not hundreds, of therapies, appliances, interventions, medications, supplements, special diets, vitamins, exercise regimens, or other treatments were effective for a relative handful of persons with AS. Out of desperation, parents of children with PDDs could spend tens of thousands of dollars trying everything, and sadly, some parents do just that.

One reason it is so difficult to sort through therapies is that we don't yet know what causes Asperger Syndrome. So it makes sense that one child may benefit significantly using the Feingold diet (which concentrates on the elimination of the artificial food colorings that many of our children react to) or a particular supplement, while another does not. Again, for parents, it is a process of trial and error.

The literature concerning children with autistic disorders is full of interesting and persuasive arguments for special diets (usually casein- and gluten-free); vitamins and supplements in dosages that far exceed the U.S. Department of Agriculture's Recommended Daily Allowances; and other therapies. Many of these therapies have received national exposure, and you may have heard of children who were seemingly cured of (or "recovered" from) their autistic symptoms through them. It is important to bear in mind, however, that the number of children for whom any of these therapies has proven completely effective is small. We hope that in the near future, science will reveal why this is so and guide the development of interventions that are more effective for more people.

We neither advocate nor discourage any of these approaches, but we do not include them in detail here because information on their efficacy for a large proportion of persons with AS is either not well established or is not widely recognized among most professionals working with AS. This is not to say that among these, you might not find one, two, or even more that could help your child. However, before proceeding, you should learn all that you can about the therapy and ask its advocates and practitioners the same questions you would ask about more established approaches.

To our knowledge, our OASIS Survey on Alternative Treatments and Interventions is the first attempt to discover which of these might be useful for persons with AS. Interestingly, though our other surveys drew upward of five hundred respondents each, the Alternative survey drew fewer than a hundred. There may be several reasons for this. Generally speaking, AS symptoms may be more readily and effectively addressed with existing therapeutic, educational, and pharmaceutical interventions than those of other PDDs. Overall, AS symptoms are not as extreme, troubling, or disruptive as those that may be found in other PDDs. It is easier perhaps to suppose that the parents of a child who never speaks or seems not to connect to the outside world in any way are more eager to try literally anything and everything than the parents of a child with AS. Whatever the reason, parents of children with AS and persons with AS appear to be less interested in these approaches. However, when we asked respondents to describe their attitudes toward alternative therapies in general, they seemed to be the type of people who would be open to trying them. Only 5 percent indicated that they did not believe alternative therapies are ever effective, compared with 58 percent who agreed with the statement "I believe that some alternative therapies are effective, but I am skeptical about some others."

Of the forty-five alternative therapies we listed, the vast majority had been tried or were being used by less than half the respondents. We asked respondents to rate their experiences with each alternative they had tried, from 1 (very satisfied; significant improvement in target symptoms) to 5 (dissatisfied; no improvement in target symptoms). Space does not permit us to delve into the theory behind every alternative approach. However, our respondents seemed to consider particularly promising the use of various nutritional supplements: calcium; DMG (dimethylglycine); fish oil; omega-3, -6, and -9 oils; Super-Nu-Thera; and vitamin B_6. Percentage-wise, the special diets (casein-, gluten-, or yeast-free) were only mildly impressive overall, but parents for whose children they were effective swear by them.

• • •

Alternative Resources

The following organizations and Web sites provide reliable information on alternative therapies and numerous links to other resources.

Autism Research Institute
This is a nonprofit organization devoted to research on the diagnosis, treatment, and prevention of autism and other ASDs.
Autism Research Institute
www.autism.com/ari

Autism Society of America
This national nonprofit organization offers information on a variety of treatment options.
Autism Society of America
www.autism-society.org

A FINAL WORD ON CHOOSING INTERVENTIONS

Do your research. Listen to everyone—including and perhaps especially those you may initially disagree with. Only you can prioritize your child's and your family's needs and decide how best to spend your time, energy, and financial resources. Given that, it only makes sense to begin with those interventions that are the most widely used (they got to be that way for a reason), best supported by research, and/or endorsed by people, organizations, or agencies with a great deal of experience in this area. Being human, we often make choices based on reasons that may have nothing to do with the actual proven efficacy of an intervention. That's especially easy to do in an area where even those methods that are widely accepted and effective have so little hard research behind them.

Once you embark on an intervention course, shift your focus from all the reasons why you like or chose that method to the results it is—or isn't—producing. Be a consumer when you make your initial decision, but be a scientist once the therapy is under way. Is it working? Is it producing any documentable, obvious improvement? If so, how much? If Jennifer tantrumed twelve times a day before the treatment, and a month later she's tantruming once every four days, you may have a keeper. Count. Keep written records. Ask others who know your child. Yes, some therapies do take time. But for certain problems—violent, self-injurious, suicidal behavior, for instance—there is no time to play around or experiment.

Chapter 7

MEDICATION

DECISIONS about using psychotropic (or psychoactive) medication are among the most difficult and confusing that parents of children with AS confront. The use of medication in children to address problems with behavior, concentration, depression, anxiety, aggression, violence, and other psychiatric symptoms is complex and in some cases controversial, regardless of the diagnosis. Add in the mysteries of Asperger Syndrome, and the decision becomes even more daunting. Nonetheless, it is a decision that at some point many parents (including those who ultimately decide not to use medication) will face.

It would be impossible to include in this chapter everything there is to know about every possible medication (and medication combination) now used for children with AS. If you are considering medication for your child, this chapter is a good place to start. We hope to give you a broad overview of the issue, general information about the types of medication most frequently prescribed, and some guidelines to help you in making your decision. The "Recommended Resources" listed on page 277 should be considered required reading.

PSYCHOTROPIC MEDICATION
FOR PERSONS WITH AS

Many persons with AS have taken or are taking medication—one study found that over 68 percent of 109 respondents had taken some psychotropic medication at some point.[1] Although many children with AS will go through life without needing it, there are those for whom medication will be indicated, either to support the child through a difficult time or a crisis or on a long-term basis to address chronic problems such as depression, anxiety, obsessive-compulsive disorder, bipolar disorder, attention deficit/hyperactivity disorder, or tics. Some situations and developmental phases can present more challenges and create more stress, such as adolescence. We also know that persons with AS—including even young children—are at higher risk than others for anxiety, depression, seizure disorders, tic disorders, and suicide, and medication can help address these problems.

When doctors prescribe psychotropic (or psychoactive or psychotherapeutic) medication, they are not "treating" AS the same way we think of "treating" diabetes with insulin or pain with morphine. There is no pharmacological "cure" or remedy for AS. However, a number of medications have been shown to be effective in addressing certain specific common AS symptoms as well as separate comorbid conditions that may exist alongside it (see chapter 3).

Comorbid Conditions Commonly Seen in Persons with AS

Attention deficit/hyperactivity disorder (ADHD)

Anxiety

Bipolar disorder

Depression

Obsessive-compulsive disorder (OCD)

Psychosis (*Note:* Persons with AS who make inappropriate comments or respond to stress in certain ways may be misdiagnosed as "psychotic" when they are not)

Seizure disorders

Social phobia

Tourette's syndrome and tics

WHAT MAKES THE MEDICATION DECISION SO DIFFICULT?

Even when medication is clearly indicated, parents may hesitate, wondering if it isn't possible that their son or daughter might not "just grow out of it" or not need it if they made certain changes at home or at school. Some would argue that except in those cases of psychiatric crisis (a child becoming a danger to himself or to others, threatening or attempting suicide), it's reasonable to try addressing difficulties through changes and accommodations in your child's life. Learning what works and what doesn't can also give you and your child's doctor additional insight into the problem. Others believe that it makes more sense to take a proactive approach long before a child's emotional state becomes a crisis.

There are legitimate concerns over the fact that the long-term safety and efficacy of most psychotropic medications for children has not yet been established. In fact, in many cases, even the pharmaceutical companies that make them cannot say with certainty precisely how many of these medications work. Later in this chapter, we address questions about FDA approval, off-label usage, and other matters.

Whatever the reason, most parents agree in theory that medication is not the best first choice, and that alternative approaches (such as behavior modification, psychotherapy, changes and accommodations at school and at home) should be tried first. In most cases, this is a reasonable approach. However, there are conditions for which medication is the first-line treatment and sometimes the most or the only effective treatment available. This is particularly true when dealing with a child who is deeply depressed or suicidal, or if allowing a behavior or mood to persist would pose a danger to the child or to others or be detrimental to the child's emotional well-being. That said, there is no such thing as a "magic bullet," a medication that can resolve your child's issues single-handedly. In virtually every case, medication along with some form of psychotherapy and behavior modification, as well as changes that provide support at home and at school, are most likely to be effective.

THE CRISIS IN CHILDREN'S
MENTAL HEALTH CARE

Contrary to what many people believe, anxiety disorders, depression, eating disorders (anorexia nervosa, bulimia nervosa), disruptive behavior disorders, schizophrenia, tic disorder, obsessive-compulsive disorder, and bipolar disorder can begin in early childhood. (Persons with AS are at increased risk of developing one, two, or more of these disorders *in addition to* having AS.) According to the National Institute of Mental Health, "Studies consistently show that about 15 percent of the U.S. population below age 18, or over 9 million children, suffer from a psychiatric disorder that compromises their ability to function."[2] Though one in ten children and adolescents suffers some level of impairment due to mental illness, fewer than half of them ever receive treatment.[3] In addition, there is concern that when children are diagnosed and treated for these disorders, they don't receive the long-term treatment they should, due to limitations imposed by health insurance companies, a lack of health insurance, or difficulty finding a qualified specialist. Another problem some families face is the high cost of some psychopharmaceuticals. A 2004 study conducted by the Pharmaceutical Research and Manufacturers Association found that prescription drugs were the "least insured of major health care services." Whereas private insurers covered more than 90 percent of hospital inpatient costs and about 70 percent of physician costs, only 60 percent of prescription drug costs was covered, leaving consumers to pay about 38 percent of these costs out of pocket.[4]

These facts seem to fly in the face of the popular perception that children today are being "overmedicated," or given psychotropic medications unnecessarily. This is not to say that children who have real, confirmed diagnoses are taking such medication "unnecessarily," although that does occur in some cases. Rather, there is evidence to suggest that one contributing factor to the rise in psychotropic medications in children is misdiagnosis. A 2000 study of five thousand children between the ages of nine and sixteen who were receiving stimulants (such as Ritalin, Dexedrine, Adderall, or Cylert) to address symptoms of ADHD discovered that only 34 percent met the diagnostic criteria for ADHD; another 9 percent were diagnosed with ADHD-NOS.[5] In other words, over half of the children in the study who were receiving stimulants for ADHD did not have the disorder for which they were being treated. On the other hand, many children who do meet the diagnostic criteria are either never diagnosed or, if diagnosed, are "undertreated," meaning they could benefit from medication but don't receive it. And then there are children who are never seen by a professional or diagnosed, whose problems are attributed to "emotional" or "behavior" issues.

Cause for concern? Certainly. However, it's equally important to bear in mind some other facts. Perhaps because it has been on the market since 1955 and is among the ten most frequently prescribed pharmaceuticals, Ritalin has become something of the stalking-horse for the antimedication faction. Critics argue that ADHD is not a "real" disorder but just "kids being kids," and point to discrepancies in the rate of ADHD diagnosis and Ritalin use along geographic, ethnic, and socioeconomic lines. And there is evidence that in some areas of the United States and among some populations, doctors may be prescribing medication for ADHD more often than is indicated. Why this may be so is difficult to establish, since so many factors determine who is diagnosed with ADHD (the qualifications and expertise of the person making the diagnosis; the ethnic, social, and educational profile of the child being diagnosed) and why medication might be prescribed. It's important to bear in mind that Ritalin is the most widely tested and safest psychotropic medication on the market today, an established fact that is often drowned out by sensationalism. And the long-term risks of untreated ADHD—substance abuse, problems with school, work, and relationships—are well documented.

Given the furor that persists around a medication with nearly five decades of safety and efficacy behind it, the controversy and confusion that surround newer, and in some cases stronger, agents isn't surprising. Reports of doctors prescribing selective serotonin reuptake inhibitors (SSRIs, which include Celexa, Luvox, Paxil, Prozac, and Zoloft) to toddlers raise a number of questions, as well they should.[6] In March 2003, the FDA issued a Public Health Advisory warning of a "possibility of suicidality associated with the use of antidepressant drug products in the pediatric population."[7] But when we question or challenge trends in psychopharmacology for our kids, we should be sure we're asking the right questions and not limit them to issues of safety and efficacy.

Many factors contribute to the rising rates of psychotropic use among our kids. Better-qualified physicians making more accurate diagnoses no doubt play a role, but ironically so do less-experienced physicians making inaccurate diagnoses. Add to this the statistical increase in diagnosed psychiatric disorders in children and adolescents, growing awareness of the dangers of untreated psychiatric disorders in children, and the relatively recent availability of pharmaceutical agents (including the SSRIs, atypical neuroleptics, such as Risperdal and Abilify, and the first nonstimulant medication approved to treat ADHD, Strattera) that target their symptoms. Clearly, there is more to the "overmedication" story than simply anxious parents and pill-pushing doctors.

Some parents and professionals (usually those who are not M.D.s) take a stronger view against medication: They simply "do not believe in" medication and may even view those who use it as taking an "easy way" out. Remember, much of what people who lack M.D.s know about psychotropic medication may be incomplete. In 2004, the Institute of Medicine reported that "nearly half of all Americans do not know how to use basic health information." The authors of the report pointed out that "health illiteracy" was common even among the most highly educated.[8] For your child's sake, and for your own, you can never have too much sound, credible information.

In our personal experience and from speaking to and hearing from hundreds of parents who have faced this decision, we know well the arguments on either side. We also know from personal experience how useless those arguments are when your child is depressed, suicidal, anxious, phobic, obsessive-compulsive, oppositional, aggressive, violent, self-injurious, hyperactive, or unable to attend or socialize to a degree that he cannot tolerate, or that you believe may ultimately be more damaging to him in the long or the short term than the possible risks of medicating. And let's be honest: Untreated comorbid conditions and behaviors like those listed above have their own "side effects," their own "risks." However, even when you make the "right" decision, you may still wonder what else you could have done to avoid facing these risks, or what the fact that your child needs medication says about you as a parent. Remember, then, that many of the behaviors, symptoms, and disorders that respond to medication arise from physical problems in the brain, namely in the neurotransmitters, the chemicals that facilitate communication between neurons. As we are learning, neurotransmitters can determine not only how we feel (in terms of mood and emotion) but what we are able to do (focus, attend, function). Medication works by chemically "normalizing" a process or reaction in the brain, either by raising or lowering the amount of neurotransmitter available—a power beyond that of parenting, therapy, and other interventions.

Debates over children and medication inevitably elicit analogies along the lines of "If your child had diabetes, you wouldn't think twice about giving her insulin." Although the comparison seems apt, it actually misses the point. After all, stabilizing blood sugar levels does not change or affect how the person on insulin thinks or feels emotionally. It might make them feel better physically, but it doesn't touch the essence of who they are. Psychotropic medication, however, is different. While we may recognize the improvements it can bring, parents are often left to wonder about immediate and long-term side effects. And by "side effects," we mean more than simply those listed on the package insert and in the *Physicians' Desk Reference.* Even when the outcome is positive, a parent may still wonder, How is this making my child feel? How is it affecting his physical, emotional, and intellectual development? Parents whose children take medication may find themselves wondering whether the medication reveals or masks who their child really is.

Finally, this is never an easy decision. Be sure that your child is seen by the best-qualified and most experienced doctor you can find. We recommend a psychiatrist or neurologist who specializes in pediatrics and, if at all possible, AS and/or other pervasive developmental disorders. Your family general practitioner or pediatrician can prescribe these medications, but you should consider consulting a specialist. In his book *Taking the Mystery Out of Medications in Autism/Asperger Syndrome,* Dr. Luke Y. Tsai, an eminent physician and researcher and the father of a child on the spectrum, writes: "I appreciate that it is often difficult for parents to find a physician who has adequate training and experience in ASD and related disorders. I wonder, however, how many parents would want a physician without adequate training and experience in cancer treatment to treat their child's leukemia or any other form of cancer. I also wonder how many family physicians and general pediatricians without [that training] would prescribe cancer medications for children with the disease."[9] This is a constantly evolving field in which a single pediatric psychiatrist may be seeing and treating more children with a particular medication than the number included in the largest study on that medication. For many children with AS who take medication, finding the right one (or ones, as it is not uncommon for two, even three to be taken simultaneously) is a process of trial and error. It is an area where professional experience is everything.

Then do your research and ask as many questions as you need to, as many times as you need to, until you're satisfied that you understand the medication your child will be taking and what you can expect. Be sure you always know and/or have written down (perhaps in your date book or on a slip of paper in your wallet) the following information:

- Correct name and spelling of each medication, both its trade name and its generic name. Be sure that you have the full name. A growing number of medications are being released in new forms. There's a big difference between Prozac and Prozac Weekly (as the name suggests, one dose lasts a full week), for instance, or Risperdal and Risperdal Consta (the latter is an injection given only once every two weeks).
- Diagnosis, condition, or specific symptom for which it is being prescribed.
- How the medication is dispensed from the pharmacy (e.g., 1 milligram tablets), a description of what it looks like ("white, oval tablet with the name JANSSEN stamped on one side") and how it is given to the child.
- Daily dosage, including the daily total (for example, 1 milligram of Risperdal) as well as the schedule of medication and how it correlates to how the medication is dispensed from the pharmacy. For example:
  .5 milligram (one half of a 1 milligram tablet) of Risperdal at bedtime
  .25 (one quarter of a 1 milligram tablet) with breakfast
  .25 (one quarter of a 1 milligram tablet) at 4:00 P.M.
- Form of medication your child is taking: tablet, capsule, liquid suspension, transdermal patch, injection.
- All possible known side effects.
- Information on how your child responds to the medication (for example, "is a little drowsy the first half hour after a dose").
- Any other medications, foods, supplements, or vitamins that are

strictly contraindicated for use with this one (consult your doctor, pharmacist, and the *Physicians' Desk Reference*).
• Any activities or situations that should be avoided.

Make copies of this information available to the school nurse, your child's other doctors and dentist, baby-sitters, any relative or friend who might care for your child in the event you are unavailable, and anyone else who may need to know (camp counselors, parents hosting a sleepover, and so on). Have copies readily available in case your child requires emergency treatment. Keep a copy in a sealed, clearly labeled envelope in your glove compartment(s), on the refrigerator, or anyplace it will be handy. Have this information with you and/or your child at all times, especially when you go away on vacation or your child is away from you.

MEDICATION AND ASPERGER SYNDROME

Categories of Medications

As you will see in this chapter, psychotropic medications are grouped under categories such as "antidepressants," "neuroleptics," and "stimulants." Many people find these confusing, because a particular medication may be prescribed to treat a range of symptoms and disorders that seem very different from those for which the medication was first created. Just remember that simply because your child's doctor prescribes an antipsychotic (also known as a neuroleptic) or an antidepressant, it does not necessarily mean that your child is psychotic or depressed. Neuroleptics have been shown effective in treating tic disorders, stuttering, OCD, and anxiety, for example, and some antidepressants also work well against OCD.

FDA Approval: What Does It Really Mean?

Many people assume that to obtain Food and Drug Administration (FDA) approval to market a medication in the United States, manufacturers must prove its safety and effectiveness in every population for every conceivable use. That is not the case. Pharmaceutical companies are required only to demonstrate a medication's effectiveness and safety when used to treat the particular condition for which it will be marketed. Once the medication is on the market, physicians may prescribe it however they see fit. FDA approval does not limit the drug's use to the condition for which it is indicated; nor does it in any way limit which conditions it may be prescribed to treat. So, for example, an SSRI that has been approved to treat depression may be prescribed to treat premenstrual syndrome (PMS). However, in order for a company to market it for that use, it would have to seek additional FDA approval based on data from studies of that medication for PMS. Most companies choose not to reinvest in further research because it is expensive and time-consuming.

How Are Medications Tested to Receive FDA Approval?

Most often the process goes something like this: A pharmaceutical company develops a promising new medication to treat a particular condition. Over the course of several years, the new drug is subjected to a series of four different types of studies, each designed to elicit different types of data on its safety and effectiveness. It is first studied and tested in the laboratory and/or in animals to establish its general safety and how it works in the body (preclinical testing), then to establish its safety in humans and to determine the maximum safe doses and schedule of administration (phase I). Next, researchers establish the medication's effectiveness and monitor side effects in phase II. The final phase, III, compares the effectiveness of the new agent against currently available and accepted treatments and monitors adverse side effects that may result from long-term use.

Many of the final-stage studies run for a relatively brief period, sometimes as short as several months. Most new medications reach the market lacking data on potential long-term effects. This is why it can be helpful to know when a medication was first approved, the indications it was approved for, how long it has been used by adults and by children, and its general safety record.

What Is "Off-Label" Use?

When a new drug receives FDA approval, the manufacturer must provide detailed information on virtually all that is known about it, including its chemical composition, dosing, results of clinical trials, side effects, and contraindications (conditions under which the drug should not be used or used with caution). Under "Indications and Usage" you will find the conditions, disorders, or diseases for which the manufacturer has established the drug's efficacy and safety. In the case of Risperdal, for example, it is "management of the manifestations of psychotic disorders." Any other use, such as to manage repetitive, aggressive, or violent behavior—for which it is commonly prescribed for persons with ASDs—is technically off-label (as of late 2004).

Using drugs off-label is not illegal, nor is it uncommon. As a drug becomes widely used among the general population, physicians and researchers sometimes notice unexpected therapeutic side effects. Some drugs developed and marketed to treat purely physical conditions turn out to have psychoactive properties; for example, Tenex (guanfacine), a drug indicated for high blood pressure, is now used to treat tics and Tourette's syndrome, as well as aggression, hyperactivity, sleep problems, and agitation. Abilify (aripiprazole), approved for adults with schizophrenia, has been found effective in children with bipolar disorder. Psychotropic medications may also be found effective in treating a wider range of symptoms than originally intended. Zoloft (sertraline), a drug originally indicated solely for depression when first approved in 1991, has since been approved for obsessive-compulsive disorder in adults (1997) and in children six and up (1998), and for posttraumatic stress disorder (1999).

FDA Approval for Pediatric Use: Why Is It So Rare?

For a drug to be approved for use in children, it must be studied in children. A placebo double-blind study—one in which half of the participants receive the medication and half receive a placebo, or sugar pill, and not even those conducting the trial know who receives which until the end—is considered the platinum standard in clinical trials. However, few are conducted on children, for several reasons. Parents' reluctance to expose their child to any medication without cause, and their unwillingness to risk getting only the placebo when their child might benefit from the medication play a role. Legally, patients enrolled in studies must give their informed consent, and some doctors and medical ethicists question if and at what age children can be considered capable of giving such consent. Finally, the number of children with AS or ASDs is relatively small, and not all who share a specific diagnosis share the same symptoms. The frequent presence of comorbid disorders may complicate attempts to discern the effectiveness of a given treatment on a given symptom.

Testing psychotropic medications on children raises many of the same questions about short- and long-term side effects parents face when considering these treatments. Understandably, pediatric volunteers for a premarketing study are rare. The result is, as Dr. Dianne Murphy, associate director of the FDA's Center for Drug Evaluation and Research, told the *New York Times,* "up to 81 percent of all products used on children have not been studied or labeled for infants and children. We're treating our children without studying the medicine to the degree that we require these drugs to be studied in and understood in adults. The laws to mandate that we study drugs were often based on terrible accidents with children. And yet children have not been studied because people wanted to protect them from experimentation. Ironically, that has led to decades-long experimentation on our children."[10] Introduced in late 2002, Strattera (atomoxetine) was one of the first psychopharmaceuticals for which children as young as six were included in the preapproval randomized, double-blind, placebo-controlled studies. Beginning in December 2000, the FDA required that any new drug that might be used by children undergo pediatric study and that manufacturers provide information on correct doses for children. In addition, under certain circumstances the FDA can require pediatric studies on a drug that has already been approved.

As the off-label use of psychotropic medications increased, officials at the National Institute of Mental Health created a model for testing medications that were already in use by children but for which there was insufficient data in safety and efficacy. The resulting Research Units on Pediatric Pharmacology (RUPP) have begun conducting clinical trials in several cities. Because of its wide off-label use in children with AS and other PDDs, Risperdal was among the first medications studied under this program.

So What Does Your Doctor Know?

When it comes to newer psychotropic medication and children, your doctor probably will be relying on findings of the preapproval studies (available in the written patient information that should come with your prescription, *The Physicians' Desk Reference (PDR),*

Web sites such as those listed on page 277, the drug manufacturer's Web site, a collection of small studies, the consensus of colleagues, and his or her own experience. Conscientious physicians stay abreast of the latest research, which for many of the psychotropics prescribed for children consists largely of studies that may be smaller and less rigorous than those required for initial FDA approval, as well as professional journal articles and letters describing case histories of children and the results of particular treatments. Although it can be argued that this type of data is not as compelling or as "scientific" as larger, more controlled studies, for some agents, this may represent the sum total of current research. This is why we cannot stress enough how important it is that your child's medication be in the hands of a pediatric specialist who has experience prescribing for children with AS or other forms of ASDs.

What Every Parent Should Know

Every medication, psychotropic or not, presents risks as well as benefits. FDA approval is based not on a "guarantee" of safety, only on the fact that the benefits of using a particular drug outweigh its known and most common risks. No one—not even the most experienced expert in pediatric psychopharmacology—can predict how your child will respond to a given medication. Generally speaking (although there may be exceptions depending on the severity of your child's symptoms), your child's doctor will opt for what is known as the "first-line" treatment, the medication that has the highest probability of being effective with the lowest level of known risk. Unfortunately, the first-line treatment isn't always the one that works for your child.

Dr. Temple Grandin, a woman with autism known for her books *Emergence: Labeled Autistic* and *Thinking in Pictures,* has written on the subject of medications and autism. She has observed, as have many parents and doctors, that some medications are more effective for persons with ASDs when given in smaller doses than those typically recommended. Of course, there are always individual exceptions, and because of differences in metabolism, some medications are prescribed for children in doses that are equal to or even higher than those for adults. With most medications, however, it is wisest to start low and build slowly, increasing the dose only after you have established that your child is tolerating it well.

Before you leave the doctor's office, be sure you have in writing (written by you or the doctor) two sets of instructions: how to start the medication and how to stop it, if necessary.

—◆◆◆—

The "Things to Know" List for Starting a Medication

- What the prescription itself is for. It should be sufficiently clear and legible so that you can read and understand it. If it's not, ask your doctor to please rewrite it. A surprising number of medications have similar-looking and -sounding names, and mistakes do happen.
- The names, both brand and generic, of the medication.
- If your doctor thinks a generic, if available, is acceptable. According to Dr. Luke Tsai, some doctors are reluctant to prescribe generic versions because of concerns about quality and dose. Consistency and reliability of a medication may be essential for some children, depending on the drug and its purpose. In fact, generics are not always simply cheaper versions of the same drug marketed under its trade name. Dr. Tsai notes that the FDA does not recognize every generic "as equivalent to its brand-name counterpart." You can find out if the generic your doctor prescribes or your insurance company insists you accept is truly equivalent by checking the FDA's so-called orange book, which is available online at the FDA's Web site.
- What the medication looks like. Ask your doctor to show you its picture in the *Physicians' Desk Reference* or on the manufacturer's Web site.[11]
- What form the medication will come in (pill, tablet, suspension, transdermal patch, etc.).
- The dose as will be dispensed by the pharmacy (important because your child's actual dose may be a half or less of a pill or tablet).
- The dose as it will be given to the child.
- The dosing schedule.
- The schedule for gradually increasing the dosage up to a target level (called *titration*).
- Anything you need to know about how the medication should be

taken: With meals or on an empty stomach? Can it be crushed and mixed into food or juice? Are there any foods or drinks that the medication should or should not be taken with? Can the pill be crushed or broken? (Some time-release medications, such as Concerta, can be ineffective if not swallowed whole. As one doctor put it, it's like "chopping a radio in half and expecting each half to work." Others, like Strattera, can cause mucosal irritation if taken broken or crushed.)

- What to do if you miss a dose.
- Any types or classes of medications—including over-the-counter medicines, herbal remedies, homeopathic remedies, vitamins, nutritional supplements, and so on—your child should avoid. Many "natural" substances react with medication, either reducing or amplifying its effect. Be sure your doctor is aware of everything your child takes, and be sure you check with your doctor before you give your child anything new, even if it sounds "safe" and "natural." Bear in mind that even seemingly "unrelated" medications can have an impact on your child. In 2002 the FDA Center for Drug Evaluation and Research (CDER) issued a warning on the popular antiacne medication Accutane, citing possible drug-related risk of neurological symptoms, depression, and suicidal ideation, attempts, and completions.[12]
- Any activities that should be avoided or that require extra caution.
- Date of your next appointment with the doctor.
- Procedure for refills (some can be called in to your pharmacy, but prescriptions for controlled substances—which include Ritalin, Concerta, and some other frequently prescribed stimulants—require the submission of a three-part prescription form that must be delivered to the pharmacy). This is especially important if you plan to purchase the prescription through an online pharmacy in the United States.[13] You may have to allow a few extra days for processing the paperwork.
- Side effects that warrant a phone call to your doctor.
- Side effects that warrant an appointment with your doctor.
- Side effects that warrant emergency treatment, including signs of overdose.
- Side effects that would necessitate stopping the medication.

KEEPING GOOD MEDICATION RECORDS

Ideally, your doctor should provide, or you can create, a form for charting your child's response. It's very easy to lose track of when a dose was increased or when a response first appeared. This information is important for you and for your doctor in making informed decisions. A sample form appears on pages 250–51.

Keep a daily log for each medication, or combination of medications, that your child takes. Communicate with the prescribing doctor. Some side effects weaken or disappear over time. The potential benefit of a medication may warrant giving the body extra time to adjust before stopping. Supplement this with a long-term summary that provides your child's entire medication history, including:

- the medication taken
- the date your child began taking it
- the dose and how it was given throughout the day
- the date your child stopped taking the medication
- general response
- side effects
- why the medication was stopped

— • • • —

The "Things to Know" List for Stopping a Medication

- Circumstances under which you might have to consider stopping this medication.
- Side effects that warrant a phone call to the doctor.
- Side effects that warrant an appointment with the doctor.
- Side effects that warrant emergency treatment, including signs of overdose.
- Whether this medication should be stopped suddenly or be slowly tapered.

- If it should be tapered, exactly what the doses, over the course of how many days, would be.
- What to expect once the medication is tapered or stopped.

MEDICATION AT HOME

All psychotropic medications can be dangerous, even lethal, if misused or taken by anyone other than the person for whom they were prescribed. They should be handled with caution at all times, from the moment you pick them up at the pharmacy.

• Try to fill all of your child's prescriptions—for everything, including antibiotics—at a single pharmacy that keeps good computerized records and has a knowledgeable pharmacist you feel comfortable talking to. Be sure that your child's prescription history is reviewed and considered when *any* prescription is filled, so that the pharmacist will be on the lookout for possible drug interactions. In addition to consulting your child's physician, also talk to your pharmacist before using any over-the-counter medicine.

• Before leaving the pharmacy, read the label and make sure it's correct (your child's name, prescribing physician, medication, dosage). In the presence of the pharmacist or other employee, open the container and make sure that the medication is in the form, size, and color you expect. Pharmacies do make mistakes, and once you open a container outside the pharmacy, they have no obligation to take it back or issue a refund.

• Keep all medicines in their original, child-resistant containers, in a safe, secure place, out of reach of all children, including the child for whom it is prescribed. Consider keeping your medication in a locked box.

• Have a daily routine for dispensing medication and stick to it. As much as possible, try to link taking the medication with an event that occurs every single day at about the same time. Bedtime is usually an easy one, but parents sometimes fall off schedule with weekend morning doses or afternoon doses that were given by the school nurse. At least for the first several weeks—and beyond, if you need

Medication Log Form
Name of medication:_____

DATE	DOSE, TIME	GENERAL RESPONSE	SIDE EFFECTS	ACTION	DOCTOR	NOTES

Here is a sample of what a Medication Log Form might look like for a child just starting Klonopin.

Name of medication: *Klonopin*

DATE	DOSE, TIME	GENERAL RESPONSE	SIDE EFFECTS	ACTION	DOCTOR	NOTES
3/21	.25 mg 7 AM .5 mg 8 PM	no change fell asleep ½ hr earlier	teacher: passing drowsiness, gone by 10	lay down for 15 min. in nurse's office		
3/22	same	less anxious about swimming lesson	teacher: less anxious during fire drill			
3/23	same		seemed tired after school			
3/24	same		seemed tired after school		called; watch for a week, after-school tiredness should pass; if not, call	
3/25	same					
3/26	same					more energy after school, back to normal
			B R E A K			
4/8	.5 mg 7 AM .5 mg 8 PM	good, no drowsiness	teacher: more willing to try new things			seems to crave more snacks

it—keep a chart on the refrigerator or someplace else convenient and mark off each dose as it is given.

• If your child is taking pills that have to be cut, ask your pharmacist to do it for you. If you do it yourself, do an entire prescription all at once. Pill cutters are handy, but they don't work for pills with unusual shapes. Try using an X-Acto artist's knife, and change the blade often, after every twenty cuts or so. Try cutting on a gel-type plastic cutting board. If your child is taking half a pill in the morning and a quarter at night, ask the pharmacist for extra bottles with child-resistant caps. Clearly label one bottle, for example, "Klonopin, .5 mg, morning" and the other, "Klonopin, .25 mg, night." Always keep the medicine in the same safe place.

• Always check with anyone else in the household who has access to the medication before giving it to your child. In the bustle of daily family life, it sometimes happens that one parent gives a dose and forgets to tell the other, who then repeats it. This can be extremely dangerous. Asking your child may not always help. One solution might be to put one adult in charge of the medication. Another solution is to say, "Whoever reads the bedtime story does the medication," or "Whoever makes the coffee in the morning gives Joey his pill." Whatever you do, find something that works and stick with it.

• Have a backup plan in case you forget a dose. First find out how to handle the missed dose. That information is usually available on the printed patient information sheet that comes with the medication. If unsure, ask your pharmacist or your doctor. In a safe, clearly labeled, child-resistant bottle, stash a couple of doses and put it in the glove compartment of every car and perhaps one in your purse. If the child is a frequent visitor at Grandma's or Uncle Jeff's, consider keeping a dose or two there as well, just in case.

• When you travel, be sure to keep all essential medications with you, in your handbag or another carry-on. *Never* pack medication in your checked luggage.

• Be sure anyone who might be giving your child his medication (baby-sitters, etc.) knows exactly what to do, is aware of possible side effects, and has access to your child's prescribing physician's phone number.

• Be sure that you are familiar with the signs of overdose or serious side effects.

• Keep your local poison control telephone number along with the name of the medication(s) posted prominently.

WHEN CAN A CHILD BE RESPONSIBLE FOR HIS OWN MEDICATION?

The older child or young adult on medication presents a real dilemma. If you assume that she is on medication because she needs it, then you understand how important it is for her to take it. But does she? As more of our children grow up and even leave home, we must find some way to teach them to responsibly manage their own medication.

Our first suggestion is to consult your doctor, who has certainly confronted this problem before. Much will depend on your child, the type of medication he is taking (for example, its potential for overdose, abuse, or serious side effects from missed doses or sudden withdrawal), and the amount of supervision he will have. (For example, if away at college, is there a trusted dorm mate or counselor who can check up on him, if needed?) If you decide to grant this responsibility in the reasonably near future, let your child start practicing while still under your roof. He should understand the medication he is taking and why, as well as have access to current versions of the charts and checklists on pages 240, 246, and 248.

MEDICATION AT SCHOOL

Parents have different views on how much of their child's personal and medical history they are comfortable sharing with his school. You may have concerns about your child being stigmatized because he takes medication or to what degree the school personnel with access to that information will honor the confidentiality that all medical information deserves.

For the sake of your child's safety, it is wise to give the school information about the type and dose of medication your child is currently taking along with his emergency contact information, at the very least. (And be sure to update this if anything changes.) In the course of receiving emergency medical treatment, your child might be exposed to other medications that could produce dangerous, even lethal complications. Anyone treating your child for any reason needs to know about any medication she takes regularly, *especially* psychotropics. Depending on the medication, you should probably alert your child's teacher and the school nurse about possible side effects and what to do if they develop. This is an especially important consideration if your child is beginning a trial of a new medication, no matter how good its general safety record.

There are other reasons to let your child's teacher and school nurse know about the medication. They are in a position to observe how your child is responding and also to make accommodations for him if necessary; for example, excusing him from gymnastics if his coordination is a little off or from a test if he's experiencing drowsiness. Many children behave differently at home than they do at school. A medication that seems to be reducing your child's anxiety at home may be making him a nervous wreck in school. These are things that you need to know. Ask your child's teacher for a brief daily report, especially when you are trying a new medication, dose, or schedule.

Some parents are attracted to the idea of turning their child's medication trial into a "scientific" experiment. They believe they'll get a more accurate "reading" on how the medication is working if they don't tell anyone at school about it. This is a really bad idea. First, your child's medication trial is not a research project. It's an attempt to find a solution to a serious problem that is not without risk. Everyone needs to be on the same page. When you opt to leave school personnel out of the loop, you remove not only an important source of information you need but a critical safety net. For example, some of the most serious side effects first appear in what seem innocuous developments: drowsiness, rashes or hives, or changes in behavior. According to Dr. Luke Tsai, "When young children take psychotherapeutic medication, behavioral toxicity often appears before any other side effect. . . . The early emergence of behavioral side effects is a warning sign."[14] The problem with school personnel not knowing to look for behavioral signs is that children on the spectrum often have mood swings and behavioral changes as a matter of course. A careful eye is needed to note what may be a warning sign.

When teachers do not know that a child's behavior may be medication-related, they may make assumptions and possibly even changes in curricular demands, behavior management, and discipline that may not be appropriate. One teacher we spoke with told us of a student whose suddenly volatile, violent, and self-injurious behavior prompted a total suspension of all academic demands and extended periods in the school psychologist's office. Looking back, she said, "If we had known what to expect and why, we could have handled it so much better. The poor kid—he was so confused and frightened by his own behavior, and the more we applied the tried-and-true strategies that usually worked, the worse he responded. By the time the parents finally told us what was really happening, two weeks later, this student was so averse to school, and embarrassed by his behavior, that they couldn't get him on the bus. Although I'd never tell the parents this, we held meetings with the principal and special education director and did consider contacting child protective services, because he was so bruised up, and recommending evaluation for placement in a more restrictive environment." As Dr. James Snyder, a pediatric psychiatrist, points out, telling teachers may help them to see your son or daughter as "a child with a problem, not a 'problem child.'"

If your child will be taking medication at school, find out what the procedure is. Usually the school nurse will require a letter from you and/or the prescribing physician that states the name of your child, the name of the medication, and instructions on doses (how much and when). State and local board of education regulations will dictate how medication is handled in your school. School policies differ regarding how large a supply the school nurse will keep on hand, who may deliver it to the school, and so on. Follow this procedure:

- Provide the medication in a clearly labeled, child-resistant bottle with your child's name, teacher's name, and doctor's name and number, as well as the name of the medication, the dose, and the form. For example, "Klonopin, .5 mg. (a half pill), after lunch."
- Provide a copy of any product information literature you receive.
- If you are required to send in a week's supply every Monday, for example, be sure your child's teacher is expecting it and that it does not fall into other children's hands en route to the nurse.
- If your child is able to open a child safety cap and/or the medication is one that might be abused by your child or others, you might consider delivering it yourself personally to the school. In some places, this is required by law.

• If it's school policy to send home empty bottles for refill, you might consider demanding (backed up by a letter) that any extra doses (due to holidays, sick days) either be kept in the office for you to pick up at a later time or disposed of so that your child's bottle comes home empty.

TELLING YOUR CHILD ABOUT MEDICATION

This is a complex, sensitive area for many parents and children. Considering the increase in children taking psychotropics, there has been surprisingly little written about it. When, how, and how much you tell your child will depend on many factors: your child's age, her level of understanding of AS and her behavior, the type of medication she'll be taking, and the circumstances under which she'll be taking it. Every situation is different, and you may wish to discuss how to proceed with your child's prescribing doctor, who, we hope, will have seen many other families through this dilemma.

Through it all, it's important to discuss this issue in a way that your child will understand. This may be easier if you and your child have already discussed his problems, whether or not you have told him about his actual diagnosis. However, simply because you have never talked to your child about some of his behaviors or told him that he has AS, don't feel pressured to do it right now. Depending on your child's age and level of understanding, it may suffice to say "I know you've been feeling very anxious lately; Dr. Townsend and I believe that this medicine might help with that."

If you are considering medication, chances are it's because your child is experiencing difficulty. In addition to the problems related to AS, your child may be experiencing embarrassment, guilt, or shame over his feelings or behavior. It's not unusual for a child who has been acting out, having trouble relating to peers, or failing in school to feel "stupid," "dumb," "bad," or worse. The idea that faulty brain chemistry beyond our conscious control is at the root of many problems can be reassuring to parents and perhaps even older adolescents ("It's not your fault; your brain works differently"). Younger children, however, may find that prospect more frightening.

Then there is the simple fact that your child will be taking medicine, and all but the very young realize that this is what you do when you are "sick" or "something is wrong." By this point, most children strongly suspect or know they are different, and different in ways that others find unacceptable. In a brief paper published in the *Journal of the American Academy of Child and Adolescent Psychiatry,* Drs. Nancy Rappaport and Peter Chubinsky write: "Even if the clinician has reassured the parents, children are also often apprehensive about taking medication and commonly believe that this is final proof that they are defective. Although they may not initially express these thoughts, many children will at some point call themselves 'crazy,' 'bad,' or 'stupid' as an explanation for why they are taking medication. Others may fear that they are brain-damaged. . . . Some children will obstinately reject medication rather than tolerate the daily reminder of their perceived defect."[15]

On the other hand, some children do see and feel the difference the right medication makes. Given the right cues by parents, doctors, and teachers, children can adapt to their need for medication without it adversely coloring their self-image. Sometimes the results of medication are so apparent to the child that the medication "sells itself."

So what do you say? First, it would be imprudent to present medication as something "that will make you feel better," "make schoolwork easier to handle," or "make you happier." The truth is, if this isn't the right medication for your child, she probably won't feel better. Making a promise that you cannot keep will only damage your child's trust in you and lay the groundwork for resistance to future medication trials.

There is also the issue of sending the right message about psychotropic medications and their legitimate uses. Parents are understandably concerned over the possible link between legitimate psychotropic medication use and the use and abuse of street drugs. However, we now know that treatment of psychiatric disorders may actually serve as a preventative. According to Dr. Timothy E. Wilens, author of the one book every parent considering medication should read, *Straight Talk About Psychiatric Medications for Kids,* "Up to three quarters of children or adolescents with a substance abuse problem may have a psychiatric disturbance in addition. The psychiatric conditions most often seen with substance problems in children are conduct disorder, ADHD, oppositional defiant disorder, depression, bipolar disorder, and to a lesser extent anxiety and panic disorders. In many cases, the psychiatric problem precedes the substance problem, leading to conjecture that many children 'self-medicate' their symptoms by using substances. In addition, children with psychiatric problems may not have the foresight or inhibition it takes to resist getting involved with alcohol or drugs."[16]

Older children and adolescents with Asperger Syndrome who have trouble being accepted by peers are known to be more susceptible to peer pressure while being less able to anticipate consequences. Sadly, this can make them attractive to peers who encourage behavior that is dangerous or illegal, such as street drug use.

WHEN MEDICATION WORKS

While no medication can cure Asperger Syndrome or address more than a few target symptoms, when the right medication attacks an especially troubling behavior, it can feel to parents like a miracle. Of course, medication alone is never the answer. Behavioral changes (yours and your child's), environmental accommodations, and other interventions all belong in the program. However, there is no denying that for a child who is anxious, depressed, self-injurious, suicidal, aggressive, violent, or explosive, simply taking the edge off can give him the space he needs to respond to everything else you do, to reclaim some self-esteem, and to focus on other things, such as school, play, and interests. It is unfortunate that so much of the discussion about children and psychotropic medication centers on "behavior management," because it shifts the focus from where it rightfully belongs: on what medication can do for your child. It is not and never should be about what medication will do for you, your family, or your child's teacher.

Adults and older adolescents with Asperger Syndrome may suffer terribly from the experience of a childhood filled with confusion, misunderstanding, and rejection. No medication is a "miracle drug," but for those children for whom responsibly prescribed medication has made a real difference in their quality of life, their self-esteem, and their happiness, its place as a treatment cannot be dismissed as an "easy way out." For some, whose symptoms are severe or disabling, medication may be the only way out. If you are a friend, family member, teacher, or anyone else who knows a child who is on medication, be understanding and supportive. Respect the difficulties such children and their families face, assume that you do not know all there is to know about the case, and think carefully before offering opinions or passing along anecdotes about someone else's medication horror story or some amazing "natural" alternative. Decisions about medication are difficult and personal. If honest, many parents will admit that they find unsolicited information and advice in this area intrusive, stressful, and awkward to handle. After enduring yet another uninformed, annoying antimedication diatribe from a friend, Patty found herself pondering the most polite way to say "Please just stop talking." Don't be that friend.

WHEN MEDICATION DOES NOT WORK

A medication that isn't right for your child usually reveals itself early in the trial, in intolerable side effects and/or a lack of efficacy. For reasons no one fully understands, some medications simply do not work for some people. It is important to bear in mind that just because a medication to treat, say, OCD fails, that does *not* mean that your child does not have OCD (or whatever condition or symptom the medication was prescribed to address).

Unfortunately, finding the right medication doesn't get you or your child home free yet. Depending on the medication your child is taking, several things could occur. He might become tolerant of the medication, requiring a higher dose, which may not be as effective or may produce other unwanted side effects. Side effects might arise months or even years after the medication was begun, necessitating a change. It is also possible that another comorbid condition could develop (such as a mood disorder, anxiety, and so on), which could make your child's current medication less effective. He may outgrow the need for one type of medication but have trouble finding a suitable medication to address new symptoms. (Conversely, sometime in the future, he may be able to tolerate and see good results from a medication he could not tolerate before.) Finally, the medication your child is on may one day simply stop working for him.

For these reasons, you and your child's prescribing doctor should always be thinking one step ahead. You should be considering not only other medications and interventions but the possibility that a particular medication is no longer necessary. Many experts suggest that periodically your child take a "medication holiday," so that you and his doctor can assess where he is developmentally and emotionally. This may not be appropriate for all children, and there are health and safety considerations to bear in mind when lowering or stopping any psychoactive medication. For instance, some studies have found that stopping a medication (such as lithium for bipolar disorder) abruptly may actually worsen the overall prognosis over the lifespan.

Always consult your doctor before attempting to reduce or eliminate a medication!

PSYCHOTROPIC MEDICATIONS

It is beyond our scope to provide everything you need to know about specific psychotropic medications. Be sure to consult the *Physicians' Desk Reference* or an equally reliable source before filling any prescription. In addition, the Medline Plus, Food and Drug Adminstration (FDA), and Mayo Clinic Web sites offer sound, in-depth information on prescription medications, including possible side effects. The FDA site also offers information on over-the-counter medications, supplements, and vitamins. The home page offers you the option of receiving the FDA's special alerts and warnings via e-mail. See "Recommended Resources," on page 277.

Regard any information from personal Web sites or those whose sponsoring agencies or organizations you do not know, online message boards, and chat rooms with caution. Although they can be good sources of general information on the experience of having children who use psychotropic medications, specific information on the medications themselves—including dosage, schedule, side effects, and so on—should never be used to make decisions for your child. *Never* make any change in your child's medication regimen without first consulting your doctor.

An emerging trend is toward prescribing more than one psychoactive medication at a time (known as polypharmacy). Often this involves using medications from different classes; for example, a neuroleptic such as Risperdal in combination with a stimulant such as

Ritalin. Other times, your child's doctor may prescribe two medications from the same class. Because many children have more than one disorder (comorbidity), they may require polypharmacy. Sometimes a second medication may be added to offset a troubling side effect in an otherwise "perfect" or very necessary first medication. In addition, some medications work better in combination, which is known as an additive effect. For example, a 2004 open-label (patients and researchers knew who was getting what) study demonstrated that approximately half of adults who had been unable to tolerate taking an SSRI were able to continue and see positive effect with the addition of the atypical neuroleptic Geodon (ziprasidone).

The following are descriptions of the types of medications most often prescribed to treat symptoms of Asperger Syndrome, high-functioning autism, and pervasive developmental disorders not otherwise specified. This is a general, basic guide. Your doctor may suggest other medications or use them to address symptoms different from those we list here.

Antidepressants

Although antidepressants are indicated for treating adults with depression, they have not been consistently effective in addressing depression in children. However, they have been found to be helpful for compulsive behavior, repetitive behavior, panic disorders, insomnia, anxiety, and other symptoms commonly seen in persons with Asperger Syndrome. Not every medication addresses every symptom.

Selective Serotonin Reuptake Inhibitors (SSRIs) (See box on page 264 for important information on this type of medication.)

BRAND NAME	GENERIC NAME
Celexa	citalopram
Lexapro	escitalopram oxalate
Luvox	fluvoxamine
Paxil	paroxetine
Paxil CR	paroxetine (controlled release)
Prozac	fluoxetine
Prozac Weekly	fluoxetine
Zoloft	sertraline

SSRIs are by far the most frequently prescribed class of medication for persons with PDDs. A survey of prescription patterns in the United States found that the use of Paxil (paroxetine) had increased by more than 113 percent in girls and by 90 percent among boys from 1998 to 2000.[17] Known as novel or atypical antidepressants, these medications work by increasing the amount of the neurotransmitter serotonin available to transmit impulses between cells. Although each SSRI works essentially the same way, there are differences in how they achieve that effect. This is why someone who cannot tolerate one SSRI may find a good match in another. Some individuals who could not take a regular SSRI may have success with one of the newer time-released or release-control forms (for instance, Paxil CR and Prozac Weekly). Because they have relatively few and minor side effects and pose no apparent risk of addiction or abuse, SSRIs are first-line treatments for depression, obsessive-compulsive disorder, and elective mutism (a rare condition in which a person does not speak, or does so under specific limited circumstances). Zoloft, Prozac, and Luvox are approved for use in children ages six and up (Zoloft), seven and up (Prozac), and eight and up (Luvox) for OCD. Prozac is also approved to treat depression in children seven and up. Since SSRIs first arrived on the scene in the late 1980s, doctors have put them to a number of "off-label" uses: for anxiety, eating disorders, panic disorder, repetitive behavior, post-traumatic stress disorder, and separation anxiety.

Unlike other antidepressants, SSRIs don't go to work immediately but instead build up to a therapeutic level in the body over the course of days or weeks. The different medications also differ in how quickly they are completely metabolized. While Prozac can remain in the body for as long as two months after the last dose, Zoloft, Paxil, and Luvox can clear the system in a day or less. For this reason, Prozac is rarely the first SSRI a doctor will prescribe for a child. (And you should consider a second opinion if your doctor suggests starting off with Prozac Weekly, which is taken once every seven days.) The most common side effects tend to be mild and may disappear over time: gastrointestinal upset, agitation, headaches, and difficulties with sleep.

One side effect that you should know about is what parents describe as agitation or disinhibition. It seems that SSRIs can induce mania in persons with unrecognized bipolar disorder. We have also come across dozens of anecdotes from parents whose children simply became "wild" on SSRIs and disinhibited, suddenly engaging in reckless, dangerous behavior or becoming uncharacteristically aggressive, even violent. This is different from the mild agitation that is a typical side effect of SSRIs and that usually decreases over time. At the first sign of possible trouble, contact your doctor. Another serious, potentially fatal side effect is serotonin syndrome. This results from either taking too much of an SSRI or from taking other medications that amplify, or potentiate, the effects of the SSRI. Headaches, confusion, sweating, diarrhea, and generally feeling agitated or nervous are all signs of serotonin syndrome and should prompt you to contact your child's physician and seek medical treatment immediately.

Atypical Antidepressants (See box on page 264 for important information about this type of medication.)

BRAND NAME	GENERIC NAME
Desyrel	trazodone
Effexor	venlafaxine
Effexor XR	venlafaxine (extended release)
Remeron	mirtazapine
Serzone	nefazodone
Wellbutrin	bupropion
Wellbutrin SR	bupropion (sustained release)

The so-called atypical antidepressants work differently from either SSRIs or tricyclics, and they also differ from one another in their uses and side effects. None require monitoring through blood tests or EKG.

Desyrel (trazodone) and Serzone (nefazodone) are used off-label for sleep problems, panic disorder, anxiety, depression, and other behaviors. They are both short-acting and may produce agitation, dry mouth, constipation, and sedation; confusion may be seen with high doses. Desyrel should be used with caution, if at all, in boys and men, since it can cause priapism (sustained, painful erection).

Early reports on Effexor (venlafaxine) indicate that it may be helpful in improving repetitive behavior, inattention, hyperactivity, restricted interests, and social deficits in persons with ASDs.[18] In addition, it is indicated for depression and anxiety. Side effects include nausea, headaches, stomachache, and agitation. Blood pressure may become elevated at higher doses. Although Effexor, like the SSRIs, affects serotonin, it may be effective for people who could not tolerate the more typical SSRIs.

Remeron (mirtazapine) is indicated for major depression but has found use off-label for a wide range of symptoms, including anxiety, sleep disorders, and panic disorder. Sedation and upset stomach are common side effects.

Wellbutrin (bupropion) is indicated for depression, but is used off-label for ADHD and other disorders. It may be helpful for children with mood swings and those "in whom there are concerns about mania or behavioral activation with a medication." Wellbutrin is short-acting and has a few potentially serious side effects: It may worsen tics and at higher doses may increase the risk of seizure (though this is very rare and is less likely to occur with extended-release preparations or lower doses).

• • •

Depression and Suicide Risk Related to Atypical Antidepressants and SSRIs

This information concerns the following medications:

Brand Name	Generic Name
Celexa	citalopram
Effexor, Effexor SR	venlafaxine
Lexapro	escitalopram
Luvox	fluvoxamine
Paxil, Paxil CR	paroxetine
Prozac, Prozac Weekly	fluoxetine
Remeron	mirtazapine
Serzone	nefazodone
Wellbutrin, Wellbutrin SR	bupropion
Zoloft	sertraline

In March 2004, the U.S. Food and Drug Administration issued a public health advisory in the wake of reports suggesting an increased rate of "suicidal thoughts and actions" in children taking these antidepressants. The FDA advised that manufacturers of the medications listed above revise their product information labeling to include a statement that "recommends close observation of adult and pediatric patients treated with [the manufacturers'] agents for worsening depression or the emergence of suicidality."[19] According to the FDA's "Talk Paper" on the subject, persons taking these medicines "should be observed for certain behaviors that are known to be associated with these drugs, such as anxiety, agitation, panic attacks, insomnia, irritability, hostility, impulsivity, akathisia (severe restlessness), hypomania, and mania, and that physicians be particularly vigilant in patients who may have bipolar disorder."[20] According to the *San Francisco Chronicle*, "The FDA estimates that nearly 11 million antidepressant prescriptions were written for children in 2002, 2.7 million of them for children under twelve."[21] While the FDA was careful to note that "it is unclear whether antidepressants contribute to the emergence of suicidal thoughts and behavior, these interim actions are intended to draw more attention to the need for careful monitoring of patients being treated with these drugs, especially at the beginning of therapy and during dose changes."[22] Some critics of the FDA believe that these recommendations and warnings do not go far enough. At the same time, some doctors who treat this population fear a future increase in suicide among children who could have been safely treated with SSRIs but were not. Parents of children taking these medications should watch for new developments (ideally, log on to the FDA's Web site and sign up for e-mail alerts). *Do not discontinue or change your child's medication without consulting his or her consulting physician.*

Tricyclic Antidepressants

BRAND NAME	GENERIC NAME
Anafranil	clomipramine
Elavil	amitriptyline
Endep	amitriptyline
Etrafon	perphenazine + amitriptyline
Ludiomil	maprotiline
Norpramin	desipramine
Pamelor	nortriptyline
Sinequan	doxepin

BRAND NAME	GENERIC NAME
Tofranil	imipramine
Triavil	perphenazine + amitriptyline
Vivactil	protriptyline

Tricyclic antidepressants are the medications from which the SSRIs stole the market for treating depression and OCD in adults. Interestingly, tricyclics were never widely used to treat depression in children because they were largely ineffective. However, medications from this class have been found effective in treating symptoms of Tourette's syndrome, tic disorder, ADHD, eating disorders, panic disorder, enuresis (bed-wetting), anxiety disorder, and, to a limited extent, depression. Anafranil (clomipramine) is approved for treatment of obsessive-compulsive disorder. Elavil and Endep (both amitriptyline), Pamelor (nortriptyline), Norpramin (desipramine), Tofranil (imipramine), and Vivactil (protriptyline) are all approved for use in children ages twelve and up for depression. Tofranil is approved to treat enuresis from age six and up and has been so prescribed since 1973.

Tricyclics are more complicated to use than SSRIs, because patients must be monitored for possible heart problems and other side effects, through electrocardiogram (EKG) and blood tests. Typical side effects include dry mouth, headaches, sedation, stomachache, blurred vision, rash, constipation, vivid dreams, and nightmares. Serious side effects include neuroleptic malignant syndrome and tardive dyskinesia (see page 270). Like SSRIs, they can also provoke a manic episode in those predisposed to bipolar disorder and also cause weight gain. Of most concern, however, is the risk of lethal overdose.

Monoamine Oxidase Inhibitors (MAOIs)

BRAND NAME	GENERIC NAME
Nardil	phenelzine
Parnate	tranylcypromine

Monoamine oxidase inhibitors (MAOIs) have been around for more than fifty years. Although these antidepressants are often effective in treating depression, anxiety, ADHD, and panic disorders, they are rarely prescribed for children and adolescents. None is approved for use in children under the age of sixteen, and they are generally reserved to treat depression that doesn't yield to other types of medication. Their main drawback is their ability to interact with a wide range of foods and medications. You may have noticed the numerous warnings about MAO inhibitors on just about every OTC and prescription label you read. That's because MAOI interactions can have serious, even lethal consequences, including liver failure and dangerously high blood pressure.

The list of foods those on MAOIs must avoid includes such kid staples as chocolate, some types of cheese, and foods containing tyramine, such as bologna, salami, bananas, and raisins, among many others. The danger of mixing alcohol or illicit drugs makes MAOIs potentially hazardous for adolescents. The inability to use MAOIs with most other psychotropic medications may mean that other symptoms go untreated. In addition, the prohibition against certain foods and psychotropic substances (including anesthesia) may persist for weeks or months after the MAOI is stopped.

Stimulants

BRAND NAME	GENERIC NAME
Adderall XR	amphetamine + dextroamphetamine (extended release)
Biphetamine	amphetamine + dextroamphetamine
Concerta	methylphenidate
Cylert	pemoline
Desoxyn	methamphetamine
Dextrostat	dextroamphetamine
Dexedrine	dextroamphetamine
Metadate ER	methylphenidate (extended release)
Ritalin	methylphenidate

Of all the psychotropic medications routinely prescribed for children and adolescents, stimulants are both the most widely used and the most extensively studied. Hundreds of randomized controlled studies have established the efficacy of the medications listed above. As a class of medication, stimulants have been used since the late 1930s, and methylphenidate—best known as Ritalin—has been on the market since 1955. It is one of a handful of psychotropic medications with FDA approval for use by children as young as age six. Stimulants are effective in between 75 percent and 90 percent of cases correctly diagnosed with ADHD. For these reasons, stimulants are considered the first-line treatment for ADHD. The arrival of Strattera (atomoxetine) in late 2002 may change that. Because it works differently in the brain, it presents a new possible alternative for those who cannot tolerate stimulants (see page 269).

Stimulants are quickly metabolized, sometimes as quickly as in one to four hours. This means that you can really target when your child uses it; for example, your child may take it only during school hours with no ill effects (like withdrawal) except the so-called rebound effect, when inattentiveness and hyperactivity seem to increase temporarily as the day's last dose wears off. Some individuals prefer time-release or extended-release medications. Concerta was the first long-acting time-release stimulant, a version of Ritalin. There are also extended-release versions of Adderall and Ritalin (Metadate XR). However, not all time-release products are created equal. Newer, advanced-release mechanisms are different and more effective than older, slow-release agents. Ask your doctor which may be best for your child.

No one knows precisely how stimulants work to calm and improve the ability to attend. The prevailing theory centers on the availability of the neurotransmitter dopamine. Neurotransmitters are chemicals that serve as "messengers" between brain cells. By making more dopamine available to carry messages, stimulants can curb or diminish inattentiveness, impulsivity, and overactivity. Though there is potential for abuse of stimulants in general, therapeutic doses are too low to produce a "high" or the sense of "being on speed." Nonetheless, some people do experience an increase in impulsivity, distractability, and hyperactivity. Often changes in the dosage, schedule, or type of stimulant can address these.

For pharmacological treatment of ADHD symptoms to be effective, it must be accompanied by behavior modification, appropriate accommodations in school, and, in some cases, psychotherapy. Medication alone will not work. However, numerous studies have shown that for many persons with ADHD (including the inattentive form without hyperactivity), psychosocial treatments alone are not effective.

You may have heard or read that stimulants can exacerbate or "bring out" tics. Stimulant use does not cause tics. What it may do, however, is exacerbate a preexisting propensity. ADHD occurs in about 50 percent of persons with Tourette's syndrome or tics. Persons with ADHD are more likely to have tics, at a rate of about 15 percent. Having TS or a tic disorder does not necessarily rule out stimulant use. Some patients have, with close monitoring, used stimulants successfully with no ill effects. Talk to your child's doctor.

Selective Norepinephrine Reuptake Inhibitors

BRAND NAME	GENERIC NAME
Strattera	atomoxetine

Approved in 2002 for use in children (as young as six), adolescents, and adults for the treatment of ADHD, Strattera is different in many ways. It was the first psychotropic medication to undergo two randomized double-blind placebo-controlled studies for each age group prior to approval. It is also unique in its action. It works by blocking the reabsorption of the neurotransmitter norepinephrine. According to Dr. Luke Tsai, "Decreased NE activity is associated with lower arousal and depression; high levels are associated with mania and increased motor activity."[23] Like any medication, Strattera is not for everyone. Unlike typical stimulants, Strattera may take anywhere from a week to a month to see the full benefit. Some patients see no benefit. Like the SSRIs, Strattera takes time to "build up" in the brain. The most common side effects are upset stomach, decreased appetite, dizziness, tiredness, nausea and vomiting, and mood swings. An allergic reaction (swelling, hives) can be potentially serious and should prompt a call to your doctor immediately. And Strattera must be swallowed whole.

Neuroleptics (Antipsychotics)

"Typical" Neuroleptics

BRAND NAME	GENERIC NAME
Haldol	haloperidol
Loxitane	loxapine
Mellaril	thioridazine
Moban	molindone
Navane	thiothixene

BRAND NAME	GENERIC NAME
Orap	pimozide
Prolixin	fluphenazine
Serentil	mesoridazine
Stelazine	trifluoperazine
Thorazine	chlorpromazine
Trilafon	perphenazine

"Atypical" Neuroleptics

BRAND NAME	GENERIC NAME
Abilify	aripiprazole
Clozaril	clozapine
Geodon	ziprasidone
Risperdal	risperidone
Seroquel	quetiapine
Zyprexa	olanzapine

Neuroleptics, also known as antipsychotics or major tranquilizers, are relatively new to pediatric pharmacology. Except in cases of psychosis and schizophrenia—the only two FDA-approved indications for this class of medications as of this writing—neuroleptics are rarely first-line treatments, due to their potential side effects. Most neuroleptics (with the exception of Abilify [aripiprazole]) work by partially blocking the transmission of the neurochemical dopamine. They can be effective in treating symptoms of Tourette's syndrome and tic disorder, dramatic mood swings, self-injurious behavior, and aggressive or violent behavior. When they work, one of the effects most parents notice immediately is the "smoothing out" of the child's temper and a rising frustration threshold. Tantrums that would normally last forty-five minutes may begin and end in less than five, for example. Unlike SSRIs, neuroleptics do not need to "build up" in the system; they take effect immediately.

All neuroleptics carry the risk of several rare but extremely serious side effects.[24] The one most mentioned is tardive dyskinesia, a debilitating, sometimes permanent series of involuntary movements. Tardive dyskinesia is progressive, beginning with facial movements such as grimacing and lip smacking and continuing on to involve the limbs in spasms. Antipsychotics can also produce other muscle problems, such as spasms, eye rolling, and tremor, among others. Another rare but potentially serious side effect is narcoleptic malignant syndrome. At the first sign of its symptoms—fever, confusion, muscle tightness, sweating, erratic blood pressure—the patient must be rushed to an emergency room. Untreated, neuroleptic malignant syndrome can result in kidney and muscle damage. Less serious but sometimes intolerable side effects include dramatic increases in appetite, weight gain, drowsiness, and cognitive blunting.

There are two "generations" of neuroleptics. The "typical" neuroleptics—Haldol, Loxitane, Mellaril, Moban, Navane, Orap, Prolixin, Serentil, Stelazine, Thorazine, Trilafon, and others—were developed from the mid-1950s through the 1990s. The newer generation, the so-called atypical neuroleptics, arrived with Risperdal in 1993. Since then, use of atypical neuroleptics in children with all forms of pervasive developmental disorders has risen markedly. The newest atypical neuroleptic is Abilify (aripiprazole). Although approved only to treat schizophrenia in adults, it has been found to be helpful among adults with bipolar disorder and is being used off-label increasingly for children with that condition, as well as those with ASDs. It is believed to work somewhat differently from the other atypicals in that it appears to both stimulate and inhibit certain dopamine receptors and some serotonin receptors as well. Early reports on Abilify have noted little or no risk of weight gain, changes in plasma glucose, increases in prolactin levels (although it may cause lower than normal prolactin levels), or cardiac effects. In some adults with bipolar disorder, Abilify produced headaches, nausea, vomiting, constipation, anxiety, insomnia, and akathisia, or motor restlessness; most of these side effects proved temporary. There are documented reports of children developing akathisia. Abilify's label also carries warnings about the risk of neuroleptic malignant syndrome and tardive dyskinesia. Because it may take weeks for Abilify to show its effects, individuals on other atypical neuroleptics (like Risperdal and Zyprexa) may need to take both (e.g., Abilify and Risperdal) for weeks or months before the "old med" can be tapered off or discontinued.

While the atypical neuroleptics as a group differ in important ways from the older neuroleptics, they are each very different from one another, both pharmacologically and in terms of their side effects.[25]

Doctors are increasingly choosing atypical neuroleptics because they appear to carry less risk of tardive dyskinesia and are effective for a wider range of symptoms. However, this should not be interpreted to mean that the new atypicals are risk-free. In early 2004 the FDA released a Safety Alert warning for all atypical neuroleptics, citing an increased risk of hyperglycemia and diabetes. Children who have hyperglycemia or diabetes or who have risk factors for these conditions (obesity, family history) should be closely and regularly monitored. These medications often produce the same increases in appetite and in weight and in some children may produce an increase in the hormone prolactin (or possible decrease with Abilify) and changes in other hormones. There is also a risk of cardiovascular effects and the rare but serious neuroleptic malignant syndrome. It is generally believed that the risk of tardive dyskinesia is dose-related; in other words, it is more likely to develop in those who have taken larger doses of neuroleptics over a longer period of time. However, there have been cases of tardive dyskinesia and other extrapyramidal symptoms (muscle contraction, slowed movements, etc.) with the atypical neuroleptics, and experts believe that we should presume there are similar risks with Abilify. Bear in mind that most atypical neuroleptics have been on the market and used in children for a relatively short time. It may be too soon to tell exactly what the risks are.[26]

Mood Stabilizers

BRAND NAME	GENERIC NAME
Depakene	valproic acid
Depakote	divalproex sodium
Dilantin	phenytoin
Eskalith	lithium carbonate
Gabitril	tiagabine
Lamictal	lamotrigine
Lithobid	lithium carbonate
Lithonate	lithium carbonate
Lithotabs	lithium carbonate
Neurontin	gabapentin
Tegretol	carbamazepine
Thorazine	chlorpromazine
Topamax	topiramate

Mood stabilizers do pretty much what you would expect from their name. They are used to treat a wide range of symptoms, including erratic and dramatic mood swings, aggressive or violent behavior, hyperactivity, and forms of depression, though not every medication is effective in treating all those listed.

The oldest among them, lithium carbonate, is approved for use in children age twelve and up to treat bipolar affective disorder. It is also used off-label to address such symptoms as aggression, agitation, and self-abuse. Lithium is the active ingredient in Eskalith, Lithobid, Lithonate, and Lithotabs.

No one knows exactly how lithium works, and anyone taking it must be monitored through blood tests to establish the correct dose. There is little leeway between a dose that is therapeutic and one that is toxic. Immediate side effects include nausea, vomiting, stomach upset, drowsiness, weakness, tremors, increased thirst, and increased urination. Because lithium is metabolized by the kidneys, it can cause kidney damage. Other effects of long-term use include weight gain, hypothyroidism (underactive thyroid), and goiter.

If your child is taking lithium, you should know the signs of lithium toxicity, a serious and potentially lethal condition. These signs include vomiting, drowsiness, confusion, slurred speech, dizziness, twitching, blurred vision, irregular heartbeat, mental dullness, difficulty walking and talking, or seeing strange colors. *If you see these signs, contact your doctor and seek emergency care immediately.*

The anticonvulsants (also called *antispasmodics*)—which include Depakote, Gabitril, Lamictal, Neurontin, Tegretol, and Topamax—are indicated to prevent seizures. The oldest, Tegretol, was approved in 1968 and is indicated for treating seizures in children age six and up. It is also prescribed off-label to address a range of symptoms, including aggression, Tourette's syndrome, and tics. Tegretol may produce gastrointestinal problems, drowsiness, dizziness, and double or blurred vision. More serious side effects include suppression of white blood cell production and bone marrow depression (which weakens immunity), liver toxicity, and severe rash. Anyone taking Tegretol must have periodic blood tests.

Valproic acid (Depakene) and divalproex sodium (Depakote) were both approved in 1978 for seizures and in 1995 for bipolar affective disorder. They have been used off-label to treat panic disorder and aggression. Because of how they are metabolized, blood tests are required to establish the correct dose and should be repeated as your doctor suggests. These medications have been used in children under the age of two, and Depakene in children as small as twenty-two pounds. Depakote may lower blood count, cause pancreatitis, and cause a mild form of hepatitis. For this reason, liver function should be tested prior to starting the medication and periodically for as long as your child is on it. More common, less serious side effects are gastrointestinal problems, headache, double vision, dizziness, weight gain, appetite suppression, anxiety, confusion, and sedation.

Newer anticonvulsants—Gabitril, Lamictal, Neurontin, and Topamax—are also being prescribed off-label to stabilize mood. Gabapentin (Neurontin) produces few immediate side effects (tiredness, dizziness, problems with gross-motor control, blurred vision) and appears to be free of serious side effects. It is the most often prescribed anticonvulsant for children. Topamax is approved to treat seizures in children age two and up; Gabitril is approved for use in adolescents (age twelve and up). Both date from the mid-1990s. Tiredness and dizziness are common side effects of both. In addition, Topamax may produce cognitive blurring, nervousness, and tingling sensations; Gabitril can cause changes in gait. Lamictal is known to produce blurred or double vision, sensitivity to light, headache, dizziness, and tiredness. *If your child develops a skin rash, contact your doctor immediately.*

Anxiolytics

BRAND NAME	GENERIC NAME
Atarax	hydroxyzine
Ativan	lorazepam
Benadryl	diphenhydramine
BuSpar	buspirone
Halcion	triazolam
Klonopin	clonazepam
Librium	chlordiazepoxide
Serax	oxazepam
Tranxene	clorazepate
Valium	diazepam
Vistaril	hydroxyzine
Xanax	alprazolam

Anxiolytics reduce anxiety and include several types of medication: benzodiazepines, antihistamines, and one (so far) atypical anxiolytic, BuSpar (buspirone). These medications have a good record for safety and effectiveness. Several benzodiazepines are approved for use in children: Ativan, Klonopin, and Librium are approved for use in children twelve and up; Tranxene, ages nine and up; Serax, ages six and up; Valium, ages six months and up. Although they are generally safe, they can be dangerous when combined with other medications—particularly alcohol, anesthetics, antihistamines, sedatives, muscle relaxants, and some prescription pain medications.

Although all benzodiazepines carry a small risk of dependence when used short term, when used for long periods, they can create tolerance and dependence. Tolerance means that your child may have to take more of the medication to achieve the same effect. Dependence can result in physical withdrawal symptoms if the medication is abruptly stopped. You may not know if your child has developed dependence, so be sure to have an adequate supply of medication on hand. Common signs of withdrawal are sweating, increased anxiety, sleeplessness, agitation, and nervousness; these aren't generally dangerous. Other withdrawal symptoms—fever, seizures, and psychosis—require immediate medical attention. However, when the medication is tapered off gradually, such symptoms can be avoided.

For the most part, the common immediate side effects of benzodiazepines—sedation, drowsiness, diminished coordination, confusion, and mental dullness—are mild and may pass as the child adjusts to the medication. Some children may respond to these medications by becoming disinhibited—overactive, silly, overtalkative, and so on—or become anxious and have trouble falling asleep. There are no known long-term side effects of benzodiazepine use.

BuSpar is a different kind of nonaddictive anxiolytic known as an azapirone. It differs from the benzodiazepines in several important ways: it seems to have a lower risk of dependence and has fewer side effects generally. (It has no relaxant, sedative, or anticonvulsant action.) However, it comes with a long list of contraindications. Immediate short-term side effects such as disinhibition, confusion, and sedation are common. Though considered generally less effective than the benzodiazepines, since its debut in 1986 BuSpar has been shown to reduce aggression and possibly be helpful for ADHD, panic disorder, and separation anxiety.

Antihistamines, which are more commonly used to treat allergic reactions, may also be prescribed for their sedative properties. Benadryl may be used off-label for anxiety, panic disorder, and separation anxiety, and Atarax for anxiety. Antihistamines are generally considered safe for children, but you should still check with your doctor before giving them to your child.

Antihypertensives

BRAND NAME	GENERIC NAME
Catapres	clonidine
Corgard	nadolol
Inderal	propranolol
Tenex	guanfacine

Antihypertensives are medications originally developed and approved to treat high blood pressure. The oldest, Inderal, has been on the market since 1967 and among this group has the highest potential for serious side effects. Today, all are used off-label in children to treat aggression, agitation, self-abuse, impulsivity, and sleep problems. Catapres (clonidine) and Tenex (guanfacine) have shown particular promise in the treatment of Tourette's syndrome and tics. Tenex is also used for ADHD. Because these medications affect cardiac function and blood pressure, periodic monitoring is necessary.

In addition, there have been reports of unexplained deaths in three children taking clonidine with other medications, particularly stimulants. There is evidence to suggest that other factors besides this particular combination of medications caused these deaths, and the combination continues to be prescribed. However, anyone taking clonidine in combination with another medication must be monitored closely. A number of health conditions contraindicate the use of Inderal (propranolol) and similar beta-blockers: heart problems, breathing problems—especially asthma—and diabetes among them.

The most common, short-term side effects tend to be mild: tiredness, drowsiness, dry mouth, trouble sleeping, headache, and sweating. You should report more serious side effects—difficulty breathing, changes in heartbeat, nausea, chest pain, dizziness, faintness, muscle weakness, pain—to a doctor immediately.

Recommended Resources

BOOKS

Luke Y. Tsai, *Taking the Mystery Out of Medications in Autism/Asperger Syndrome: A Guide for Parents and Non-Medical Professionals* (Arlington, TX: Future Horizons, 2001).

Timothy E. Wilens, *Straight Talk About Psychiatric Medications for Kids,* Revised Edition (New York: Guilford Press, 2004). If your child is currently on prescription psychotropic medication, or if you are considering it, this easy-to-read, informative book is a must.

WEB SITES

Food and Drug Administration
http://www.fda.gov/

MayoClinic.com DrugInfo, http://www.mayoclinic.com

Medline Plus, http://www.nlm.nih.gov/medlineplus/ druginformation.html

Medscape Drug Database, http://www.medscape.com

Physicians' Desk Reference Information for Consumers, http://www.pdrhealth.com

Chapter 8

SPECIAL EDUCATION BASICS

You cannot discuss special education without talking about special education law and the "alphabet soup" of acronyms that quickly become the shorthand second language of parents of children with special needs (see the OASIS Web site for a listing of common acronyms and other abbreviations). Special education is governed by a host of federal, state, and local laws and regulations and then shaped by the individuals—educators, administrators, and officials—charged with carrying them out. Because, by definition, special education is tailored to the individual, there is often a wide variation in the type and quality of services and/or accommodations from student to student.

Here we present a basic overview of the role of special education in the lives of students with Asperger Syndrome. In "Recommended Resources" (page 325) we list a relative handful of the hundreds of books that have been written on the subject of special education and a mere sampling of the countless Web sites devoted to this cause. We urge you to read at least one, if not all, the titles listed, to familiarize yourself with the state and local regulations that apply to your child and, whenever necessary, to seek help—from another informed parent, an advocate, an advocacy organization, or an attorney who specializes in special education. If at all possible, make time to attend a conference, seminar, or talk on the subject.

It is impossible to generalize about the educational needs of children with Asperger Syndrome beyond saying that each child is unique. Appropriate placements range from self-contained special education classrooms and schools dedicated to AS and/or related disorders to regular mainstream classrooms. Some students with AS will go through their school years without ever needing to be identified officially as "a child with a disability" requiring special education and/or related services. However, even those who, academically speaking, are star students will often benefit from accommodations, special education, and/or related services.

Special education–related services that a student—even one who is academically successful—who has AS might receive include but are not limited to:[1]

- Speech and language therapy
- Occupational therapy
- Audiology services
- Physical therapy, adaptive physical education, or other therapies
- Recreation, including therapeutic recreation
- Orientation and mobility services
- Services from a school psychologist, counselor, or social worker
- Services from an aide or paraprofessional
- Services from a consultant knowledgeable about AS to work with your child and the school staff
- Services from a reader, scribe, typist, interpreter, or Braillist
- Medical services, for purposes of diagnosis and evaluation, and school health nurse
- Counseling and training for parents
- Resource centers
- Transportation
- Vocational education
- Assistive technology, such as voice-activated software, laptop computer, or books on tape

In addition, a student with AS who does not qualify for special education and/or related services may need accommodations and considerations: for instance, more time to get from one class to another; an aide or fellow student to help her organize and pack the right books to bring home each afternoon; transportation in a smaller school bus; or extra time or access to a word processor for written tests.

As students near adolescence, you should look closely at what skills or support he or she may need to succeed at college, in job training, or at work. Before your child leaves elementary school (yes, we said elementary school), speak with your district's special education department and start networking with parents of older students with similar needs, support groups, and local, county, and state agencies that provide services and job training for individuals with disabilities. Do not make the mistake of assuming that just because your child is on an academic track and destined (at least on paper) for the school of his choice that such programs have nothing to offer him. Find out. Your child may need an IEP to access some of these services.

Also, keep your eye on the calendar. It's very important that accommodations be in place and official long before you request things like extended time for SATs/ACTs. That is because the College Board requires up-to-date documentation and will not allow for accommodations that are not already in use in high school. Colleges will also require documentation of disability and up-to-date reports.

IS THERE A "RIGHT" EDUCATION FOR STUDENTS WITH AS?

Although many children with AS share certain types of strengths and deficits in learning-related skills and abilities, there is no single educational "profile" for AS. In addition, it is common for persons with AS to have other comorbid conditions that affect learning, such as ADHD, OCD, and nonverbal learning disability (NLD or NVLD). As a result, there is no single program, method, or technique that works for every student. A child with AS can be academically gifted or beset by multiple learning disabilities—or both. (See box on page 396 on giftedness.) Most often, children with AS display a mixture of strengths and weaknesses. Jessie, who has been reading with comprehension since age three and can do long division in her head, is so severely dysgraphic that her test scores are always very low and written assignments go undone. Eric, who has an above-average IQ, has been diagnosed with dyslexia and dyscalculia (see page 78). Assessments indicate that Kevin probably would be an average to above-average student academically. However, his multiple sensory issues and difficulties with pragmatic speech make every school day torture.

Students with AS can work well in a range of educational situations, provided, of course, that each is in the setting that best addresses his particular and unique needs. In our OASIS survey of 439 parents of children with AS, over 80 percent had Individualized Education Programs (and half of those students had IEPs in place prior to diagnosis), and about 15 percent had Section 504 plans. More than 70 percent of all students attend regular public school (including self-contained special education classrooms and special education programs within the regular school); less than 10 percent are placed in a special education school or facility. Of the students who attend regular (non–special education schools), we found that:

- Only 19 percent were in self-contained (i.e., containing only special education students) classrooms for all or part of the school day.
- Nine percent were in inclusion classrooms with pull-outs for services and/or resource room, and 1 percent were in inclusion classes without any additional services.
- The remaining 72 percent were placed in regular, mainstream classrooms with extra services or supports divided almost evenly among:
  - No extra help or support
  - No extra help but pull-outs for services and/or resource room
  - A one-on-one aide or paraprofessional

In the past several years, a number of programs and schools designed to serve students with AS (and, in some cases, related disorders) have opened across the country. They are still relatively few, and their educational philosophies vary. (For the latest information, visit the "Schools and Camps" section of the OASIS Web site.) Don't forget to look in your own backyard, and your neighbors'. Some school districts that have one or two students who could benefit from a specially designed classroom or a program may pool resources with other districts to create something together none of the districts could set up, support, or fund on their own. For example, Patty's son Justin attends an Asperger classroom in a regular public school. He and his classmates have the best of both worlds: a small learning environment tailored to their needs coupled with access to and involvement with typical peers when appropriate. No district could maintain such a classroom for one or two students, but by accepting students from several neighboring districts, this one has allowed Justin and his classmates to have a highly individualized program in the least restrictive and most socially appropriate environment.

Here again, networking pays. School districts do not always advertise such programs, and you might be surprised to discover how little your district special educators know about what's going on even around the corner. You are not limited to only what your district has to offer. If you find a public school program that you believe might suit your child's needs and is within a reasonable distance (your local regulations may have something to say about how far or how long a child can travel), ask your special education administrator to apply to that district or program on your child's behalf.

WHAT IS SPECIAL EDUCATION?

Special education is more than extra help. According to the Individuals with Disabilities Education Act, "The term 'special education' means specially designed instruction, at no cost to parents, to meet the unique needs of a child with a disability, including—(A) instruction conducted in the classroom, in the home, in hospitals and institutions, and in other settings; and (B) instruction in physical education."[2]

Prior to 1975, when Congress passed Public Law 94-142, the Education for All Handicapped Children Act, special education as we now know it simply did not exist. The federal government had no statutes affirming the legal right to public education for children with disabilities. These children had no protection from being refused admittance to school on the grounds that they were unable to learn or would disrupt or distract teachers and other students. Where so-called special education classrooms did exist, they often segregated disabled children from their peers in classrooms that were inferior—both physically and academically—from those of nondisabled students. Just six years prior to the passage of Public Law 94–142, school authorities in North Carolina could have a parent arrested for attempting to enroll a disabled child the authorities had previously refused to take.[3]

In the wake of the 1954 U.S. Supreme Court decision in *Brown* v. *Board of Education,* a movement among parents of disabled children took root. In finding that racially segregated schools could not be considered "equal" and that segregation violated students' rights to equal protection under the law, the U.S. Supreme Court in *Brown* looked closely at the impact of segregation on students. Interestingly, the decision spoke of the public schools' crucial role in preparing students for life beyond the schoolhouse and mentioned the psychological impact of segregation on "their hearts and minds." "In these days, it is doubtful that any child may reasonably be expected to succeed in life if he is denied the opportunity of an education," the Court wrote. "Such an opportunity . . . is a right which must be made available to all on equal terms."[4]

Public Law 94–142 (which was renamed the Individuals with Disabilities Education Act when it was reauthorized in 1990) established the right of every child to receive a "free appropriate public education." Further, it charged the individual states and local educational agencies with the responsibility for carrying it out. Over the years, IDEA has been revised, in 1990 and again in 1997. The 1997 revisions, which were published in their final form in early 1999, substantially expanded the rights and protections of parents and students, particularly in the areas of parent involvement, and discipline, suspensions, and expulsions.

In its findings, however, Congress stated clearly what many parents of children in special education know too well:

> Since the enactment and implementation of the Education for All Handicapped Children Act of 1975, this Act has been successful in ensuring children with disabilities and the families of such children access to a free appropriate public education and in improving educational results for children with disabilities. However, the implementation of this Act has been impeded by low expectations, and an insufficient focus on applying replicable research on proven methods of teaching and learning for children with disabilities.[5]

IDEA AND CASE LAW

Although IDEA is a revolutionary, landmark piece of legislation, it is, like most laws, open to interpretation. The interpretation of a specific point is as much determined by case law as by the law itself. The most recent standing decisions within your federal circuit usually prevail. Only rulings made by the United States Supreme Court apply in every U.S. jurisdiction. Legal counsel on both sides of a dispute should always have one eye trained on ever-evolving case law.

If you reach a point where you believe that your school district is in violation of IDEA or other relevant statutes and regulations, we suggest you consult a professional advocate or an attorney who specializes in special education law before proceeding with mediation, an impartial due process hearing, or a lawsuit.

IDEA AND YOUR STATE REGULATIONS GOVERNING SPECIAL EDUCATION

In shaping special education, IDEA does not stand alone. Every state has its own department of education regulations regarding special education. State regulations must meet the requirements set forth in IDEA. A state must grant students with disabilities who qualify for special education under IDEA or under the state's own eligibility requirements what is mandated in IDEA. Your state is free to exceed IDEA in terms of procedural matters, eligibility, and services, but it cannot offer less than IDEA mandates. A state may mandate specific services not included in IDEA. New York, for instance, requires that for children classified as autistic "provision shall be made for parent counseling and education for the purpose of enabling parents to perform appropriate follow-up intervention activities at home."[6] In addition, an individual school district, school, or program may provide services that exceed what is required even by its state. Your state may set student-to-teacher ratios for self-contained special education classrooms at 10:1 but your local school district may decide that a ratio of 8:1 is more appropriate.

IDEA does not address the specific components of an effective IEP, nor does it require that any student receive the "best" education, only one that is "appropriate." IDEA does not mention specific teaching methods, even though it is well established that certain methodologies have been demonstrated to be more effective than others and that IDEA requires schools to "apply replicable research on proven methods of teaching and learning for children with disabilities."[7] IDEA also requires that staff have adequate training, a crucial provision for students with AS, since so few educators have had such training. What that means in practice may vary from district to district. In one district or school a special education reading teacher may be certified in the Orton-Gillingham method (a highly specialized reading method developed specifically to address dyslexia) or the school psychologist may have experience in using applied behavior analysis with children with AS. For students who would benefit from these approaches, they are invaluable. However, it is a mistake to assume that simply because one method or approach would be the most effective for your child it will be available or provided automatically. For various reasons we'll explore in this chapter, special education programs are not—and should not be—uniform. In fact, parents should always remember that the *I* in IDEA stands for "individuals" and the *I* in IEP stands for "individualized." Special education should be "custom tailored" for each and every student, not simply taken "off the rack."

While IDEA stands as the overriding law of the land, the policies and "traditions" of your state and your school district (in IDEA terms, your "local education authority," or LEA) can have a profound impact on the quality of special education your child receives.

• • •

A Political Moment . . .

A newer element in the special ed mix is the 2002 reauthorization of the Elementary and Secondary School Act (ESEA), which provides federal funds to public schools. Dubbed this time out No Child Left Behind (NCLB), this act applies to all public schools that receive certain types of federal funds. While NCLB has been hailed for establishing a system of stricter accountability for student performance, emphasizing adoption of proven educational methods, expanded parental choice in schools, greater control at the local level, and extra help for students who need it—all good things, and, some argue quite persuasively, good for students with special needs, too—it is not without its critics. Objections to NCLB have come from state and local elected leaders and officials, school administrators and teachers, and parents over many points. One aspect of NCLB that has received the most criticism, even from those who support the act's overall objectives, is that in demanding these changes without providing the funds to carry them out, the federal government has placed an unfair financial burden on states and local school districts.

What does this have to do with IDEA? One thing parents learn quickly is that in most areas of the country, funding for special education and related services is not what it should be. When IDEA was originally passed in 1975, Congress promised to provide to local school districts 40 percent of the cost of providing the education and services IDEA mandates (or requires). As we near the thirtieth anniversary of the passage of the act we now know as IDEA, Congress has yet to provide even half the share of funding it promised. In fact, the closest it has ever come is 17 percent.

Now that your local school district is faced with meeting a mandate for all students, one cannot help but wonder what may be in store for students who receive special education and related services under IDEA. What does this have to do with you and your child?

In 2002 the House and the Senate began working on reauthorizing IDEA. In the process of reauthorization, changes can be made, and in the past, these changes were overwhelmingly positive: requiring preschool and early intervention services, for example. The last time IDEA was reauthorized, in 1997, the results were a clear win for parents and children: increased parental involvement in the IEP process; required transition services to help students prepare for life after high school; and special disciplinary procedures that protected students with disabilities. Through the 2003 and 2004 sessions of Congress, some of these proposed provisions of IDEA have come under attack from several fronts. Among the most vocal opponents to particular sections are school administrators and educators who believe they should have more discretion in handling the behavior issues of students with disabilities and more leniency (i.e., less frequent reporting) on children's progress. (To be honest, the paperwork connected to special education can be daunting, and it does consume surprisingly large amounts of teacher time.) Many child advocacy groups believed that the Senate version of the bill was preferable to the House version. In the end, though, there was no dispute: both versions weakened or removed important protections for parents and students. As of this writing, a "new" IDEA is in limbo, and the 1997 amendments remain in force.

It is impossible to say what the new IDEA will look like. Keep abreast of developments, and let your representatives at every level of government know your views on the legislation that affects your family. For better or worse, it too often comes down to politics. It is outrageous to think that such basic protections and rights remain subject to the whims of party politics and the invisible hands of special interest groups. As an important first step, we should all demand that our representatives support full funding of IDEA.

WHAT WILL SPECIAL EDUCATION MEAN FOR YOUR CHILD?

Parents new to the world of special education often hear the well-meaning doctor, therapist, regular education teacher, friend, or family member saying, "Go to your school district. You have a right to get all the services and help your child needs." That sounds great, but it betrays some common misconceptions about special education. One is that any student who is behind his peers academically, developmentally, or socially is entitled to receive services.

First, let's look at what your local school district must do, by law.

- At a parent's request, it must provide for a full assessment of a child at no cost to parents. (See chapter 3.)
- At a parent's request, it must provide for an independent or private assessment of a child if the parent disagrees with the original assessment. This must be done at no charge to the parent and must be done in a timely manner. Unfortunately, some parents

encounter resistance from their school districts on providing an independent educational evaluation (IEE) and are forced to pursue the matter in an impartial due process hearing.

- It must meet with the parent to discuss the findings of the assessments and determine whether or not that child is eligible for special education and related services (under IDEA) or accommodation (under Section 504; see page 293).
- If your school district determines that your child is not eligible for special education and related services or accommodations (or if the school district finds your child eligible for accommodations without special education and related services), you may request an independent, impartial hearing.

Even if your child has a diagnosis or has been evaluated in the past, he can be considered for special education services only after he has been assessed by professionals qualified to administer recognized, validated tests. No federal statute specifies precisely what degree of disability must be shown for eligibility under IDEA, although some states do have guidelines that address this in terms of degree as measured by standardized assessments (for instance, a twelve-month delay, a 33 percent delay, or a score of 1.5 or 2 standard deviations below the mean). It is imperative that parents have a basic working knowledge of the terminology and concepts behind the tests and measurements used in special education. The best source for this information is the Wrightslaw Web site.[8]

As important as standardized assessments are, a child's eligibility cannot be determined based on a single test or the impressions of a single evaluator, no matter how experienced. This is why IDEA requires that eligibility be determined by a multidisciplinary team. Further, that team must assess the child "in all areas of suspected disability." According to attorney Lawrence M. Siegel, author of *The Complete IEP Guide: How to Advocate for Your Special Ed Child,* that includes, "health, vision, hearing, social and emotional status, general intelligence, academic performance, communicative status, motor abilities, behavior and cognitive, physical and developmental abilities."[9] In addition to whatever assessments your school district plans to administer, it must also consider information from a wide range of sources: parents, teachers, doctors, and others familiar with your child as well as previous assessments.

The tests administered must be given in your child's native language. They must also be valid, which means that they are the appropriate instruments for measuring specific abilities and disabilities. For example, an evaluator cannot conclude that because your child's IQ tested in the normal or above-normal range she does not have a problem with pragmatics or adaptive social skills. These tests must be administered and scored only by persons qualified to do so. Publishers of standardized assessment instruments (tests) clearly spell out in their instructions who may administer a test. If anyone else gives a test, the results are automatically invalid. Under IDEA, it is illegal for, let's say, the school's speech therapist to give your child a test that is designed to be used only by a psychologist or psychiatrist.

WHO IS ELIGIBLE?

Simply having a disability doesn't automatically entitle a student to special education under IDEA; nor does the fact that a student theoretically could "do better" with extra help obligate your school district to provide that help. Conversely, simply having an average (or higher) IQ doesn't automatically exclude a child from qualifying for services or accommodations under Section 504 or IDEA. This is important for parents of children with AS to understand: we've heard from probably hundreds of parents through OASIS whose school districts have attempted to discourage them from obtaining evaluations or services by telling them, in effect, "Your child is too smart for special ed." There are numerous state and federal laws that address the rights of disabled persons. IDEA is unique and the focus of this chapter because it mandates a "free appropriate public education" (FAPE) for any child with disabilities from birth to age twenty-two who meets its eligibility requirements.

Here are two important legal definitions, from IDEA:

> Child with a Disability—The term "child with a disability" means a child—(i) with mental retardation, hearing impairments (including deafness), speech or language impairments, visual impairments (including blindness), serious emotional disturbance (hereinafter referred to as "emotional disturbance"), orthopedic

impairments, autism, traumatic brain injury, other health impairments, or specific learning disabilities; and (ii) who, by reason thereof, needs special education and related services.[10]

Of interest to parents of children who have any form of PDD or other disability is this additional definition:

Child aged 3 through 9—The term "child with a disability" for a child aged 3 through 9 may, at the discretion of the State and the local educational agency, include a child (i) experiencing developmental delays, as defined by the State and measured by appropriate diagnostic instruments and procedures, in one of the following areas: physical development, cognitive development, communication development, social or emotional development, or adaptive development; and (ii) who, by reason thereof, needs special education and related services.[11]

Specific Learning Disability—The term "specific learning disability" means a disorder in one or more of the basic psychological processes involved in understanding or in using language, spoken or written, which disorder may manifest in imperfect ability to listen, think, speak, read, write, spell, or do mathematical calculations. . . . Such term includes conditions such as perceptual disabilities, brain injury, minimal brain dysfunction, dyslexia, and developmental aphasia. . . . Such term does not include a hearing problem that is primarily the result of visual, hearing, or motor disabilities, of mental retardation, of emotional disturbance, or of environmental, cultural, or economic disadvantage.[12]

• • •

Early Intervention and Preschool Services

As IDEA evolved, its coverage expanded to include special education and related services for infants and toddlers (mandated by 1991) and preschoolers, ages three to five (mandated by 1994). Now that children on the spectrum are being diagnosed at earlier ages, and some are even receiving an AS diagnosis before kindergarten, early intervention (EI) and preschool services will play a larger role. If your child is under age three, discuss your concerns with your pediatrician, who can help arrange an evaluation through a state or local agency at no cost to you. Also contact your municipal, county, or state departments of health and education. Every state sets its own policies regarding approved providers and costs to families. You do not access preschool services the same way you would if your child were school-aged. Your district, however, probably can direct you to the agency that will provide a full evaluation, determine eligibility and/or services, and provide those services (usually through outside agencies that specialize in this work). Infants, toddlers, and preschoolers receive services in a wide array of settings: home, early intervention classroom, family child care, hospital (inpatient), outpatient service facilities (such as an occupational therapist's office), and regular nursery school or child care settings, among others. For many children on the spectrum EI services are provided in the home; in other words, special ed teachers and other therapists come to you. However, it is highly individualized, and where your child receives services may depend not only on his particular needs but on what may be available. Your area may have a shortage of teachers and therapists for home work, but a very good EI center–based program or preschool, or vice versa. Depending on your child, you may be able to arrange for him to receive occupational therapy at his regular preschool or for your child's ABA therapist to work with the staff of his day care center to help him develop more appropriate play skills.

One cornerstone of both EI and preschool services is parental involvement. As with IEPs, parents have input into the development of the IFSP (Individual Family Service Plan). If your child's teachers and therapists are coming to your home, you will have a chance to see firsthand what is involved, and training for parents is a key component in good EI and preschool programs, regardless of where your child's services are delivered.

If you have any concerns about your child's development, or another professional suggests that he or she does, contact your local health department, your pediatrician, and your school district right away and get this process in motion. (Even though your school district has no direct involvement in EI, someone on staff should be able to point you in the right direction.) Especially when children with AS are young, they may not always appear to be "that different" from their peers. Especially if your little one seems advanced in certain areas and has hit or beat most developmental milestones, it can be difficult to fully accept that he or she needs help and tempting to stick with the regular child care, nursery school, or preschool arrangements you now have. (The usual argument for this is access to typical peers and social development.) If you find yourself confronting this dilemma, please consider EI and preschool services. For children on the spectrum, there is no doubt that earlier treatment is better than later. Despite their kind intentions, most regular nursery school and preschool teachers are not qualified to provide these children much more than tolerance and support.

For more information on EI, see "Early Intervention Services for Children Birth Through Age 2," at www.thearc.org/faqs/early.html and DisabilityResources.org's "Early Intervention" at www.disability/resources.org/EARLY/html.

IDEA has evolved over time. Until 1990, autism was not among the disabilities specified in IDEA. Recently, ADHD was added to the list of disabilities, but students with conditions such as Tourette's syndrome and obsessive-compulsive disorder are not specifically mentioned. Students for whom these conditions adversely affect their ability to learn may be eligible for special education and/or related services but be classified as disabled under "serious emotional disturbance" (SED) or "other health impaired" (OHI).

SECTION 504 ACCOMMODATIONS

Sometimes the adverse affect of a disability is not considered to impede the ability to learn sufficiently to warrant an IEP even though it clearly has some impact on the student's access to regular education. Instead, the school district may offer what are commonly known as "504 accommodations," after Section 504 of the Rehabilitation Act of 1973. The resulting document that specifies the accommodations and/or services a student may receive under Section

504 is known as Section 504 Services and Accommodation Plan (or "504 plan"). The Rehabilitation Act of 1973 is a civil rights law, not an education law, designed to "empower individuals with disabilities to maximize employment, economic self-sufficiency, independence, and inclusion and integration into society."[13] Its definition of an individual with disability is far broader than IDEA's, and the rights and protections that it grants are far more limited.[14] Renowned special education attorney Peter W. D. Wright illustrates the difference between IDEA and Section 504 in this analogy:

> A handicapped child is in a wheelchair. Under Section 504, this child shall not be discriminated against because of the disability.
>
> The child shall be provided with access to an education, to and through the schoolhouse door. However, under Section 504 there is no guarantee that this wheelchair-bound child will receive an education from which the child benefits. The child simply has access to the same education that children without disabilities receive. Now assume that the child in the wheelchair also has neurological problems that adversely affect the child's ability to learn. Under IDEA, the child with a disability that adversely affects educational performance is entitled to an education that is individually designed to meet the child's unique needs and from which the child receives educational benefit.[15]

You may be advised—by educators, doctors, friends, and others—to avoid an IEP and go for Section 504 accommodation instead. The reasoning is that in order to qualify for an IEP and the resulting special education and related services, a child must be identified (or "labeled") as a child with a disability. Some parents feel that this is stigmatizing. Others believe that a Section 504 accommodation plan is essentially "IEP lite," a nicer, less time-consuming, less exacting instrument. As one OASIS visitor posted, "I went for the 504 because I figured, why use a hammer when a chisel would do." This may seem a reasonable approach, but only if you are fortunate enough to have a child who needs minimal accommodation (not services) and live in a school district where the chisel can do the job. However, in the end, an IEP is unquestionably the superior instrument in terms of the range of services and the rights it protects.

Plus, eligibility under IDEA automatically entitles a student to protections and rights under Section 504.

Parents may also be under the common misperception that having an IEP automatically relegates a student to a special education program (such as a self-contained special ed classroom). This is not true. As Sheri Taylor-Mearhoff, from Amicus for Children, says, "Special education is a service, not a place." A child with an IEP can be fully mainstreamed in a regular classroom if such placement satisfies two key tenets of IDEA: The placement serves his individual educational needs and it is the least restrictive environment (LRE).

Even though a child may seem to require only accommodations, a full evaluation is strongly recommended for a child with or suspected of having Asperger Syndrome or any PDD. Though few parents or children could be said to look forward to the evaluation process, there are a few things to consider. Asperger Syndrome is a neurologically based disorder with a full range of possible comorbid conditions, including learning disabilities or differences in styles of learning. Some of these are blatantly apparent and may seem to have always been present; others seem to crop up only when academic or social demands tax a particular weakness. So though your child's dysgraphia may have always been apparent, his problems with pragmatics may suddenly seem more glaring when he's called on to analyze what he reads or to think more conceptually.

There are some circumstances under which 504 accommodations are recommended; for example, if a student is doing well in a regular education classroom but needs to be seated at the front of the classroom because of mild problems with attention, vision, or hearing. You should know, however, that some school districts do provide special education and related services to students who are, technically speaking, eligible only under Section 504. This may be the result of state or local policies.

Daylong seminars and towers of books and legal decisions address the differences between IDEA and Section 504. You need not become a legal scholar, but you should know the pros and cons of each. The following table offers a brief overview of both and highlights their key differences.

If your child is found to qualify as a child with a disability under IDEA, he is also automatically eligible for accommodations or related services under Section 504. You might then decide which

Comparing IDEA 1997 and Section 504

ISSUE	UNDER IDEA 1997	UNDER SECTION 504
What is the purpose of the statute?	To provide individualized special education and related services to children with disabilities; these services may be in addition to those provided to students without disabilities.	To eliminate barriers that prevent persons with disabilities from fully participating; to prevent discrimination in any area—employment, housing, etc.—based on disability. The goal of Section 504 for students is to ensure that children with disabilities have the same access to education that children without disabilities have.
Through what means are the individual statutes' purposes achieved?	By designing, providing, and carrying out an Individualized Education Plan (IEP) that specifies the special education and related services tailored to meet each student's specific needs and work toward specific goals. By definition, a free appropriate public education (FAPE) is one from which the student will benefit.	By making modifications and accommodations within the realm of general, regular education. Section 504 does not require that the student receive any benefit from the education provided, only that he have the same equal access to that education.
To whom does this law apply?	Persons with specific categories of disability: "mental retardation, hearing impairments (including deafness), speech or language impairments, visual impairments (including blindness), serious emotional disturbance . . .	Any person who has a physical or mental impairment that substantially limits one or more major life activities; any person who has a record of having had such an impairment; any person who is regarded to have such an impairment.

ISSUE	UNDER IDEA 1997	UNDER SECTION 504
	orthopedic impairments, autism, traumatic brain injury, other health impairments, or specific learning disabilities" (outlined on page 290).★ ADD and ADHD are now considered within the category of "other health impaired."†	Note for the purposes of IDEA, "impairment" is not the same as a "disability." Some examples of conditions that may be addressed through a 504 plan are ADHD, oppositional-defiant disorder, obsessive-compulsive disorder, and posttraumatic stress syndrome. In some cases, depending on the severity of the condition's impact on the student's ability to learn, that student might qualify as being "other health impaired" or having an "emotional disturbance" and qualify under IDEA.
How is eligibility determined?	By the degree to which the disability has an adverse effect on a student's ability to learn or educational performance.	By the presence of a physical or mental condition that "substantially limits"—permanently or temporarily—a student's learning.
My school district has just notified me that my child should be evaluated for special education and related services or	Until your child's evaluation is complete, you may not know whether he or she will be eligible under IDEA or Section 504. You should know that both IDEA and Section 504 charge school districts with the obligation to find and identify all children—from birth to age twenty-two—who may have a disability. You can refuse to allow the school district to evaluate your child. However, your school district has the right to pursue the matter	

★Individuals with Disabilities Education Act, 20 U.S.C. §1401(3).
†Individuals with Disabilities Education Act, 34 C.F.R., section 300.7 (c) (9).

ISSUE	UNDER IDEA 1997	UNDER SECTION 504
accommodations. What are my rights?	through an impartial due process hearing.	
What type of educational evaluation will my child undergo?	A multidisciplinary evaluation that assesses the child "in all areas of suspected disability," using validated tests and other evaluation materials administered by "trained and knowledgeable personnel." Your school district must also consider any private evaluations and must also consider "information provided by the parent."	The school district can decide the extent of the evaluation it conducts, and it must use validated tests and other evaluation materials administered by trained personnel. The school district is not required to consider information provided by parents, nor that derived from private evaluations.
Who will be making the decisions regarding my child's eligibility for services and placement?	"A team of qualified professionals and the parent of the child." In addition, your state may require the presence of others; for example, a parent member of the committee who is not related to the student but who has a child with a disability. Parents may also invite whomever they choose to attend (friend, family, legal counsel, advocate, etc.).	Your school district can decide who makes decisions regarding your child's eligibility and placement. There is no requirement that the district consider information from a variety of sources, nor is there any requirement that a meeting take place prior to a change in placement.
Can a child be placed without parental consent?	A child cannot be classified or placed without parental consent. Parents are entitled to an impartial due process hearing.	Parents are entitled to an impartial due process hearing.
What recourse do I have if I believe that the school	The school district must provide an independent educational evaluation at no cost	None specified. There is no legal obligation to provide an independent

298

ISSUE	UNDER IDEA 1997	UNDER SECTION 504
district's evaluation results are incorrect or incomplete?	to parents (at public expense). (See answer to next question.)	educational evaluation at no cost to parents (at public expense).
What if my school district refuses to provide an independent educational evaluation after I request it?	Your school district cannot deny your child an independent educational evaluation without first going through an impartial due process hearing.	Independent educational evaluations are not covered under Section 504. Any further action is at the discretion of your school district.
Must a child receive a special education classification? (The actual categories for classification may vary from state to state.)	Yes. This means that your child will be identified as a child with a particular disability.	No.
Is this statute funded? In other words, does the federal government provide states and school districts with the funding to implement this statute?	Yes, though at an average of just over a third of the "40 percent of the average per-pupil expenditure in public elementary and secondary schools in the United States" promised in IDEA.	No.
What are the requirements	Both IDEA and 504 require that tests and evaluations be given in the student's native	

ISSUE	UNDER IDEA 1997	UNDER SECTION 504
of evaluations?	language; validated and proven to accurately assess the factors it is intended to measure; administered by trained personnel; and used to determine specific educational needs.	
Can my school district test or assess my child for possible special education and related services without my permission?	No. Parental consent is required for testing. However, if a parent denies consent to have a child tested, a school district may seek the authority to do so through an impartial hearing.	Yes. Parental consent is not required.
Are there any mandated deadlines for a school district completing evaluations and IEPs or 504 plans?	No. However, your state special education regulations do set forth clear timetables for procedures beginning the day you formally request an evaluation.	
Will my child receive an IEP that sets forth his present level of performance, type and frequency of special education, and related services, with the goals of such education and services stated in measurable terms?	Yes.	No. However, your child would be entitled to a 504 plan.
How often will my child's	IDEA requires that this be done annually.	No frequency indicated.

ISSUE	UNDER IDEA 1997	UNDER SECTION 504
IEP or 504 be revised?	However, parents may request changes and revisions as frequently as they see fit.	
How often will my child be reevaluated?	A multidisciplinary evaluation must take place once every three years.	No frequency indicated.
Who draws up my child's IEP or 504 plan?	Parent(s) of the student with disability; at least one regular education teacher (if the child is or is expected to be participating in a regular classroom); at least one special education teacher; a representative of the school district who is qualified to participate (as outlined in IDEA); a person qualified to interpret the instructional implications of evaluation results; at the parent's discretion, other persons who have knowledge or special expertise regarding the child; if appropriate, the child.	Whomever the school district designates. Parents need not be included.
How does each define "free appropriate public education," or FAPE?	The provision of special education and related services.	The provision of regular education services or special education services.
Does my school district have any obligation to provide an education from		

ISSUE	UNDER IDEA 1997	UNDER SECTION 504
which my child will benefit?	Yes.	No.
Must we as parents be consulted if the school district decides to change my child's placement?	Yes.	No.
What recourse do I have if I think my child is not benefiting from his current educational placement or if I believe my child's rights under this statute have been violated?	An impartial due process hearing (usually referred to simply as an "impartial hearing"), at which you and your school district present your arguments before an impartial hearing officer. If you prevail, your school district must reimburse you for the cost of reasonable attorney's fees. Once you have exhausted remedies under IDEA (i.e., gone through an impartial hearing), the law also grants parents the right to bring a civil action in any state or federal district court.	None specified. However, some states do follow IDEA procedures for 504 cases. Check your state regulations.
Who is protected under these statutes?	IDEA covers persons with specific disabilities from birth to age twenty-two, or graduation from high school.	Section 504 covers persons with disabilities across the lifespan.

ISSUE	UNDER IDEA 1997	UNDER SECTION 504
Will my child be provided with vocational training?	IDEA requires that by the age of fourteen (your state may set an earlier age, though not a later one), a child's IEP must provide for transition services. These are defined as "a coordinated set of activities for a student with a disability that are designed within an outcome-oriented process, which promotes movement from school to post-school activities, including post-secondary education, vocational training, integrated employment (including supported employment), continuing and adult education, adult services, independent living, or community participation." These must be "based on the individual student's needs, taking into account the student's preferences or interests," and "include instruction, related services, community experiences, the development of employment and other post-school adult living objectives, and, when appropriate, acquisition of daily living skills and functional vocational evaluation."★	No provision.

★Individuals with Disabilities Education Act, 20 U.S.C. §1401(30).

ISSUE	UNDER IDEA 1997	UNDER SECTION 504
What happens if my child is suspended or expelled from school due to behavior?*	A student has a right to continue receiving a free appropriate public education, even if she is expelled.	Section 504 does not require free appropriate public education for expelled students.
Does it matter that my child's behavior results from his disability?	Yes. However, IDEA sets forth a strict procedure your school district must follow (a manifestation determination review) in the event your child is suspended or expelled.	Yes. A child whose behavior is determined not to be disability related can be expelled.
Can my school district change my child's placement because of his bad behavior?	Yes, but only after the completion of a functional behavioral assessment (FBA) and a behavior intervention plan (BIP). Ten business days after the eleventh day a student has been removed from school (even if it is for a portion of a day), both the FBA and the BIP must be complete.	Yes. There are no requirements for FBA or BIP.

*If your child is facing suspension, expulsion, or other serious disciplinary action, we strongly suggest you seek outside advice from an advocate, advocacy organization, or special education attorney. These provisions are relatively new to IDEA, and not all school districts are following them as strictly as the law requires. In the post-Columbine surge toward "zero tolerance" disciplinary policies, students whose behavior is not fully understood may be singled out for disciplinary measures.

course is best for your child. The reverse, however, is not true. Eligibility under 504 does not make one eligible under IDEA.

There are exceptions to every rule, and different school districts go about things their own way. Some school districts will provide specific services under a 504 plan; others will do so only under an IEP. Remember, a 504 plan offers only accommodations and access to the same regular education that nondisabled students receive. Also bear in mind the training and experience of the educational staff who will be working with your child.

Generally speaking, though, you should consider an IEP if:

- Your child's requirements go beyond simple accommodations and involve services (occupational therapy, physical therapy, speech and language therapy, an aide or paraprofessional, etc.)
- You believe she would benefit from a smaller than average class size; placement in a special education classroom, program, or school; one-on-one teaching or assistance
- You have reason to think your child's disability may contribute to behavior that could result in disciplinary measures, such as suspension and expulsion
- You have concerns about your child's academic abilities because she has a learning disability or because her style of learning is different, unique, or not well understood
- You have concerns about your child's academic abilities because of AS-related difficulties with sensory integration, fine-motor skills, and/or emotional and social difficulties
- You have reason to believe that your school district is less than cooperative, compliant, or dedicated to special education in general or to students with disorders similar to your child's
- You have concerns regarding your child's ability to cope with attending college or postsecondary training, finding and holding a job, or living independently, which could be addressed by transition services.

A GREAT IDEA: THE IEP

The heart of the IDEA is the IEP, or Individualized Educational Plan, which must be created for every child who is eligible to receive special education services. Although the process of determining a student's needs and formulating a written plan to provide special education and/or related services seems straightforward enough, there are many different views on how to craft the best IEP. There are a number of books on the art and science of the IEP, and we recommend that you read at least one. Although IDEA sets forth what an IEP should contain, it's up to individual states and school districts to develop their own formats. Early in the evaluation process, before you begin work on your child's Section 504 plan or IEP, ask your school district for a blank IEP form so you can familiarize yourself with the format.

● ● ●

Key Components of an IEP

The format, style, and content of IEPs vary widely from school district to school district. Some are highly individualized, while others are "cookie cutter" productions in every sense of the term. One school district may take pains to craft a plan specifically to a child's needs, while others choose descriptions of a child's needs from an IEP program, complete with bar codes or a standard checklist (methods that some special education advocates consider inherently inferior). In the end, how the IEP plan looks isn't as important as what it contains and how well it is implemented by the educators who work with your child. As we have mentioned, there are dozens of books and Web sites devoted solely to the art of the IEP. According to the Learning Disabilities Association (LDA), here is a general overview of what you should find in your child's IEP:[16]

- A statement of your child's educational performance level
- A statement of annual goals, including short-term instructional objectives
- Specific special education and related services to be provided and a statement of the extent to which your child will participate in regular education programs
- The dates for initiation of services and the anticipated duration of services

- Appropriate objective criteria and evaluation procedures and schedules for determining at least annually whether instructional objectives are being met
- All accommodations and modifications necessary for participating in regular classroom education programs
- A statement of the least restrictive environment

•••

Understanding Goals and Objectives

In IEP terms, a goal takes a broader, long-range view of a student's development in a particular area. The objectives are the skills or behaviors the student must master for him to reach that goal. Goals are viewed as being long term; objectives as relatively short term. You should look to see relationships between goals and objectives: If the goal is the fruit at the top of the tree, the objectives are the rungs on the ladder your child will climb to reach it. Objectives should state clearly what your child will learn to enable him to reach his goals.

According to Robert F. Mager, whose *Preparing Instructional Objectives* is a classic on the subject, "An instructional objective is a collection of words and/or pictures and diagrams intended to let others know what you intend for your students to achieve." Objectives consist of three key elements:

Performance: what the student is expected to do (write a three-paragraph book report using correct grammar, spelling, and punctuation; or orally answer three questions about a book he has read; or write a book report that is punctuated to the best of his ability)

Conditions: under what conditions he will do it (in class, in the cafeteria, on the playground, in speech class, in gym; every day, when requested, three times a day, ten times a day; with his teacher, classmates, staff people; and so on)

Criteria: what constitutes acceptable performance, mastery, fluency, or completion. This can be described in terms of the task

(David will cut the shapes star, square, and heart within an eighth of an inch on either side of the line) or percentage of correct answers (answer twenty daily math problems at 80 percent accuracy) or occurrences (appropriately line up going to and from lunch three days a school week; work independently without talking out for a minimum of two minutes). The objective should define what constitutes "appropriately lining up" (independently walking to line without talking out, crying, or engaging in stereotypies) or working independently (the aide is at least four feet away, the student is engaged in work). In addition, the objective should state what constitutes mastery: achieving the stated criterion for ten days, for three days in a school week, for three consecutive days? While Scott probably has mastered fractions if he is correctly answering thirty questions at 90 percent accuracy every day for five days running, Kara's not talking out for two minutes over five days probably does not mean that that problem is fully under control.

All of these elements must be concrete and measurable. What does that mean? First, keep in mind that if you cannot see or observe something, you cannot measure it. If you cannot measure a behavior or performance, you cannot accurately track how a student is doing. While we may all feel comfortable with statements such as "Robert is doing much better in math" or "Sally seems to be able to read much more easily," those are not acceptable for gauging progress or for making decisions regarding educational programs or placement.

Unfortunately, experts in special education have countless horror stories about poorly written objectives and their effect. There is no way to observe or measure whether or not Ashley:

1. *improves* her social skills
2. *understands* borrowing when subtracting numbers
3. *comprehends* the meaning of idiomatic expressions
4. *increases* reading comprehension

However, we can determine whether or not Ashley:

1. independently and appropriately *greets* her teacher and a minimum of two classmates each morning with 100 percent accuracy. (Her aide observes her and tallies up greetings each morning.)
2. *correctly answers* twenty written math problems requiring borrowing at 90 percent accuracy without use of a calculator, number line, or other device. (Ashley takes a weekly written math test.)
3. *accurately explains, orally or in writing,* the literal and the pragmatic meaning of five idiomatic expressions at 80 percent accuracy after they are presented verbally and visually in speech class. (Ashley's speech teacher records Ashley's responses and tallies up her score.)
4. after reading a chapter in a fiction book at Ashley's current reading level, she will *correctly answer* three questions, chosen from among these categories: a character's actions, words, motivation, and thoughts; the background or history of the setting. Where appropriate, Ashley will predict what might occur next. (Ashley receives a written test every day after reading a chapter.)

So we know that Ashley has improved her social skills because we can see that she is greeting her teacher and classmates. She demonstrates her understanding of borrowing by correctly completing math problems, and so on.

Good objectives clearly spell out the criterion for performance, not only what the student will do but the level of accuracy required. What constitutes acceptable performance, or criteria, really depends on what the student is learning. Eighty percent accuracy in correctly answering social studies questions is fine, but 80 percent accuracy in decoding is not (imagine not being able to decode every fifth word).

The must-have resource for parents is Diane Twachtman-Cullen and Jennifer Twachtman-Reilly's *How Well Does Your IEP Measure Up? Quality Indicators for Effective Service Delivery* (see "Recommended Resources," page 325). This is essential, because it explains the process of writing goals and objectives specifically for students on the autism spectrum. This is important because most of the IEP goal banks that school districts use to generate goals and objectives are not specifically geared toward students with ASDs and may be especially lacking when it comes to those goals and objectives dealing with behavioral, social, and emotional concerns.

DEVELOPING A PARTNERSHIP
WITH YOUR SCHOOL DISTRICT

We started this chapter with a glimpse of the many strengths and weaknesses children with AS bring to academic life. Now let's consider the strengths and weaknesses of school districts and educators, particularly the administrative division responsible for special education. You may find professionals in a range of different specialties, with varying levels of understanding about AS and related ASDs. Again, there is no widely accepted profile defining what constitutes an effective program to address the needs of children with AS. The willingness and ability of your particular school district to accommodate your child and provide appropriate support and services are also highly variable. On one end of the special ed spectrum, you find administrators and teachers who are well informed, take an active role in educating themselves or staff to work with AS, and subscribe to no particular educational ideology beyond providing the program most appropriate for each individual student. At the other, you find administrators and educators who flatly refuse to entertain the notion that a child with multiple speech and OT issues whose aptitude test scores are in the 98th percentile needs any "special help," or who view your child's social difficulties as psychological and emotional problems rather than the manifestations of a neurological disorder.

Based on what we have heard from parents across the country through OASIS, the vast majority of school districts fall somewhere between these poles. For reasons we'll explore further in this chapter, a host of factors determine your local school district's ability to meet your child's school-related needs. Some are concrete: state special education regulations, money, staffing, facilities, local access to quality out-of-district or private schools, professional staff, and consulting experts. Others, while less obvious, may be more influential: personal attitudes of special education *and* regular education administrators and teaching staff toward students with disabilities like AS or ASD, or the school's prevailing culture when it comes to persons who are different. As a result, local school districts and special education programs do not always fulfill their obligations to our kids.

— ● ● ● —

Is Inclusion for Everyone?

IDEA and state special education regulations require that children with special needs be educated in the least restrictive environment (LRE). The belief that every child with the ability to learn within a regular education setting should be allowed access to it has driven the special education movement from the start. In fact, in certain quarters, it's considered politically incorrect even to suggest that some children might fare better in environments that are more structured, more sheltered, less stimulating, and less populated than a regular classroom. At the same time, educators are being pressured to move children out of special education classrooms and into the mainstream for a number of reasons: to save money, to make space for other children with special needs, or to lower the percentage of special needs students being educated in more restrictive environments.

Most parents and most special education professionals view inclusion in a regular education classroom as the most desirable learning environment, because it offers the most access to the general curriculum. (Unfortunately, many special education curricula are watered down, although there is no justifiable reason why this must be so for all students.) In addition, the regular education classroom is often simply assumed to offer superior opportunities for socialization and social acceptance.

Unfortunately, for some children with AS, the regular education classroom is a less than ideal setting. While it's possible to address many special needs through services and supports, schools don't always succeed in managing the environmental and social challenges these children face. When a school fails to address these issues, you must consider alternatives. Your child may need less exposure to the regular classroom, more time in smaller group settings, or home schooling. The general emotional well-being of your child should be considered first and foremost. (For more, see chapter 10.)

BECOMING YOUR CHILD'S BEST ADVOCATE

In 2000, the National Council on Disability released its report on the state of special education, "Back to School on Civil Rights." It found, among other things, that "Federal efforts to enforce the law over several administrations have been inconsistent, ineffective, and lacking any real teeth." One result that the report found, which many parents can attest to, is that "enforcement of the law is the burden of parents who too often must invoke formal complaint procedures and due process hearings, including expensive and time-consuming litigation, to obtain the appropriate services and support to which their children are entitled under the law."[17]

This does not mean that your school district will fail your child. In fact, there are school districts and individual schools across the country that are providing quality special education. However, it is also true that even good school districts sometimes lack the experience and knowledge to meet the needs of students with AS. In school districts that are not meeting their obligations to special education in general, the student with AS may face a particularly tough time.

It is "parent nature" to protect and defend a child, and AS probably makes most of us more protective and more defensive than we might otherwise be. For most parents, the entire special education process is fraught with uncertainty and anxiety. School is the social world of childhood, and it may be difficult even for those who accept their child's disability to see her differences made "official." Many of us carry our own strong emotions about our school experiences, good and bad.

Although as parents we are, legally, equal partners with those responsible for our child's education, in reality many of us do not feel like equals in the process. Yes, you are the expert on your child; you may even be better informed about AS than some of the professionals. Yet in the crucial details that make or break an IEP or Section 504 plan—assessment, placement, programs, related services, accommodations, and so on—we are novices, no matter how much we research beforehand. The process demands parents do two seemingly contradictory things: advocate passionately for one of the people we love most in the world while dispassionately participating in a complex (and for most of us, alien) legalistic exercise. A classic example of that tension: You want what is best for your child, but legally your school district is not required to provide it. In fact, special ed experts and advocates advise parents never to request what is "best," only what is "appropriate."

If this seems counter–"parent" intuitive, it is. However, learning to work effectively within the special education framework often requires the discipline to separate your emotions from the process. Under "Recommended Resources" at the end of this chapter we have listed books covering every aspect of special education law from basic guides on writing good IEPs to sophisticated strategy manuals. Depending on your experience, you may find room for one or all of them on your shelf. Here, our focus is on the "inner parent" and the attitudes and actions that inform true, effective advocacy.

Understand and deal with the system as it exists, not as you believe it should be. Entering the special education process is like joining a long, complex board game already in progress that most of the other players have played hundreds of times. Even if you come to the game having memorized the written rules, your fellow players have a great advantage in their understanding of the strategies and philosophies behind how those rules are actually applied. Unlike you, they also have the power to influence that.

If the special education process is like a game of Monopoly, how it is played will depend on where you live. Every game of Monopoly comes with a set of written rules, yet you probably had one friend who insisted that all the fines went to the Free Parking kitty, another who eliminated singles from the bank, and another who permitted loans to bankrupt players to extend the game.

Learn how your school district plays the game. Before you even contact your school district about eligibility evaluation and certainly before your first meeting with them, find and talk to people who have had experience with your district's special education personnel. Other parents whose children are receiving services in your district are an obvious source, but also be sure to contact:

- Local special education advocates, advocacy organizations, and attorneys in your area. When speaking to a professional who charges for his services, state your intention, be brief, and express your appreciation for his input. You may be calling on him again.
- Local chapters of disability rights organizations, including those

who represent persons whose disabilities are different from your child's. Hint: Autism and AS organizations are obvious choices, but ADHD organizations are a good place to start, since they represent a relatively large population that is routinely served in both special education and regular schools and classrooms.

- Any professionals who have treated or evaluated your child or consulted on her case.
- Any professionals you know socially who work in education. It's a small world, and teachers, therapists, and consultants often have colleagues in other districts.

Don't be surprised (or shocked) to hear someone tell you that your district is not as good as it could be. If a parent or a professional offers you an emotional account of a horror story, try to focus on the facts, not the emotion. There are two sides to every story. Bear in mind that when you're talking to parent and professional advocates, special education attorneys, and other professionals, their job is dealing with difficult situations. Few people call in the experts when things are going well. Some people feel they have an obligation to prepare you for the worst-case scenario. Again, listen and file it, but don't take it to heart. There's a real danger in bringing to the process heightened suspicion and distrust before it's warranted in your case. It increases your own anxiety, diminishes your ability to think and advocate clearly, and serves no one.

On the other hand, make note of recurring themes, such as a district's or a school's tendency to miss procedural deadlines, direct students with disabilities to restrictive environments, or create one-size-fits-all, cookie-cutter IEPs. Many school districts are less than fully compliant, and your school may be one.

Establish a relationship away from the meeting table with the key special education staff. Prior to any evaluations or meetings, ask to meet with or at least speak to the senior administrator who will be in charge of your child's case. Use this time to introduce yourself and your child. Discuss your concerns about your child (*not* the special education process itself yet) and what you may have done to date to address these, such as consulting specialists, pursuing independent evaluations and diagnosis, and any therapeutic interventions you have initiated, including things you do at home on your own (using charts, schedules, or Social Stories, for instance). Offer a succinct history of your child's experiences in school and school-like settings, at home, and in other settings (play dates, church or temple, dance class, sports activities). Be sure to give equal time to the positive as well as the negative.

Send the right message. Remember that one of your goals in having this conversation and all of your dealings with your district is to leave the impression that you are a reasonable, capable, informed, and committed parent. Try to send the right message. Even if you know that your child's last teacher was incompetent or that the inflexibility of the three nursery schools he attended contributed to his being asked to leave them all, be judicious and impersonal without deflecting blame on either your child or yourself. You may say, "Everyone at the last school agreed that David probably needs to have a teacher with special education training," not "His last teacher really didn't know what she was doing." Or "The nursery schools Alexis attended weren't structured to accommodate a child with her behavioral issues," not "There were other kids in those schools who were real brats, but they just wanted to get rid of Alexis because she required more attention."

Be careful that the explanations you offer for your child don't sound defensive. Some professionals who work with children with disabilities reflexively view as "denial" a parent's insistence that behaviors have broader explanations or that the child has strengths in addition to weaknesses. Be clear in acknowledging that your child has or may have a problem. To do otherwise is to give your school district the impression that you are uncomfortable facing your child's disabilities and may be satisfied with less help than your child may need or be eligible to receive.

Even if you have specific ideas about placement, objectives, and educational methodology for your child, keep them to yourself until all the evaluations are complete and you've had a chance to consider the possibilities. Unless you've been through the special education process before, chances are you may not be aware of the full range of available options. Your child is unique. The inclusion program or the private special education school that worked well for someone else may not be right for your child. You may be encouraged by a special education administrator to look at different classrooms, perhaps even different schools, before a placement decision is made. On the positive side, you'll have at least an image of each place and some sense of what it's like beforehand.

On the negative side, at least for some parents considering more restrictive settings (self-contained special education classrooms, specialized schools, etc.), is the realization that your child may require such help or that his classmates may also have some degree of disability. You are not less of a parent for secretly wishing that your child didn't have to be there. Acknowledge your feelings, but try to see the situation objectively. Focus on what a particular program or setting is, not what it isn't. At the same time, communicate to the special education staff and teachers that you view special placements as stops along the line to a more inclusionary setting, if that's possible or desirable for your child. Special education should function as a greenhouse, a place to shelter and nurture children as they gain skills, not a warehouse.

Which will be the best decision for your child? There is no one-size-fits-all solution. Yes, in the best of all possible worlds, children with ASDs would find a place—a comfortable place where they were actually learning—in a regular classroom or a less restrictive environment. And, of course, there are many experts out there who advocate just—and only—that. But remember: No one whose book you're reading or whose conference you attend knows your child or what your local district's resources might be. Is your child with special needs better off in a regular classroom where he is completely dependent on an aide and socially isolated from classmates because there is no school psychologist available to create a social skills curriculum for your child and the class? Or are his immediate and long-term needs better served in a smaller classroom where he can do more things independently and have more structured opportunities to interact with classmates? Ideally, the members of your IEP team will be able to answer all your questions and discuss the pros and cons of each possible choice. Bear in mind throughout that nothing said or done is ever etched in stone. Until the evaluations are complete and your child has spent a reasonable amount of time receiving special education and related services, no one truly knows what's most appropriate for him.

Another word of warning: As much as we would all like to see our children included and their deficits overlooked, be judicious about how you express this. Parents who trumpet their absolute belief that their child must be mainstreamed or "really doesn't have that big a problem" play nicely into the hands of those school districts that are more than happy to do less than what your child's needs require. Don't let educators "flatter" your child out of services (as in "He's too smart for the resource room" or "She's too high-functioning for behavior modification or ABA"). If you are distressed or appalled by the possibility that your child might "be special ed," keep that to yourself, too. School districts have been known to dissuade parents from seeking expensive (for the district) special education and services by playing to parents' fears of stigmatization. One parent told us of a school psychologist who warned her away from a self-contained kindergarten class she felt would be perfect for her daughter by saying "You don't want her in with those kids. They're all doped up on meds." Another was dissuaded from seeking an IEP by several committee members who mentioned several times that to be eligible, her daughter would have to be "labeled."

Be a professional parent. Regard your involvement in your child's education much the same way you would a business, and your relationship with the school district as a business partnership.

• Take the time to learn the laws, regulations, and school policies that apply to your child. You don't have to become a legal expert, but you should understand your basic rights and obligations as well as those of the school district.
• Obtain, organize, and update your child's school, medical, and other relevant records. Request a full set of your child's school records from your school district. Keep these, along with report cards, written communications with teachers and the district, copies of evaluations and other reports, copies of IEPs, notes and tape transcripts from meetings, and anything else you believe is important in a readily accessible file. Under IDEA, your school district is obligated to provide you with a full and complete set of your child's records. They may charge you a reasonable fee for photocopying. However, if you cannot afford the fee, your district must provide you the copies free of charge. Also know that you have the right to have included in your child's file your written objections, corrections, and clarifications to anything you find therein.

• Get into the habit of writing letters. A letter not only communicates, it becomes part of your child's official record. Contemporaneous accounts of events are invaluable, especially if you find yourself pursuing mediation, an impartial hearing, or a lawsuit down the road. Write to express concerns and ask questions. Write to restate what was said during a recent telephone call or conversation. Write to clarify your position, follow up, and confirm that promised services are being delivered. Familiarize yourself with the basic writing guidelines for "A Letter to a Stranger," which you can find at the Wrightslaw Web site (www.wrightslaw.com). The premise of the "Letter to a Stranger" is that you'll use your letters to put down in writing the key facts and events in your child's school history in such a way that the reader will consider you a fair, rational, and knowledgeable parent. Needless to say, letters that are sharply worded, confrontational, insulting, or accusatory don't make the grade. (Granted, you might feel great writing them; if so, write them, then throw them away.)

• Take notes during any telephone conversation you have about your child. Note to whom you spoke, the date, the time, and the gist of the conversation, then include a brief summary of the conversation in a follow-up letter.

• If possible, try not to attend meetings alone, unless you are comfortable doing so. We encourage the participation of fathers not only for the obvious reasons but for the fact (alas, sexist but true) that the paternal presence has been known to color the tone of meetings in a positive way. There is nothing wrong with bringing your friend or your mother, but it might be better to choose someone who can be more than simply a witness. Depending on your situation, another parent who has experience with special education, a lay or professional advocate, or, if the going gets rough, a special education attorney might be better choices.

• Approach any meeting with your school district, especially IEP meetings, like a business meeting. Come prepared and on time. (In the busier seasons, school districts often schedule meetings back to back.) Be sure you leave with a record of what was said, either by having someone along taking notes for you or, preferably, your tape recording of the meeting.[18] (And don't forget to transcribe it immediately, lest you forget an important point or have additional questions.) Be sure that you fully understand what your district proposes for your child, and precisely how it plans to implement that program. For example, who will be providing speech therapy, when, where, and how often? Also, be sure that you understand the district's reasoning behind all of its decisions, those in your favor and those not. Finally, never feel pressured to agree to anything about which you're uncomfortable. *If you have reservations about anything in your child's IEP, don't sign it.* Inform your school district that you need a few days to consider their recommendations and ask to schedule another meeting. And, of course, follow it up within a few days with a letter outlining your understanding of what occurred in that meeting.

• Remember, your child's IEP is not a "package deal." You have the right to accept some components and reject others. It is a good idea to spell out in writing which parts of the IEP you accept and which you are rejecting.

• Your child may be eligible to receive services during the summer vacation. Ask your district about extended school year (ESY) services.

• Join your local Special Education PTA (SEPTA) or other support or advocacy organization, if available. These not only can be excellent sources of information, they can also provide a sense of community and understanding.

• Study up on the art of negotiation. Special education attorney Peter Wright recommends Gerry L. Spence's *How to Argue and Win Every Time: At Home, at Work, in Court, Everywhere, Every Day* and Roger Fisher's *Getting to Yes: Negotiating Agreement Without Giving In* and *Getting It Done: How to Lead When You're Not in Charge.*

WHEN PROBLEMS ARISE

In the best of circumstances, with accurate information and the best intentions, parents and educators can disagree. When you believe that your child's education could be improved by a particular teaching method or access to a specific service, it can be difficult to hear that your school district disagrees or that your child is deemed ineligible. When the IEP you so carefully crafted hasn't been read or implemented by the third week of school or when you continue to see the outbursts you know could be curtailed or eliminated by basic behavioral techniques the teacher "doesn't believe in," it may be difficult to maintain your "professional parent" cool. Another potential trouble spot is the provision of special education or related services over the summer vacation.

You may have other parents, your spouse, and your friends encouraging you to go after your district, make a big stink, and "show them." The latest outrage may be the first or it may be just the last in a long history, and parents easily fall into a cycle of replaying past injustices, great and small.

Righteous anger is a powerful feeling and, to be honest, can be a refreshing break from the doubt, uncertainty, and anxiety many of us experience at times. But the sense of empowerment you feel is a false one. You may feel that your case and your cause are as unique as your child, when the truth is, educators have seen this all before. If you've ever marveled at how easily some special education professionals resist being persuaded by emotionally overwrought parents, consider how much practice they've probably had. Part of being professional, for them, is maintaining a caring yet neutral demeanor. Parents who routinely become extremely emotional, make threats, become verbally abusive, or attempt to dominate the proceedings probably will not get the "rise" out of professionals they would like. Some interpret this as professionals being callous and uncaring. No doubt there are some who are, but more often than not, the professionals are just being professional. The fact is that parents have a far greater investment in these outcomes than anyone else. And, besides, imagine your next district meeting with your child's teacher verbally abusing you or your chairperson pounding on the table. (If that happens, by all means, get help. That behavior from professionals is inappropriate and unacceptable.)

TRY TO WORK IT OUT

Ultimately, many decisions about accommodations, special education, and/or related services sometimes boil down to judgment calls. It may well be impossible for a parent to know the true reason why a child is being denied a one-on-one aide in a mainstream classroom, for example. You may be told it is because an aide is not warranted for your child, or that an aide would foster more dependence rather than independence, or that the presence of an aide would stigmatize your child in the eyes of her peers.

Your school district must give you prior written notice of its decision, and that should include an explanation of the decision. Bearing in mind that there may be cases in which those objections would be correct, ask your school district to explain the decision in terms of your child specifically. A reasonable explanation of a decision not to hire a one-on-one aide for Sam might be: "In Sam's basic academic subjects, he's been doing above-average work without extra help, but we do see the anxiety and related behaviors at less structured times, such as lunch and recess. We believe he warrants closer supervision or a quiet place to go to, if he wishes, during those times only." In contrast, "We find aides often create more problems for the children than they solve" or "This isn't how we do things" are not reasonable explanations, because they don't address your child's unique, individual needs.

You may never know what invisible (to parents, at least) factors may be shaping your child's education. In the case of an aide or paraprofessional, it may be district resistance to hiring additional personnel, or a classroom teacher's reluctance to accommodate a child with special needs, or her refusal to add the supervision of that aide to her duties, or the long list of other parents making the same request who have been denied and probably will restate their demands when they learn that your child got the aide. You may be told by your school district that they have had "bad experiences" with aides, because "good people are hard to find" or because "there is always a lot of turnover." That may well be true. However, a district's past failure to provide aides with better training and better wages, or to treat them as important members of the education team, does not excuse it from the obligation to provide a suitable aide for your child today.

In these situations, arguing from a moral or ethical perspective about what is "right" or "best" for your child is often ineffective. Pointing out your district's policy shortcomings may not help, either. In the best of all worlds, your child's education should not become a battleground (although you should not let that discourage you from taking up the cause in letters to your board of education, superintendent, local elected representatives, and local support organizations). Keep your focus trained on the needs of your unique child, and force your school district to do the same by asking (repeatedly, if necessary) for the reasoning behind the decisions.

In every exchange with your school district, try to bring something to the table: input from other professionals who know your child, information on a behavioral approach that worked, new findings about AS that may play a role in your child's problems, or informative books, articles, or tapes. Be knowledgeable, but avoid giving the impression that you're a know-it-all. Carol Gray, the creator of Social Stories, suggests that parents try to avoid stating the problem and offering the solution in the same conversation. Some teachers and educators may feel self-conscious or embarrassed that they do not have the same information you do.

BE REALISTIC ABOUT WHAT YOU— AND THE LAW—CAN AND CANNOT DO

Perhaps in the future, our legislators will see fit to make states, school districts, and educators fully and immediately accountable for the quality of education our children receive. At the moment, oversight is lax and accountability spotty. The rewards for a school district conscientiously following the law, adopting the most effective methods, and providing the education from which our children can derive the most benefit accrue to children and parents, not school personnel. In fact, there may well be budgetary and other pressures that work as disincentives to your school district's doing its job as well as it could and should.

At the same time, school districts know very well how slowly the procedural wheels turn. The penalties school districts, schools, and educators theoretically face for failing to meet their obligations are so rare and distant as to be nonexistent. Though every parent has the right to a fair and impartial due process hearing (and you may represent yourself, as some parents do), special education professionals know that relatively few parents have the resources to pursue it for all but the most egregious violations. Some subtly and not-so-subtly let it be known that activist advocate parents are not smiled upon and that professional advocates and special education attorneys create an "adversarial" atmosphere. (What is often conveniently overlooked is which side struck the adversarial pose that got you to this point to begin with.) This is why school districts don't always respond automatically to parental threats of reporting procedural violations or pursuing legal action the way a poorly run department store jumps when you threaten to contact the Better Business Bureau. They know from past experience that the percentage of parents who actually do follow through is relatively low.

Your goal, then, should be to take charge and steer your child's journey through what one author calls "the special education maze" with an eye to avoiding whatever problems you can and responding rationally but assertively to the first signs of trouble. The wheels of bureaucracy turn slowly, and it may be weeks or months before changes can be put in place. In the interest of maintaining a good relationship with teachers and their district, parents may feel uncomfortable pressing for quick responses or pursuing a matter on the next administrative level up. At the other end of the spectrum are parents who believe it's best to resolve matters quickly. They have no qualms about reporting problems to state and federal authorities or calling in a professional advocate or special education attorney early on. Neither approach is right or wrong. How you choose to deal with your school district will be influenced by your child, your school district, the problem at hand, and your own personality.

WHEN TO CONSIDER GETTING HELP

Most parents think of getting outside help only after they believe they have exhausted all of their options or have become too emotionally overwrought to be effective. In fact, you may consider bringing in a professional advocate or special education attorney at any point in the process. We tend to think of advocates and attorneys as a last resort, but some parents find it helpful to have them on their team from the beginning. Contrary to the belief that advocates and attorneys "create" an adversarial environment, in fact, their presence may help prevent the situations that demand such a posture later on. For some parents, using an advocate or attorney is simply a matter of practicality, because they lack the time, the energy, or the inclination to be as effective an advocate as they believe their child deserves. Also, you can learn a lot from a professional advocate or attorney, and this can improve your own advocacy skills.

To find an advocate or attorney, ask around for references. Special education attorneys are rare in some parts of the country, and you may find a lay advocate who has had extensive experience dealing with your school district. If, however, you have reason to think you may be pursuing an impartial hearing or other legal action, consult a special education attorney as early as possible. With any luck, doing so might force a change that would make such action unnecessary.

Before hiring anyone, be sure you understand and agree not only on the nuts and bolts of fees and scheduling, but also on the advocate's attitude toward the process and your school district. One parent we know consulted an attorney who advised her that the best way for her to obtain one special service by winning at a future impartial hearing was to "reject the entire IEP"—despite the fact that the IEP was satisfactory in every other aspect. Further, that IEP allowed for her daughter's placement in the perfect AS program in a private school. Had she followed that attorney's advice, she might have won the sought-after service (probably months later), but her daughter certainly would have lost her place in the very small and in-demand program. Remember, whomever you hire will be speaking for you and acting on your behalf. Just because you have hired someone to speak for you does not absolve you of your responsibility to know what is going on. If anything, that responsibility may even increase. If you have questions or problems concerning how an advocate or attorney sees your case, your district, or a strategy, feel free to consult with another advocate or attorney for a second opinion, if possible.

HOW YOU CAN MAKE A DIFFERENCE

Now, for some good news. Schools—public, private, charter—across the country are meeting the challenge of educating children with AS. Parents can and do make a difference.

What can make a difference for your child? Closest to home, if you have a kind thing to say about any of your child's teachers, aides, therapists, or other school personnel, say it. Be sure that your district superintendent, building principal, board of education, special education administrator, and anyone else in a position to help, support, or promote those who have helped your child know all about it. Write letters, arrange a brief meeting, even consider standing up and speaking for three minutes at your next open school board meeting.

When special education, understanding, and a little bit of extra effort work, everyone needs to know. More informally, the occasional note, a bouquet cut from your garden, a batch of cookies, or a special favor from you never hurt, either.

What else can make a difference? An active (and, some would say, activist) local parent organization—preferably one that includes you; administrators and teachers who are willing to learn about AS and try new approaches; and finally, parents who have the savvy to truly be their child's best advocate and who recognize when they need outside help. Ultimately, the success of your child's educational program is the result of teamwork. Taking an active role in your child's education also means taking the time to develop relationships with teachers, therapists, administrators, and others who know your child. For additional information on dealing with AS in the classroom, see chapter 11.

Recommended Resources

BOOKS

Lawrence M. Siegel, *The Complete IEP Guide: How to Advocate for Your Special Ed Child* (Berkeley, CA: Nolo, 1999).

Diane Twachtman-Cullen and Jennifer Twachtman-Reilly, *How Well Does Your IEP Measure Up? Quality Indicators for Effective Service Delivery* (Higganum, CT: Starfish Specialty Press, 2002).

Peter W. D. Wright and Pamela Darr Wright, *Wrightslaw: Special Education Law* (Hartfield, VA: Harbor House Law Press, 1999) and *From Emotions to Advocacy: The Special Education Survival Guide* (Hartfield, VA: Harbor House Law Press, 2002).

WEB SITES

Special education law is an ever-evolving field. We strongly recommend that you subscribe to the free e-mail newsletters and alerts some of these sites provide.

Amicus for Children, www.amicusforchildren.org

Council of Parent Attorneys and Advocates (COPAA), www.copaa.net

Wrightslaw, www.wrightslaw.com

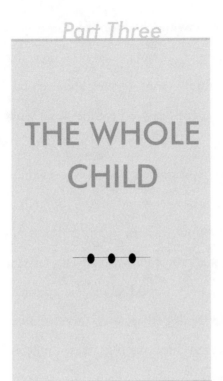

Part Three

THE WHOLE CHILD

● ● ●

As parents of children with Asperger Syndrome, we know how it is to feel like the ringmaster of a three- (and sometimes six-, or ten-) ring circus. In one ring is the school district you struggle to train to toe the line. How easily that goes depends on whether you inherited the dancing bears or the man-eating lions. In another, you (we hope with some professional help) are facing the day-to-day (sometimes moment-to-moment) challenges with the flexibility of a contortionist and the aplomb of the world's greatest magician (all the while making a mental note to start working on your mind-reading skills). In the next, you juggle the competing demands each day brings. Some days you're catching the cream pies; others the flaming swords. Meanwhile, high on that tightrope, under the spot-light, with all eyes on him, your child is inching ahead. You hold your breath as he fitfully stops, teeters, and even takes a step back. But then you hold your heart as he glides for a while with grace and confidence. Sometimes, he falls. Through it all, though, you never stop looking up, and you never let go of the net.

Until now, we've concentrated on the different "rings" the AS circus plays in. Now we turn our attention to the practical issues of parenting its "star," the child with AS. It may seem an obvious point, but how we help our kids manage emotional, social, and educational challenges is perhaps even more important than the other interventions they receive. We are, for now, the constant, and these years provide infinite opportunities for the "teachable moments" that can make such a difference in how our children understand, respond to, and cope with not only themselves but also the world.

Perhaps equally important, how well we parents learn to anticipate and handle the many difficult moments of our children's lives helps us, too. Unraveling the small knots saves your personal resources for bigger tangles. Ironically, it is in understanding your child, accepting her limitations, and applying basic "Asperger sense" and sensitivity that you—and she—make the first crucial steps forward.

The Essential Meditations

• **"I can make a difference."** The parent-teacher conference, the birthday party, the supermarket, inside your own home—is there no end to the many opportunities we share for having our parental self-esteem crushed? (This is a rhetorical question; please don't start counting.) To survive, and for your child to thrive, you have to have faith in your ability as a parent. No one is as interested, concerned, or as invested in your child as you are.

• **"My child with AS is my child first."** Especially in the time immediately following diagnosis, you may worry that you're seeing or responding to your child's AS first and the child himself second. Even in those moments when it feels as if "addressing the AS" is consuming every moment, stop and remember your child for the person that he is, not the disability or the diagnosis that he has. Make a conscious effort every day to look for and celebrate the humor, the wisdom, the joy, the affection, and the fresh worldview that is your child's gift to you.

• **"My child will grow up."** Time passes for everyone. Although it is likely that his development will be uneven and he may not always seem to be keeping pace with his same-age peers, your child will mature—intellectually, emotionally, and socially, as well as physically. With support, he will become more patient, more thoughtful, more responsible, more capable, more independent—in a word, more grown up—than he is today.

• **"I am a capable parent and person, but I am not perfect."** No one is perfect. The fact that you're facing extraordinary challenges doesn't automatically bestow upon you boundless patience and infallible judgment. (But if it's true that "practice makes perfect," you may be getting closer to perfection than you think.) Don't undermine what you realistically can do by not forgiving yourself for what you cannot.

• **"It is never too late for my child."** Rather than anguish over how late your child was diagnosed, learned to ride a bicycle, or showed an interest in making friends, look ahead. Although AS may have placed your child on a different route, with a different schedule and different stops, he is still on the journey, and it is not all one-way. There is no time limit on when he can acquire skills, abilities, and understanding. Early intervention is not the only intervention. We are all capable of learning throughout our lifetimes. People with AS are no different.

• **"It's okay to be sad, angry, afraid, apprehensive, or uncertain."** You and your child will have bad days and rough patches. There will be times you will curse this disorder and everything it brings. And there will be times when that is the only healthy, rational response. You are not a "better" person for denying those feelings or a "worse" person for wishing that life would be easier for your child. Also, don't be afraid to validate these feelings in your child. Respect his feelings.

• **"I can change the world, if only a little bit at a time."** Through simply loving and supporting that remarkable, unique person who is your child, you have already begun. Everything you do for your child and every contact you make on his behalf will make a difference not only for him but for those families who come after you. When you advocate for him, you advocate for everyone. Without even realizing it, you and your child will change the world.

• **"I am not alone and neither is my child."** There are thousands upon thousands of children and adults who are diagnosed with Asperger Syndrome. Although the AS community is smaller and initially may be somewhat hard to find, it is here for you and your child. It truly understands. And it needs you as much as you need it.

Chapter 9

YOUR CHILD'S EMOTIONAL LIFE

MANY children with AS will experience what would best be described as "emotional difficulties." We use this term with some trepidation, since too often people who don't understand AS assume that it's simply an "emotional problem." When we talk about emotional difficulties, challenges, and problems, we are speaking of those that seem to arise from the AS itself (such as difficulty regulating or modulating behavior, low frustration tolerance, or rage) and those that develop in part as a response to the challenges of AS (depression, anxiety, low self-worth, and so on).

Although social difficulties often prompt concern, the first bell ringers many parents, family members, friends, educators, and doctors notice are problems with self-regulation, frustration tolerance, and extreme or unusual expressions of anger, sadness, confusion, depression, or anxiety. In most cases, the child behaves in a manner that is considered "immature" for his age or "out of proportion" to the circumstances.

The ability of the person with AS to learn to understand and appropriately express powerful emotions is the cornerstone of several other important life skills. Socialization, maintaining friendships, and working with others in school and, later, at work all depend on learning to recognize, self-monitor, and modulate emotional responses. Ironically, by the time many parents reach the point of diagnosis, their child may have developed a repertoire of emotional responses that create obstacles to effective discipline, socialization, education, and therapy. These difficult behaviors also give our kids the unfair reputation as lazy, stubborn, spoiled, rude, selfish, self-centered, or attention-seeking. Such labels—spoken or unspoken—can take an inestimable toll on our kids' self-esteem. They can also have an adverse impact on how we feel about ourselves as their parents.

As parents, we spend more time with and exert a greater, more consistent influence over our children than anyone else. Ultimately, teaching our children to cope with their emotions falls to us, no matter how many other professionals we rely on. To some extent, virtually every moment is "a teachable moment," an opportunity to explicate and illuminate the world our children can find so confusing.

FACTORS THAT MAY CONTRIBUTE TO EMOTIONAL DIFFICULTIES

Developmentally related emotional immaturity. For various reasons, children with Asperger Syndrome appear to be less socially mature than their chronological age would suggest. Generally, it is believed that children with AS are, on average, about three years "behind" in terms of social and emotional development. One team of experts contends that between the ages of nine and nineteen, a child with AS has the emotional maturity of someone two-thirds his age. (For example, a nine-year-old has the maturity of a six-year-old.) Compared to same-age peers, they may seem more naive, more emotionally volatile, and less in control of themselves. Those whose problems with motor planning, motor skills, executive function, central coherence, and other abilities go unrecognized may develop a dependence on others for the most basic activities (such as getting dressed, bathing, finding things, and so on). Children with autism spectrum disorders often don't let parents know that they no longer need assistance the way typically developing children do. For example, most typical children will hit a phase where they revel in taking off their own clothes, which signals to parents that they can begin teaching dressing and undressing, and helping them to another stage of independence. However, a child with AS who has motor skills deficits usually cannot remove her own clothing spontaneously, therefore "missing" the chance to develop an important, independence-building skill in a developmentally appropriate time frame. At the same time, in the absence of this important signal, her parents miss out on a chance to nurture that independence by stepping back. Years of well-intentioned "help" can result in learned helplessness and an unhealthy overdependence on the prompting, direction, reminding, nagging, and presence of others. When combined with low frustration tolerance and AS's hallmark avoidance of the new, novel, or untried, learned helplessness can result in a child who seems unable to do much for himself and is "unwilling" to try.

Low frustration tolerance. Particularly as they grow older and realize that others are more capable, our kids can become frustrated and angry struggling over zippers, handwriting, and basically just knowing what to do or where to go.

Difficulty beginning and ending activity or behavior. Persons with AS often struggle with two "bookend" difficulties: starting and stopping. Some of the problems with initiation may lie with deficits in executive functioning and the inability to plan the steps of something like gathering all the books and notebooks for tonight's homework. Over time, a child may become so used to making mistakes in carrying out the simplest activities, such as getting a snack from the refrigerator or getting the right materials on her desk for the test, that she may fall into the habit of not even trying or performing tasks with a lack of mastery and fluency and/or an unacceptable number of errors. As a result, she needs more prompting. At the other end, it's hard for persons with AS to quit an activity at the appropriate time. Part of this is probably related to difficulties with transitions or change, and children who are obsessive, compulsive, anxious, or perfectionistic may have additional difficulty recognizing when "enough is enough."

Deficits in theory of mind. Despite our ability to "read" the minds of others who think like us, we are often woefully inadequate to the task of understanding the person with AS. Not only do persons with AS have problems with "automatically" understanding that other people have thoughts, feelings, and desires that are different

Actual Situation: Mummy has an apple for Tracy's lunch.

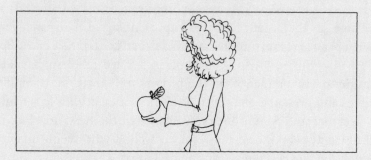

This is Tracy. This picture [below] tells us what Tracy wants.
Desire: Tracy wants a banana.
This picture [below] tells us what Tracy thinks.
Belief: Tracy thinks Mummy has an apple for her.
DESIRE QUESTION: What does Tracy want?
prompt—look, this picture tells us what Tracy wants.

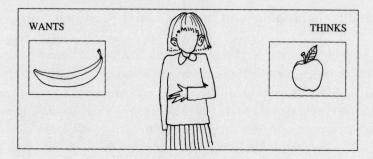

BELIEF QUESTION: What does Tracy think?
prompt—look, this picture tells us what Tracy thinks.
EMOTION QUESTION: Tracy wants a banana. Tracy thinks Mummy has an apple for her. How does Tracy feel?
prompt—does she feel happy/sad?
JUSTIFICATION QUESTION: Why does she feel happy/sad?

Outcome: Mummy gives Tracy the apple for lunch.

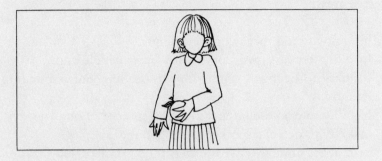

DESIRE QUESTION: What does Tracy want?
*prompt—look, this picture tells us what
    Tracy wants.*
EMOTION QUESTION: How will Tracy
    feel when Mummy gives her the
    apple for lunch?

prompt—will she feel happy/sad?
JUSTIFICATION QUESTION: Why will
she feel happy/sad?

This series of three pictures from *Teaching Children with Autism
to Mind-Read* illustrates an exercise in helping a child understand "belief-based" emotions. In this advanced mind-reading
exercise, the child is asked to determine how Tracy feels based
on what Tracy believes to be true and why she believes it. To
do this, a child with AS or another ASD must put herself in
Tracy's shoes, so to speak, and imagine how Tracy might
feel—a difficult feat for someone with mind-blindness. (From
Teaching Children with Autism to Mind-Read, Patricia Howlin,
Simon Baron-Cohen, and Julie Hadwin [Chichester, England:
John Wiley & Sons, 1999]. Reproduced by permission of
John Wiley & Sons, Limited.)

from their own, they are often at a loss as to what constitutes a correct response in a given situation.

In their essential *Teaching Children with Autism to Mind-Read*, Patricia
Howlin, Simon Baron-Cohen, and Julie Hadwin state, "Mindblindness has far wider implications for development than experimental
studies alone might indicate. Such difficulties continue to affect social

and communicative functions well into adult life." They then list ten affected areas:

1. Insensitivity to other people's feelings
2. Inability to take into account what other people know
3. Inability to negotiate friendships by reading and responding to intentions
4. Inability to read the listener's level of interest in one's speech
5. Inability to detect a speaker's intended meaning
6. Inability to anticipate what others might think of one's actions
7. Inability to understand misunderstandings
8. Inability to deceive or understand deceptions
9. Inability to understand the reasons behind people's actions
10. Inability to understand "unwritten rules" or conventions[1]

Deficits in central coherence. According to educational psychologists Val Cumine and Julia Leach and teacher Gill Stevenson (authors of *Asperger Syndrome: A Practical Guide for Teachers*), central coherence is "the tendency to draw together diverse information to construct a higher-level meaning in context."[2] Neurotypical people get the "bigger picture" without thinking. Without any conscious effort, you know that the real meaning of words and events derives from their context. You probably know that when the movie hero's love interest says she's going to "slip into something more comfortable," it has an entirely different meaning than when your mother says it coming through the door after a long day of work. The words are the same, but the context—and thus the meaning—is different. That essential contextual information is what many persons with AS cannot access without a great deal of training and concentration.

In every situation, your brain automatically sorts and prioritizes incoming information, so that when someone on the street screams at you "Look out!" you don't stop to note the color of his shoes. You understand automatically what's important and which details you must attend to in order to understand. If two people are talking, you listen to what they say but you also note their nonverbal language, how they respond to each other, and so on. You don't focus on the Coke machine behind them or the fact that today is Thursday and your dog has a vet appointment. Someone with Asperger Syndrome, however, might do just that.

Problems with central coherence are believed to manifest in such behaviors as insistence on sameness and routines, perseverations, obsessions, and, oddly enough, the development of special abilities. Sometimes a child with AS will seem to hear only part of what you said, focusing on a word with particular meaning to him to the exclusion of all else. If you say, "We may have time to go look at the model trains after dinner," your child may hear that as meaning that you are going to look at model trains.

Deficits in executive functioning. As discussed earlier (see page 56), executive function is essentially the ability to "prepare for and execute complex behavior, including planning, inhibition, mental flexibility, and mental representation of tasks and goals."[3] EF deficits are also at the core of the motor-planning difficulties many persons with AS have, as well as problems with understanding emotion and imitating the behavior of others and engaging in pretend play.

Self-consciousness, embarrassment, fear of making mistakes. Sooner or later, a person with AS begins to notice that he is different from his peers. Typically, this occurs in early adolescence, but it can happen far earlier. Children who are prone to emotional outbursts, social faux pas, teasing, bullying, or ridicule may realize this sooner. Unfortunately, many people consider people with AS "aloof," "oblivious," or "absentminded" and assume that they simply don't notice the behavior of others. As most parents can attest, that is hardly true. The pain and humiliation children with AS feel is acute and real. Unaddressed, it can lead to further avoidance of potentially difficult situations, anxiety, depression, misplaced anger, and other problems.

Difficulty with attribution. How we perceive, respond to, and later think about our experiences plays a significant role in how we see ourselves and the world. Attribution is a fairly complex psychological concept that, in its simplest terms, describes our ability to understand "the causal judgments that individuals use to explain events that happen to themselves as well as social and physical domains of life. . . . Such causal attributions are frequently answers to 'why' questions."[4] No doubt, how you perceive and make sense of, for instance, the rowdy adolescent who accidentally bumped into you on the line in the supermarket or the teacher who chose to confer the special privilege of caring for Tommy Turtle over the holiday to another classmate determines how you feel about what occurred and how you feel about yourself. If you have functional theory of mind, you can be annoyed at the rambunctious kid in the supermarket while knowing somehow not to take it personally. This kind of thing rarely happens and it had nothing to do with you personally. You can figure out from observing that kid for ten seconds that he would have bumped into anyone; you just happened to be standing there. Similarly with Tommy Turtle. Most neurotypicals would not have failed to notice that Deidre, who will be Tommy's guardian over the break, has seemed a bit sad lately because her pet frog Herman died. They would not have difficulty understanding why Deidre is getting Tommy this time. They would know that it has nothing to do with them, nor does it mean that they will never be chosen to care for Tommy in the future.

But what would these situations—and the hundreds like them we make attributions about every day—be like for a child with AS? Theory-of-mind deficits can and do result in major errors in attribution. If you cannot accurately assess the kid on line at the supermarket, what would stop you from believing that he chose you and you alone to bump into? Or that his intent was not to hurt or to anger you? Or that if he bumped into you, who is to say someone else might not do it? Or that he will do the same thing if he sees you again? When you cannot assume another person's perspective, make even a decent guess as to their possible motives, or take in the many circumstances that might contribute to a given situation, you are left with just the observable facts. Your interpretation of the situation cannot help but be in some way flawed. When persons with AS act out on flawed assumptions—in this example, say, express anger toward or even shove the bumping boy—problems can arise.

First, it is important to understand the different domains of attribution. We can view events or situations in terms of their causality (internal or external), control (stable, unchanging over time, or unstable, changing over time), and generality (global, whose effects are broad and influence many things, or specific, related only to a narrow, specific area). When you view causality as internal, you operate from the premise that you can exert control over a situation. Conversely, when you view causality as external, you assume that you exert no influence. When you view control as stable, there is no hope of change; what occurred yesterday will occur today and tomorrow as well. When you see it as unstable, there is the chance that situations might change. Just because this kid bumped you in the supermarket does not mean he or anyone else will bump you again. Finally, a global sense of generality means the rainstorm this morning that canceled the softball game has ruined the whole day. If you look at it more specifically, the rain ruined the softball game. Period. Neither way is right or wrong. What constitutes a healthy, appropriate response depends almost entirely on the situation. It's probably a good idea to regard the weather or your boss's whims as beyond your control. But it would be detrimental to your ability to function if you viewed keeping the car gassed up, getting to school on time, or seeing the dentist regularly in the same light.

Studies of typical children have demonstrated a strong relationship between attributional style and self-esteem, academic achievement, perceived loneliness, social success, and goal-directed behavior after failure, or the willingness to persist, to try again. So-called attributional abnormalities are also related to depression, anxiety, and paranoia. We know that persons with Asperger Syndrome make flawed attributions, for many reasons: lack of social understanding, problems with central coherence, deficits in social understanding.

Dr. Brenda Smith Myles, who has made landmark contributions to our understanding of children with AS, and her colleagues have studied attribution in students with AS. They found among thirty-three adolescents with AS a relationship between one having depressive symptoms and one attributing "social failure to their ability and the sum of their ability and effort."[5] The authors write, "An internal explanation or taking responsibility for negative events is associated with a loss of self-esteem."[6]

When you discuss social situations and problems, listen carefully to what your child says. What some would call "paranoid thinking" among those with AS is probably an example of flawed attribution writ large. Get into the habit of listening not only to what your child says happened or may happen but their reasoning of why they believe that. Make sure to pinpoint what kind of attributions your child is making in every emotional or social situation and be prepared to explain the correct one.

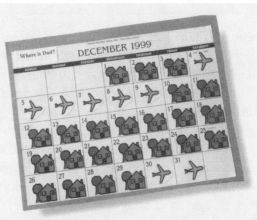

Children with AS and other ASDs often have difficulty conceptualizing time. As a result, they may become anxious when a parent or family member is away from home. This calendar was designed to answer the question "Where is Dad?" Houses are used to show the days that he will be at home; airplanes to indicate the days that he is out of town. (From Jennifer L. Savner and Brenda Smith Myles, *Making Visual Supports Work in the Home and Community: Strategies for Individuals with Autism and Asperger Syndrome* [Shawnee Mission, KS: Autism Asperger Publishing, 2000]. Reproduced by permission of Autism Asperger Publishing Company.)

CREATING STRUCTURE AT HOME

Having regular daily routines for things like meals, homework, and bedtime can have a positive emotional impact on a child with AS. Ironically, many of us find that, prediagnosis, we've developed "antiroutines." Many children with AS never got the knack of putting themselves to sleep as babies, so we end up with an eleven-year-old who falls asleep wherever, whenever, if ever. Homework, another common battleground, may be put off, avoided, or abandoned because parents and children alike succumb to anxiety and frustration. Ironclad resolutions to leave on time for school, work, and other appointments are blown to dust by unpredictable and inexplicable responses to transition. And so on. Especially before parents learn to understand their child's AS-related behaviors, family routines suffer from stress and unpredictability.

We've heard from parents who prefer not to set routines because

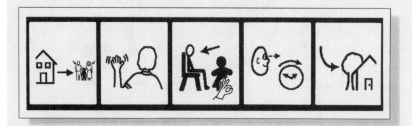

Using a simple "comic strip" format, parents illustrate for a child what will happen tonight: Mom and Dad will go out, everyone will wave good-bye, the baby-sitter will be there to care for him, Mom and Dad will return home. Having information presented visually can help a child better understand what is going to happen and when. Parents can review this information prior to going out, and the child can refer to this visual support as often as he needs to feel comfortable. (From Jennifer L. Savner and Brenda Smith Myles, *Making Visual Supports Work in the Home and Community: Strategies for Individuals with Autism and Asperger Syndrome* [Shawnee Mission, KS: Autism Asperger Publishing, 2000]. Reproduced by permission of Autism Asperger Publishing Company.)

it simply doesn't fit their lifestyle. They may believe that their kid should have greater latitude in making his own choices or is "happier doing his own thing"—even if that means staying up past midnight on school nights playing video games, skipping meals, or neglecting basic hygiene. Some reason that because their child is subject to so much structure in school, she needs or deserves a break from routine. In fact, persons with AS usually benefit from routines. Generally, they need more predictability, structure, and certainty, not less. For children who have difficulty conceptualizing time, as many persons with AS do, set routines can serve as "landmarks" (before dinner, after homework).

Another way parents can provide structure is by being consistent about household rules. Even if you felt stifled by your own parents' rules as a child, bear in mind that for the child with AS, consistency means less stress and confusion. For parents who feel they spend more time than they like watching, instructing, and correcting their children, basic rules can help to reduce their "active" involvement.

Children with AS often find comfort in rules. Having rules for everyday activities—say, for example, dirty clothes go immediately into the hamper, not on the floor, before bath time—eliminates the occasions when your child will have to wonder what to do next. Each time he puts his clothes in the hamper, it is one more opportunity to praise, one less occasion to correct, reprimand, remind, or scold.

Rules about behaviors can present a little more of a challenge, because children with AS may have difficulty understanding how to handle inconsistency. Many families find that trouble often starts with the "this time only" exception to an otherwise ironclad rule; let's say jumping on the bed, riding the scooter without a helmet, or walking the dog without his leash. Where typical children might be able to see the bigger picture and how circumstances and judgment may make it okay to bend or break a rule now and then, a child with AS might see it differently. Once you break that rule, the genie may be out of the bottle and you may find it difficult to put it back. To minimize confusion at her house, Patty developed the "always/never standard" for most situations. In other words, if it's okay to eat pizza in the den, it should always be okay; if it's not okay to eat pizza in the den, it should never be okay.

This worked fine when Justin was little, but now he is an adolescent. He needs to practice exercising good judgment, making decisions, and dealing with the consequences. It has to become his job (not Mom's or Dad's) to ask himself, *What kind of food is okay to eat in the den? Where in the den should I eat it? What should I do if I make a mess?* (He has to clean up any mess he makes.) It's time to change the pizza rule. Of course, there will always be exceptions, but sticking to a set of rules for most everyday matters will greatly reduce the number of situations open to debate and misunderstanding.

USING LISTS, VISUAL STRATEGIES, ACTIVITY SCHEDULES, AND OTHER "REMINDERS"

Deciding to have rules and routines is great. The problem sometimes arises when a child with AS knows there is a rule or routine but lacks the organizational skill or initiative to follow through. Some parents and teachers resist the idea of making lists, visuals, or activity schedules for children with AS. They mistakenly assume that these are really only for children with more difficulties and fewer cognitive strengths. That's simply not so. Remember, there are characteristics of ASDs that "cross" every diagnosis. One is difficulty attending to appropriate cues. Most of us without an ASD depend on a countless array of environmental cues to get us through our day, so that we are basically responding to a series of elaborate cascades of cues for such seemingly simple activities as getting ready for school or making dinner.

We know that persons across the spectrum have a tendency to underattend to or miss relevant cues and to focus instead on irrelevant cues. For children with AS, problems with executive functioning, possible attention deficits, anxiety, and central auditory processing issues—the list goes on and on—can turn the simple "It's time for your shower" into nothing short of an attempt on Everest. Sometimes the problem is not that our kids don't know what to do; they do. They may not know precisely how, or in what order, or what to do now after they have done whatever came before. Or they may need to have a clearer, more concrete picture of the sequence of events than they can generate internally.

An activity schedule is "a set of pictures or words that cues someone to engage in a sequence of activities. . . . Depending on the child, the activity schedule can be very detailed—breaking a task into all of its separate parts—or it can be very general, using one picture or symbol [or in the case of students with AS, words] to cue children to perform an entire task or activity."[7] Activity schedules promote independence, because your preteen son's being able to refer to a chart listing the sequence of events that should occur during showering does not need you outside the bathroom door reminding him what to do or later reprimanding him because he forgot to wash his hair. In this case, you could type up a list of steps (turn on shower, wet hair, shampoo, rinse, etc.), laminate the sheet, and place it in the bathroom. For a younger child, you might draw and laminate a basic body form and number the areas to wash in order. As time goes by, and your child becomes more independent—the ultimate goal of using tools like these—you can change the list or schedule from, say, pictures to words, or from full sentences to single words. The goal is to gradually fade the cues until the routine is so well established that the activity itself provides the cues your child follows.

TANTRUMS AND RAGES

While not every person with AS experiences tantrums and rages, this behavior is far and away the most often cited "problem" behavior parents face. "Tantrum" is as apt a description as any, but it sounds babyish after a certain age. "Rage" is often the correct term, but many of us recoil from its connotations. "She totally melted down," "He blew up," and "He spun out of orbit" seem fit to describe anger that goes "from zero to sixty in a second," "is off the charts," and "out of control." We also have heard from parents who opt to use less descriptive, more neutral terms, such as "neurological episode" or "frustration response."

Regardless of why your child is experiencing outbursts, it is important to always remember—and to remind others—that this reaction is not as volitional or subject to the degree of self-awareness and self-control that the neurotypical person possesses. The more emotional your child with AS becomes, the less able he will be to reason, apply skills he does have, and control himself.

These outbursts are more likely to occur in situations in which the person with AS feels emotionally stressed, which may include such public settings as school, the playground, the shopping mall, the birthday party, and other environments that put his behavior "on display."

WHAT PARENTS CAN DO
TO HELP WITH EMOTIONAL
DIFFICULTIES

Regardless of the source of your child's emotional issue or its manifestation (crying, tantruming, withdrawal, depression, and so on), your responses must be shaped by the realities of dealing with Asperger Syndrome. These "realities" probably don't include "tough love"–style approaches, inflexibility, or the well-intentioned advice of anyone who doesn't understand AS (including family members, professionals, friends, neighbors, and strangers). One of the biggest challenges for many parents is that the best, "AS-correct" response often demands from us qualities like patience, reason, and perseverance, plus the emotional distance to maintain them. These may be sorely tested at the height of your child's meltdown, no matter how well you understand the disorder.

Difficult as it may be, you must train your focus on managing the outburst itself, *not* on addressing its causes, the manner in which your child is expressing himself, or expressing your disapproval or distress over the event. This is a tall order for those of us who would feel oddly unparentlike if asked to dispense a Band-Aid without the accompanying "How many times have I told you not to skate without your knee pads?" After all, as parents we're practically programmed to serve up, with the best of intentions, a side order of guidance, correction, advice, admonition, or warning with every dish of help, instruction, or support. For typical children, this may be effective. For children with AS, however, it may be disastrous, exacerbating tempers, fueling self-blame, and adding more confusion and anxiety to the mix.

We may feel compelled to get in that all-important "last word," but as Dr. Brenda Smith Myles and Jack Southwick, authors of *Asperger Syndrome and Difficult Moments,* perceptively point out, "It is not important to have the last word, but it is imperative that parents have the LASTING word [emphasis in original]. In this way, children will learn to understand that they can count on parents to help set boundaries for them and enforce limitations." They present four basic steps for coping with the potentially interminable debates parents and children with AS are prone to:

1. Say what you mean—mean what you say.
2. Say it only twice in a calm voice.
3. Verify the child's understanding. If the child processes information visually, you may need to choose your words carefully. Consider using icons or pictures to facilitate understanding.
4. Stop talking and take action.[8]

Although the steps are simple, following them through in the midst of a crisis isn't always so. The key to managing outbursts productively—that is, so your child emerges from the experience with more self-control and self-esteem—is first controlling your own responses. We each have different capacities for coping with emotionally charged situations. Parents who are naturally uncomfortable with confrontation, who feel it is inappropriate to express strong emotions such as anger, or who have been traumatized by physical or emotional violence, may have an especially difficult time dealing with rage. If you have problems maintaining self-control on a fairly consistent basis or if you find yourself avoiding the issue (and letting your child become increasingly out of control), consider seeking professional help to address your feelings. Remember, your child's sense of the world as an unpredictable place is a key component of his anxiety and possibly his outbursts. What could be more frightening than a parent out of control or unable to reestablish control? Enough said.

SUPPORTING A HEALTHY EMOTIONAL ENVIRONMENT AT HOME

Conflict is a natural part of growing up and learning to separate from one's parents. The challenge facing parents of children with AS is that the nature of the conflict is significantly more complex. All children need discipline and a sense of limits, and children with AS may need them even more. You probably watch your child with AS more closely; her vulnerabilities may make you quicker to intervene, to correct, to explain. Add to this your child's limitations in social understanding and emotional awareness and it's hardly surprising that misunderstandings, arguments, and outbursts occur. When it comes to preventing and responding constructively to emotional outbursts, most of the dos are actually don'ts. Here is a list of what *not* to do:

• **Don't believe that tantrums and rages "come out of nowhere."** They don't. If you look carefully enough, you will probably be able to identify the trigger or the antecedent of your child's outbursts. It may not be the same for each one, but it will usually follow a pattern that involves sensory issues and other environmental factors, anxiety, misunderstanding, social difficulties (teasing, bullying, rejection), fatigue, or stress, to name a few possibilities, or some combination of these.

• **Don't assume that there is "nothing" you can do.** It's true that there is nothing you can do to "stop" a rage cycle in progress, but you are in control of many other important factors. You can be sure that your response serves to defuse rather than exacerbate the situation. You can remove your child to an environment or situation conducive to better control. You can study the situation for information that will help you prevent or better manage future outbursts.

• **Don't ignore the warning signs or the conditions that you know may prompt an outburst.** The signs appear as ominously as dark clouds before a storm. Some kids whine, complain, repeat the same questions anxiously, or become unusually quiet. Others engage in "nervous" habits: toe tapping, finger tapping, pacing, nail biting. Their tone of voice may change; they may appear tense; they may grimace, roll their eyes, or use other facial expressions to convey their discontent. You can divert a tantrum before it explodes in a number of ways. Each child is different, and what works for one may not work for others, but try redirecting your child's attention, using humor, asking him to engage in something of special interest to him, gently directing him to a familiar, routine activity, or removing him from the situation in a calm, neutral way ("Let's go inside" as opposed to "Let's get away from that noisy lawn mower"). Some children respond to touch or a mutually agreed upon nonverbal "secret signal" that lets them know you know they're uncomfortable. In one family's house, this "rumbling" stage, as one expert terms it, has often been short-circuited with the simple "Do you need a hug?"

• **Don't respond to the behavior; respond to your child.** Communicate to your child, verbally and nonverbally, that you are there for her, that her behavior will not drive you away, and that you are her ally—not her enemy—in the fight for self-control. Don't say anything about how the outburst is making *you* or others feel.

• **Don't use too many words.** Considering that words are, according to Dr. Fred R. Volkmar of the Yale Child Study Center, the "lifeline" through which persons with AS understand the world, it is little wonder that parents sometimes feel compelled to talk a child through a tantrum and end up making a bad situation worse. In the moment of rage, words are just more sensory static, irritating and distracting. The more you say, the more likely you are to provoke further anger and frustration. Sometimes it's best to say nothing.

• **Don't say what you don't mean or fail to do what you say.** When you do speak, say less, but mean it more. In other words, strip your language down to the basics, then, at the first sign of a possible storm, be prepared to act. You could respond to the classic toy store meltdown with "Okay, well, if you're going to get so upset because you don't want to share trains here at the train table, I'm afraid that we're going to have to leave," then watch your child throw himself to the floor. Or you could simply say, "We are going now," take your child's hand, and leave the store—even if that means your nephew's birthday present is left in the shopping cart, your child is screaming bloody murder, you have to pick him up and carry him to the car, and everyone in the store is looking at you. No bargaining ("If you want to try one more time, and if you can behave, we'll stay"—honestly, how many times has that ever worked?), no cajoling ("If you stop crying now, I'll give you a cookie"), and no permitting the situation to deteriorate because you must finish shopping or you refuse to let these tantrums run your life. Someone must be in control, and it has to be you.

• **Don't expect your child to handle situations that you know are beyond him without support and an escape plan.** Sometimes as parents, our wishful thinking gets the best of us. We may know that Jeremy hates hearing children singing "Happy Birthday" and that Sarah panics inside movie theaters. Yet sometimes we are persuaded to "give it another try" by our fears that they may never learn to adapt, the influence of others, and sometimes even our children's desire to do certain things. It is important to help your child expand his repertoire of life experiences. You should encourage new experiences, but treat them like "experiments" and don't burden your child unfairly with responsibility for the outcome. If Jeremy wants to attend his best friend's party, have a plan to take him for a walk outside the party room during the singing. Go over with Jeremy what's going to happen as many times as it takes, then be sure you see it through, even if it requires that you be the only guest's parent who stays for the party. If Sarah is determined to try to go to the movie all the other kids are talking about (and any indication that your child wants to be part of the crowd should be supported), try to determine what caused problems in the past. Was the sound too loud? The theater itself too large? Too crowded? Did she feel trapped because those she was with wouldn't leave at the first signs of her distress? Is she worried she may have to use the automatic hand dryer in the restroom? The list goes on and on. Be a detective and do your research. If your child can tell you what bothered her the most, perhaps you can find a solution: a quieter theater (sometimes older neighborhood theaters that haven't been modernized with state-of-the art sound systems are more tolerable), going at a less popular time (weekday afternoons as opposed to Saturday afternoons), wearing special earplugs, going someplace where there are paper towels (or, better yet, packing a few in her pocket), letting her know that if she is uncomfortable, you will leave immediately. No matter what the outcome, praise your child for her courage, point out everything that she did manage to handle, and let her know that you are proud of her and willing to try again when she is. One mother we know estimates she spent over a hundred dollars just buying snacks and sitting through previews before her daughter could finally manage a whole movie. But it was worth it. Most important, ask your child what she thinks would make the experience a better one next time.

• **Don't expect your child to read, understand, or respond appropriately to your body language or facial expression.** Don't depend on nonverbal communication to carry important messages such as "I am becoming annoyed," "Your behavior is inappropriate," or "I am losing my patience." At the same time, be on guard for the negative, antagonistic messages you may be sending through rolling your eyes, frowning, crossing your arms in front of your chest, turning away, and so on.

• **Don't ask rhetorical questions.** This staple of many parents' crisis repertoire—"What were you thinking?" "Don't you know better?" "What do you want me to say?" "Can't we go to the supermarket once without you making a scene?" "Is it too much to ask that I can finish a phone conversation without being interrupted?"—can be very threatening to a person with AS. He may feel pressured to actually answer a question that (a) has no answer, and (b) is only adding to the verbal barrage.

• **Don't make generalizations.** Statements like "You always do this" and "You never do that" are provocative and beg to be argued (something some of our children seem all too adept at).

• **Don't use sarcasm, hyperbole, or gentle teasing to make your point.** Even persons with AS who can understand your real meaning when they're relaxed may not be able to do so when they're upset.

• **Don't issue ultimatums or say you will do something that you cannot or will not follow through on immediately.** Ultimatums such as "If you don't stop screaming, I'll leave the room" may be effective if your child has not been swept away by a full-blown outburst and is simply in the habit of yelling to get your attention. (Remember, always determine the purpose of your child's behavior before deciding how you will address it.) Under "non-rage" conditions, there's nothing wrong with teaching the art of negotiation ("If you can sit quietly through the rest of your sister's recital, you can have some extra time on the Game Boy"). Once your child has lost self-control, however, any "deal" that demands he control what he obviously cannot will only add to his already overwhelming stress and anxiety. In fact, the prospect of future unpleasant consequences may make it harder for him to regain control, not easier.

• **Focus only on the present moment and the issue at hand.** Disconnect your child's present behavior from the past or the future. Neither he nor you can control either, and recalling past "failures" or predicting future ones undermines your child's ability to regain control and his self-esteem.

• **Don't teach, preach, or explain until your child is safely out of crisis.** Practically speaking, it's a waste of breath, because your child simply will not be able to take it in and process it in any useful way. Extra verbiage only adds to the "noise" and the stress of an already difficult situation. Later, when your child has recovered and is in a calm, receptive mood—and that may be fifteen minutes later or days hence—you should revisit the situation with him, propose reasonable ways that he might handle it differently next time, and let him know that he will have support if he needs it.

• **Don't outnumber and overwhelm your child.** If you can keep your crisis interaction to a one–on–one exchange, so much the better. Sometimes parents and family members can develop a good "tag team" strategy that plays to their strengths. Mom may be good at weathering the outburst calmly as Dad delivers the recovery hugs. Since there may be times when you need backup (the other parent, a family member, a friend), be sure ahead of time that everyone understands the rules of engagement. It's not unusual for a child to "re-explode" when third or fourth parties, well meaning though they may be, toss in their two cents by repeating what you may have already said, asking their own questions, or attempting otherwise to help. One mother told of her child spinning further out of control when, after saying "I hate myself!" his grandmother insisted, "No, you don't! What a terrible thing to say! It breaks my heart to hear you talk like that." Sometimes a person with AS simply cannot handle being spoken to by even one person, much less a chorus. If you see that someone else's involvement is causing distress, use a silent signal or simply say "I am handling this. Please leave." Do not explain, debate, or argue then, but later do make sure that everyone understands how to respond in the future.

• **Don't let your words or actions have any point or goal beyond helping your child regain his emotional equilibrium without feeling guilty, "bad," or in any way diminished in your eyes or his own.** When it's over, be supportive and loving. Try to arrange for him to have some quiet downtime, be alone, or do something he finds relaxing. Let him know that you understand how difficult it is for him. Although it may feel strange to offer compliments on your child's behavior during a meltdown, if there is any way in which your child has exhibited improved self-control—say, by not using foul language, by letting someone know he was feeling stressed before the outburst, by not hitting or throwing things, by regaining control more quickly—praise him explicitly and generously.

● ● ●

What to Do in Case of Personal Crisis

Unfortunately, despite everyone's best efforts, children with AS sometimes reach a point of emotional crisis. This can be due to severe depression, anxiety, or another disorder; adverse reaction to prescribed psychotropic medication or alcohol or illicit drugs; or a tantrum or rage cycle that has gone far out of control. Other crises may occur because a child is experiencing suicidal or violent thoughts and impulses, which he may attempt to act upon. As the parent of a child with AS, it's easy to feel that no one—not even the professionals—understands how to handle AS. As a result, some parents are reluctant to seek emergency medical help or the aid of law enforcement to help bring a rapidly deteriorating situation under control. Sometimes a crisis arises out of another crisis—for instance, a child runs away and hides during a house fire because he's afraid of sirens, or bolts from an emergency medical technician despite the fact that he is bleeding profusely from a cut.

Every child is different, and the resources in your community are different as well. So while we cannot offer a one-size-fits-all step-by-step guide, here are some suggestions for coping with crisis.

• Be prepared. The first thing you do after closing this book should be to learn what you can do in your community to protect your child in the event of a crisis.

• Before the crisis, establish a relationship with a psychologist, psychiatrist, or physician in your community who is knowledge-able about your child and the impact of AS on him. This way you will have a professional who can speak for your child in the event other medical professionals or law enforcement personnel become involved.

• Educate your local law enforcement officials about the fact that you have a child with an ASD and guide them to the resources available (see "Encounters with Law Enforcement and Other Authorities," page 465). Before the crisis, pay a personal visit to your local police precinct and ask to speak with someone there about your child and AS.

Dennis Debbaudt, the father of a child with autism and a private investigator who is an authority on law enforcement issues and ASDs, also recommends that parents and adults with ASDs consider carrying with them at all times a small card, which you can type up and have laminated, that includes the following information: the person's name, the diagnosis and its basic symptoms and behaviors, medications he may be taking, your name and numbers as well as those of his doctors and school personnel who are familiar with him, particular sensitivities or extreme reactions (panic when touched, fear of sirens, and the like). It should also indicate that persons with AS may have diffi-culty understanding their legal rights, and that if arrested, they must be protected from the general jail population. Teach your child that if he is approached by a law enforcement officer, firefighter, emergency medical technician, or other community helper, he should immediately tell the person that he has Asperger Syndrome (or other ASD) and/or ask permission to hand that person the card.

• Before the crisis, contact the local chapter of the Autism Society of America, any other autism- or mental health–related support group, and your local mental health department. Some organizations, institutions, and government offices can provide "crisis teams" of personnel especially trained to deal with persons in psychiatric crisis. Find out if such an organization exists in your community, contact them, and talk to them about your child.

• Find out from your child's doctor the name of another doctor who could talk to authorities or medical personnel in the event that he himself is unavailable.

• Find out which organizations and hospitals in your area have knowledgeable personnel on staff in the event that your child's doctor isn't available. You might want to contact the head of a local children's hospital or the pediatric department of a local mental health center, then speak with someone about your child and whether they would be willing to respond to other medical and law enforcement personnel in the event of an emergency.

• During a crisis, keep calm and call for help the moment you sense the situation is veering out of control. If at all possible, try to make contact with the local mental health center, your child's doctor, or a representative from a local autism or mental health organization before dialing 911. Try to have someone at your side who will be able to work as a liaison between your child and law enforcement or medical staff, if the need arises.

• Some localities offer 911 identification systems, so that if you do need to call 911, those responding will be notified that your child has an autism spectrum disorder. If your community has such a system, have your child's condition entered today.

• Always have a brief written description of your child's condition, medication he may be taking, and situations or behaviors he may react adversely to. Remember, you may not have an opportunity to discuss these points clearly in an emergency situation.

• If your child is removed from your home or from school, try to accompany him and explain his disorder and its ramifications to everyone directly involved in his care. Be very vocal and clear about the fact that your child's ASD and related conditions may place him at high risk for adverse reaction to psychotropic medication. Before anyone tries to "give him something to calm him down," demand that they first contact your child's doctor or another physician familiar with the disorder. This is especially important if he is currently taking or has recently taken psychotropic medications—both prescription and illicit.

• If your child is held in a hospital under psychiatric observation, impress the need, with the help of your child's doctor, therapist, or teacher, to make the environment as therapeutic as possible. Dr. Brenda Smith Myles suggests that familiar teachers can play an important role by spending time with the child and being part of the treatment team.

• If your child is arrested, contact agencies and organizations for support and for referrals to attorneys who specialize in handling such cases. Again, your child's doctor should be involved, as should anyone who knows your child and can explain his behavior.

• If you have a personal attorney, make sure that he is aware of your child's disability. It is better that your lawyer or someone in his or her firm be educated about Asperger Syndrome before a crisis occurs.

• If your child will wear it, consider getting her a MedicAlert bracelet or pendant. For a minimal cost (currently $35 for the first year, plus $20 for each year thereafter), you receive a bracelet or pendant with basic contact information—child's name, list of medical or psychiatric conditions, allergies, medications—plus the MedicAlert ID number health care or law enforcement personnel can give at the service's toll-free, twenty-four-hour number to obtain more details. In addition, MedicAlert, in conjunction with the American Academy of Pediatrics and the American College of Emergency Physicians, offers a special service designed for children with special health care needs. Once a medical professional contacts MedicAlert, a detailed form that you and your child's doctor fill out and submit to MedicAlert is faxed out immediately. You can contact MedicAlert by phone at (888) 633-4298 or on the Internet at www.medicalert.org. This Web site includes a special section about autism.

WAYS TO INCREASE
EMOTIONAL AWARENESS

Most people who don't have AS paint their emotional self-portraits and landscapes from a full palette. Not only can we automatically access dozens if not hundreds of shades of happiness, sadness, anger, joy, disappointment, fear, and surprise (to name only a few emotional states), but we can mix them and qualify them in infinite combinations to precisely describe our experience to ourselves and to others. Most of us understand the concept of having mixed feelings. We can be thrilled at the prospect of a new job yet reluctant to leave coworkers who have become friends. We are able to hold in our minds responses that, on the surface, seem to be in conflict, like the classic "love/hate" relationship. For a person with AS, the relationship between those two emotions is more often than not an either/or proposition.

In comparison, persons with AS seem to have a far more limited emotional spectrum, with most of the shades concentrated at either end and few representing degrees of feeling that fall in between. As a result, the child with AS may respond to situations and people in ways that seem extreme, out of proportion, or inappropriately intense. Though no one has determined precisely why this occurs, experts agree that helping persons with AS learn to recognize, understand, modulate, and express their emotion more appropriately is crucial.

There are many ways to teach a child with AS about emotion and to expand his emotional palette. Social Stories and Comic Strip Conversations, as well as social skills training and cognitive behavior therapy, can all help. Using pictures, photographs, and a mirror, you can teach your child not only how to read the facial expressions and gestures of others but how to mimic them appropriately. Through role-playing and watching and discussing videos, movies, or television programs, you can increase your child's understanding of tone of voice and body language, as well as broaden his understanding of how others think, feel, and may be expected to act. For children who have difficulty modulating their responses, creating an "emotion scale" that uses objects, symbols, numbers, or words to convey different degrees of, say, happiness or frustration can be very helpful.

— ● ● ● —

Henry's Anger-mometer

Children with Asperger Syndrome often have difficulty identifying, modulating, and expressing their feelings in a manner that is appropriate to a given situation. Devices like this anger scale can make the idea that there are different levels of any emotion concrete for children. It can also help them identify the conditions that warrant one degree of intensity as opposed to another.

CONDITION	HOW ANGRY AM I?	IT WOULD BE SMART TO (Choose all that you need!)
Red	I feel like hitting someone or something or running away.	Ask for time out in a safe place right now.
Orange	I feel like screaming or calling someone a bad name.	Ask for help right now. Take deep breaths.
Yellow	I felt like screaming for a moment, but I feel less angry now. I'm still thinking about it.	Sit down and try to remain quiet. Tell someone how I feel right now.
Green	I wish it didn't happen, but it won't ruin my day.	Talk about it later.
Blue	All calm. I was annoyed for a minute, but it's over. I'm okay now.	Ask to talk with Mom or Dad. Draw a comic strip or write a Social Story with someone now. Draw a comic strip or write a Social Story with someone later. Think about my dog Bert. Think about my favorite movies. Imagine resting safely in my underground secret laboratory (my bedroom).

This scale was developed for Henry, a nine-year-old fan of science fiction disaster movies, who has assigned color-coded "condition" levels to his angry emotions. Henry also needed some reminders of what he could do to bring the "alert level" back down. There are a dozen options available to Henry at every alert level, and he is responsible for choosing which he needs in any given moment. He may need more than one; for example, he may have been taught to stop and practice deep breathing whenever he feels angry. If he's feeling in the "blue zone," that may be all he needs. This scale also recognizes that some choices may not always be available (for instance, Mom and Dad may not always be available to talk, or Henry might be somewhere without a designated safe place to go to). For children who need more guidance, you might want to pair up just one or two possible actions they can take with different condition levels. Be sure, of course, that all of the activities, persons, or situations listed are available. You can also make one using photographs of your child playacting different emotions.

Be your child's "emotional guide." Get into the habit of narrating and explaining your own emotional and social behavior. Telling a child who is inconsolable over the restaurant being out of chocolate mousse that he is "overreacting" teaches him nothing. However, you can use your own disappointment in a similar situation to teach. Instead of ordering blueberry pie when the waiter tells you the mousse is gone, let your child know what you're thinking. You might say to your child in an upbeat tone, "I was looking forward to the chocolate mousse, so I'm a little disappointed, but I'm glad they have blueberry pie. I like that, too. Sometimes restaurants and stores run out of things we want and we get the chance to have something else that we like. I know I'll get to have the mousse some other time."

Let your child know when you're faced with situations that are problematic for him—handling a change in plans, disappointment, or misunderstandings. Expressing anger inappropriately is a common problem for children with AS. Beyond the obvious—not modeling behavior you don't want your child to copy, like slamming down the phone or shouting—you can narrate the thoughts, feelings, and decisions that help you handle your own reactions. "I'm sorry that your sister broke that special plate, but I know it was an accident. She said she was sorry, so I know that she feels bad about dropping it. Sometimes accidents happen to people even when they're being very careful. Accidents aren't anyone's fault. I wish the plate hadn't broken, but I'm not upset about it."

Remember the importance of generalization and how difficult it is for many of our children to "carry over" skills from one environment or situation to another. Your child may be learning a range of skills in different areas: how to greet friends in socialization, how to organize himself for work in school, how to tie his shoes in OT. Still, he needs you to help him learn to use them in the real world. Stay on top of what he is being taught and find out from his teachers, doctors, therapists, and others what you can do to help him practice his new skills and apply them more widely. Never underestimate the reinforcing power of small, everyday activities. For a child with problems with visual discrimination, that could mean being given the "job" of finding his favorite flavor of ice cream in the supermarket freezer. One with fine-motor issues can get in a lot of practice just opening food packaging while you cook dinner or buttoning his little sister's coat after he buttons his own.

Teach independence—which is the true root of lasting self-esteem—at every opportunity. Hard as it may be to do, resolve never to do for your child what she can do for herself, even if that means taking three minutes to put on a pair of socks or ten minutes to set the table. Do whatever you must to help your child become more self-reliant. Give your child ample opportunities to practice making decisions, dealing with consequences, and managing emotions. When faced with a difficult situation, run down a mental checklist and determine how your child views the situation and what specific deficit or deficits might be at work. If the problem is executive function, then you need to focus on organization. If the social misunderstanding arises from an erroneous attribution, get out paper and the markers and draw that Comic Strip Conversation. Anxiety about Mom's upcoming business trip? Make a calendar like the one on page 340, or visit Web sites that might show the hotel where she will be staying or some of the places she will be going. Show your child that you have Mom's phone numbers and can reach her. Make a tentative schedule for calling her or plan to send an e-mail to her every day she is away. Write a Social Story explaining why moms make business trips, stressing that she will be available and she will come home.

A FINAL WORD

It is not always easy to set clear priorities when it comes to addressing the many issues related to AS. However, regardless of how much your child may need this service or that treatment, your first priority should always be his mental health and emotional well-being. Free your child from the worries, anxieties, fears, and difficulties that you can. Teach him to understand, to cope, and to compensate for those you cannot. Show him through your words and your actions that you not only love him, but that you respect him, enjoy him, and value him. Let him know that he is a person who deserves the respect and the affection of others. Help him to build a foundation of self-esteem and confidence from which he can one day venture into the world on his own.

Chapter 10

YOUR CHILD IN
THE SOCIAL REALM

ULTIMATELY, for all children and adults with AS, social skills and social difficulties will have a profound effect on virtually every aspect
of their lives. When most of us think of "social skills," we think in
terms of our child learning to get along with others and to have personal relationships. In addition, social ability colors virtually every
other experience. We have heard from many parents of children
with AS and adults with AS whose opportunities for satisfying,
meaningful education, employment, and recreation are often severely undermined by their poor social skills. Social skills difficulties
have other repercussions. They make our children more vulnerable
to those who would take advantage of them or do them harm; they
render our children open to unpleasant, even dangerous "misunderstandings"; and they make it easier for them to retreat from even
positive, rewarding social interactions and relationships. According to
Dr. Tony Attwood and Carol Gray, "A recent study examined the
perceived quality of life of high-functioning adults with autism and
Asperger Syndrome, and only one variable, 'hours spent with
friends,' was able to significantly predict the scores on any of the
quality-of-life measures. These adults valued and desired friendships
more than anything in their lives, yet few had the ability to maintain
acquaintances, let alone friends."[1]

We do not mean to devalue time spent in other pursuits or to say that our children or adults with AS must become social butterflies. But most children with AS *do* desire friendships yet are weak in the types of skills that, in most cases, lead to the development of these types of relationships.

Clearly, children with AS need specific, explicit instruction in developing social skills. Participation in structured social skills group training and one-on-one cognitive behavior therapy can be extremely valuable, as can using tools such as Social Stories, Comic Strip Conversations, visual strategies, and theory-of-mind exercises. More than anything, however, our children need practice in social skills across as broad a range of experiences and situations as possible. We must aggressively capitalize on every opportunity to teach, reinforce, practice, and increase our child's social ability.

That sounds great, right? However, when it comes to teaching someone social skills, most neurotypical people find themselves at a loss. We can figure out how to teach a child how to read, ride a bike, or tie his shoes because these are skills we ourselves were taught by someone else or that we learned by observing others. There were certain steps involved, seemingly natural abilities already in place, prerequisite skills we developed from infancy on because we could observe the behavior of others and apply our native theory-of-mind skills to understanding what we saw, and we tapped these to develop ever more complex and sophisticated skills. Most of us feel, understandably, that social skills came naturally, and in a sense they did. If asked to explain what you observed that led you to assume that your best friend was reluctant to discuss her latest date or how you figured out that the telephone solicitor's promise of a free Caribbean cruise was a scam, you would probably say, "I could just tell." But how? You probably don't know how you know, or if you do, you would need a few minutes just to explain it.

Our minds automatically take apart every life experience and "file" its components—the thoughts, actions, emotions, and attitudes of ourselves and of others—for future use. Even more important, and amazing, these components can be recombined in infinite combinations. We can apply what we learned about the bully on the elementary school playground to dealing with our boss, our experience of being a child to the experience of raising a child, our grief to comfort another. Or we can call upon information learned outside our own direct experiences to guide our responses. Even if we have never encountered the specific situation—for example, attending a religious ceremony that is different from our religion—we are able to draw on information we have read or heard about to help us know what to do. Even more important, we are able to look around the room and see how others are responding and adjust our behavior, attitude, tone of voice, facial expression, body language, and the words we use and how we say them accordingly.

To varying degrees, persons with AS lack those abilities, so that what is observed and retained (which may be limited to begin with) remains a discrete, unique event whose social and emotional components are neither broken down nor retrievable in "pieces." In cooking terms, it would be like amassing a pantry Martha Stewart would envy yet being unable to conceive of using the flour, sugar, eggs, milk, vanilla, baking powder, and salt in anything but a particular sugar cookie recipe.

Barb recalls a time when one of her son's classes was temporarily held in another part of the building. After class was over, he asked his teacher where he should go to wait for her. She gave instructions, which he thought he was following. However, when he went to what he thought was the right hallway to wait, he discovered that he was alone. He lacked prior experience or knowledge of the hallway, and he'd never been in a situation in which he was lost in the school. The biggest problem, however, was that he didn't look to see where the rest of the class was heading.

A SPECIAL CHALLENGE FOR PARENTS

Since the social skills arena is usually the one in which our children's differences and deficiencies are the most glaringly obvious to others, if not ourselves, we—and our kids—may harbor painful memories of their social failures. At a certain age, children may also be reluctant to venture into those social spheres that have been difficult for them. One mother we know says, "As much as I believe Sam could benefit from spending time on a quiet playground with a few good friends, we have such a history of 'disasters' there, he avoids it. And, if I'm honest, I admit that I'm secretly relieved. Just recalling the looks we got from other parents and kids, and the terrible meltdowns Sam had there through the years is enough to make me cry even today."

Encouraging children to participate in building social skills isn't always easy, either, and it's not hard to understand why. For someone with AS, it's difficult, frustrating work. It demands that they think and behave in ways that are counter to their natural social instincts, and that alone can be anxiety-provoking. Most of all, though, the process of practicing social skills may be, from your child's point of view, a high-risk venture. Just as more social exposure increases the chances for success, it also increases the opportunities for misunderstanding, embarrassment, and rejection. While it's never too late for a person with AS to benefit from social skills training, older children may be more resistant to starting therapy than younger ones.

Though most parents can understand the need for expanding a child's social repertoire, some feel conflicted. As one father observed, "My twelve-year-old daughter says that she doesn't want or need friends. She says that she prefers to be alone. Part of me sympathizes with her and agrees that maybe this is just who she is. Another part of me, however, is always looking ahead and wondering. Does she prefer to be alone because it's so hard to be around other people? Or does she really want to have a friend or two but is afraid of trying?" Again, the familiar questions arise: Is AS something to have or someone to be?

Teaching a child with AS about social skills requires a clear-eyed assessment of where he stands today. Understanding why your seven-year-old dominates the few play dates he has or why your preteen cannot talk to his peers without talking *at* them is useful only insofar as it leads you to the most appropriate intervention. If you find yourself saying "Well, that's just the way she is" or "She has AS, and that's part of it," remember that "the way she is" without intervention may not be the way she "is" at all. It may be "the only way she knows how to be" at present. Social skills are learned.

BASIC SOCIAL SKILLS

For most parents, the greatest advantage of developing social skills is the ability to participate comfortably among peers and, they hope, to have and to become a friend. Though there are many components of what we term *social skills* (see chapter 6), and educational and therapeutic interventions should all involve some degree of social skills training, here we will focus on what parents can do.

Reinforcing Social Skills in Daily Life

In addition to Social Stories, Comic Strip Conversations, social skills training, and cognitive behavior therapy (all discussed in depth in chapter 6), there are other tools and techniques you may find helpful in building social skills.

Visual strategies. You can use drawings, calendars, charts, schedules, photo essays, and other visual tools to "show" as well as tell. You might, for example, use a circle to indicate which people in your child's life are "close family," "family," "close friends," "friends," "neighbors," and "strangers" and describe what types of greetings, physical contact, or topics for opening conversation are appropriate for each.

Playing board games. Board games are fun and can provide good practice in basic social skills such as turn taking, listening, observing cues (e.g., whose turn it is to roll the dice), planning, and motor planning, among others. Cooperative, as opposed to competitive, games require that two or more players work together toward a common goal. Some wonderful examples of these types of cooperative games are made by a company called Animal Town; Save the Whales, for example, is a game in which players work together rather than against one another. In a simple game of checkers, developing a defensive strategy demands some degree of perspective taking ("What will my opponent do if I do this?") and consideration of what your opponent may be thinking.

Movies, videos, television programs. Movies and television programs—particularly those on video, which can be paused, stopped, rewound, and repeated—can be used to draw your child's attention to and discuss many social skills–related topics. For younger children, programs such as *Sesame Street, Mr. Rogers' Neighborhood, Blues Clues,* and *Thomas the Tank Engine,* as well as films such as the *Toy Story* series, *The Iron Giant, Lilo and Stitch,* and others offer ample fodder for discussions about understanding the behavior, feelings, and thoughts of others. Because the narrative is often simple and the characters' facial expressions exaggerated, children with AS may find them easier to follow. For older children, just about anything that is not excessively stimulating, violent, or otherwise inappropriate may be rich with discussion possibilities.

Reruns of programs such as *Third Rock from the Sun, The Beverly Hillbillies, Mork and Mindy, Mr. Bean, My Favorite Martian,* and similar "fish out of water" comedies base their humor on the premise that characters lack necessary social skills for the environment in which they find themselves. Not surprisingly, persons with AS are often drawn to fictional characters struggling to understand an "alien" culture: Mr. Spock from the original *Star Trek* and Data from *Star Trek: The Next Generation,* as well as characters from other classic science fiction TV series such as *Dr. Who, Babylon 5, Star Wars, Hitchhiker's Guide to the Galaxy, The Prisoner,* and others. The current flood of movies and television series about comic book superheroes (*Smallville, The Justice League, Teen Titans, Spider-Man, X-Men*) often depict characters whose specialness is a double-edged sword and who work hard to make sense of the mere mortals whose world they must share. The Harry Potter movies (and books) provide many examples of characters who are not what they seem or whose motives are questionable. You can watch or read along and ask your child what makes him think Gilderoy Lockhart is not really brave or Professor Snape is not really pleased to see Harry back at Hogwarts. Beyond discussing the obvious (the plot, the characters), you can also draw your child's attention to and talk about what a character means when he shrugs his shoulders or the different ways in which different characters greet each other. You can explore questions surrounding a character's thoughts, motivations, and feelings. How can you tell someone is lying? Why do you think she did that? What is that character "saying" without talking? What might happen next?

If possible, seek out videos and DVDs that touch on or include something of your child's special interest. Documentaries on even the most technical subjects, such as the development of the jet fighter or the history of the personal computer, usually have some human interest angle worked in. You can talk about what those involved in developing technology thought or felt about what they were doing.

Mirror work; audio and video recording. In a safe, relaxed at-mosphere, working with your child in front of a mirror or recording and playing back his voice and/or image can help him get a sense of how he appears and sounds to others. With practice, children can be taught to modulate their voices and use an appropriate style of speech. You might practice how to say "no" to a friend's offer of ice cream, your brother's daring you to jump on the new couch, or a stranger's inappropriate advance. You can also teach and practice appropriate fa-cial expressions, such as accompanying most greetings with a smile or using gestures appropriately with and without words. There is one "yuck" face appropriate at Grandmother's when the brussels sprouts get passed around that is quite different from the one you make when your brother puts a worm in your ice cream. There is one hello for friends in church, another for those same friends out on the play-ground; one "excuse me" for politely interrupting a conversation, another for accidentally breaking Mom's favorite vase, and so on.

Mirror work and recording are also good for learning to express and interpret the different meanings of the same sentence when you change the volume, cadence, tone of voice, stress, and facial expres-sion. For instance:

I didn't know you wanted the red apple today.
Meaning: You are mistaken. You didn't tell me that you wanted the red apple today.

I **didn't know** you wanted the red apple today.
Meaning: I really didn't know you wanted the red apple today; I'm not lying.

I didn't know **you** wanted the red apple today.
Meaning: I'm sorry I gave it to Suzy. I didn't know you wanted it.

I didn't know you **wanted** the red apple today.
Meaning: I didn't think you cared whether you got the red apple or not.

I didn't know you wanted the **red** apple today.
Meaning: I thought a green apple or a yellow apple would be okay; you didn't tell me the apple had to be red.

I didn't know you wanted the red **apple** today.
Meaning: I thought you wanted the red grapefruit or the red pear.

I didn't know you wanted the red apple **today.**
Meaning: I planned to go shopping tomorrow; you didn't tell me that you wanted it for today.

Regular comic strips and comic books. Because they tell a story with visuals as well as words, comic strips and comic books can also be used in teaching some social skills. In our OASIS survey we discovered that the highly visual Japanese animé comics are very popular among older kids and adults with AS. Unlike movies and television programs, comics have the ability to show what a character is thinking and saying and doing in the same "frozen" frame. Obviously, some comics are more suited to this than others, depending on your child's age, reading ability, interests, and so on. If your child has anger management issues, you might steer clear of comics that contain violence or feature characters whose behavior you do not want to see imitated. Patty has used *Batman* comic books from the 1940s and 1950s to help Justin understand the relationship among thought, word, and action because they are graphically less impressionistic and less violent than later versions. (Another added benefit: a surprisingly rich vocabulary and the frequent use of colorful appositives—something persons with AS have trouble with—such as "mirthful menace," "killer clown," "grim jester," along with "villain," "criminal," and "nemesis," for the Joker.)

Novels, short stories, some journalistic accounts. Both fiction and nonfiction can be used as springboards for discussions about emotions, thoughts, feelings, and beliefs. Because prose usually lacks accompanying visuals, it may not be accessible to all children. However, for children who have sound comprehension skills, any well-told story can be explored in terms of perspective taking and point of view, the relationship between what characters mean and what they say, what they think and what they do, and so on. Reading aloud stories that are rich in dialogue and "acting out" the lines is another way to sharpen speech skills, particularly when it comes to tone of voice, stress, and volume. For younger children, you can contrast the imperious attitude and voice of Yertl the Turtle to the growing frustration of the otherwise mild-mannered Mack in *Yertl the Turtle,* or use the Mr. and Miss Books series (*Mr. Silly, Mr. Grumpy, Mr. Sad*). For older kids, characters in Harry Potter books, Judy Blume books, the Wayside School series, the Encyclopedia Brown series (there's always a bully and good guy), and the Box Car children are good choices.

Music. Good music of any genre can inspire emotions and thoughts. If your child likes music, view it as another platform from which to launch discussions about feelings and ideas. If it's instrumental music, explore what your child thinks the music is "saying" or what story it's "telling." If the music has lyrics, talk about what the song is saying, how it says it, what the singer may be thinking or feeling. Is it the same as the words she sings? Or is it different? How can you tell? If you can, try presenting your child with two different versions of the same song and talk about what makes them sound and "feel" different. Or take a simple song your child knows well and ask him to sing or hum it "happy," "angry," "disappointed," or "scared," even if the words don't fit.

BREAKING DOWN BASIC SOCIAL BARRIERS

All the world is a stage, and we are all players. While great minds ponder the true and many meanings Shakespeare intended, for parents of children with Asperger Syndrome, it really boils down to scripts and rehearsal. It may take a highly structured approach to teach certain social skills. However, once your child begins to get it, you should work equally hard at helping him learn to generalize what he has learned and apply it to many different situations.

Most of us recognize the need to prompt and prepare children for events outside the daily routine: birthday parties, vacations, doctor's appointments, the first day of school. Beyond giving a general rundown of what will happen, it's equally important to talk about where and when the event will occur, who may be there, and who your child can go to if he has a question or needs help, and to address any specific concern your child may have. (Does the place have a restroom? An alarm system in case of fire? Food? A water fountain?) Be sure to ask specifically, "Is there anything you feel you need to know about the party?" You may be surprised by what you hear. One mother told us that her son Zack avoided birthday parties through the third grade. She assumed the noise and commotion were simply too much for him. One day he said, "I would like to go to Kari's party, but I hate pepperoni." It took his mother a few minutes to make the connection. When he was five, they served pepperoni pizza at the last party he attended, and since then, he has assumed that all birthday parties serve pepperoni pizza—and that he has to eat it. No wonder the Social Stories his mother wrote and the explanations she offered him about balloons, clowns, candles, and kids screaming "Happy Birthday" hadn't worked.

When you prepare your child to go somewhere, keep details that are subject to change general. Say "Many of your classmates will be at David's party," rather than "Joey and Sam will be there," or "The party will end sometime in the hour after four o'clock," rather than "The party ends precisely at four."

Once again, we turn to our old and constant friend, the teachable moment. A mother who often took her daughter Cindy out for lunch started with teaching her how to ask the waitress for the check—which requires looking for the waitress, waiting for her to approach and ask if you would like anything else, and then pausing—and to say "Thank you" (preferably while making eye contact). Once Cindy mastered that, her mother taught her how to order. Again, it was a great minilesson in watching another person for the cues that signal "your turn," listening for and responding to questions about the order, saying "thank you," and so on.

Cindy became a favorite at one restaurant, with staff and strangers commenting on how polite and well-mannered she was. That became a lesson in recognizing, accepting, and acknowledging compliments. One day her mother was pleasantly surprised to hear Cindy say to the waitress, "Thanksgiving is next week. Are you going to spend it with your family?"

"Why, yes," the waitress replied. "How about you?"

"Oh, I'm going to my grandmother's. She makes pumpkin pie. Do you like pumpkin pie?"

"I sure do."

"Okay." Then after a few seconds of silence, Cindy looked up again and chirped, "Have a nice Thanksgiving!"

"You, too."

Once Cindy became comfortable with the "restaurant routine," her mother helped her adapt it to the doughnut shop, the pizza parlor, the bakery, the ice-cream store, and the fast-food place—each of which presents its own variations on the basic theme. Next on Mom's agenda: paying for the food, waiting for change, saying "thank you" again; after that, counting out the money and checking the change.

◆ ◆ ◆

Bullying and Teasing

Persons with AS and related disorders are even more likely to be targets of teasing, harassment, and bullying of both a verbal and physical nature. There is truth to the saying that there is "safety in numbers." Victims of bullying and teasing are likely to be those children on the perimeters of social groups, the loners, the children who don't fit and are perceived by their peers as being "different." There are certain times and areas where teasing and bullying are much more likely to occur—unstructured and less closely supervised times at school such as lunch, recess, in school hallways, in bathrooms, in locker rooms, and on the bus; anywhere your child might be perceived by his attacker as "alone" or without help. For example, some students find the walk to and from school the worst time of day. Too often school districts take the position that what happens "off school property" is not their responsibility. These are the times when most children with AS face the greatest challenges socially and are the most vulnerable, emotionally and physically.

Most OASIS parents report that their children who are harassed on a regular basis are painfully aware of the abuse inflicted on them, though others report that their children don't even understand that they are being teased, threatened, or made fun of. Although there seems to be a greater awareness of the dangers of allowing teasing and bullying to continue, OASIS parents report that a "kids will be kids" attitude prevails. Too often teachers, family members, and friends seem to believe that children with AS will learn appropriate social behavior if they find themselves shunned or teased by other children.

One mother reported that when she told her son's teacher about an incident in which a bully called her son a "retard" and pushed him on the playground, the teacher first refused to believe the incident had occurred, then added, "Well, your son *is* different and it bothers the other children." Other parents have reported numerous occasions in which the response to their complaints about teasing have amounted to blaming the child with AS for "bringing it on himself" by essentially being who he is. None of these responses are acceptable—from children or adults—or should go unchallenged.

When bullying and teasing are not addressed appropriately (i.e., stopped), the child with AS may be provoked to respond in kind or be forced to physically defend himself. Unfortunately, the chances are good that the person(s) provoking your child are socially savvy enough to "hide their tracks," so that all a teacher or other witness sees is your child responding, not the provocation. The child with AS who does fight back may be viewed as the aggressor and not the victim.

In today's school climate of "zero tolerance," a child who in frustration does fight back or act out risks suspension, expulsion, and perhaps even involvement of law enforcement officials (see box "Zero Tolerance Policies in Schools," page 399). When older children are bullied in junior high and high school, quite often the bullying goes unreported, out of fear that "telling" will make the abuse worse.

We know of families who have opted to home school rather than continue to subject their children to constant harassment from bullies. While incidents of both verbal and physical bullying occur at all grade levels, parents of children with AS report that incidents seem to peak during the junior high school years. This is not to say that bullying stops at high school, but parents report that it's much more likely that their teen is teased and rejected than physically attacked.

Unfortunately, bullying and teasing aren't confined to peers. All too often, children and adults with ASDs are subjected to teasing and harassment from adults, teachers, coaches, friends, and family members who persist with the misguided belief that they can embarrass or shame someone into "acting normal." Siblings of children with disabilities are often teased as well.

It is *imperative* that our children and their siblings be protected from both physical and emotional abuse from anyone. One hundred percent of the adults with Asperger Syndrome who have participated in the OASIS message boards or contacted Barb through the Web site report the devastating effects these kinds of incidents had on their lives. Parents can attest to the pain and suffering their children feel as a result of being bullied by their peers.

How Parents Can Help

- We urge all parents to have an IEP or Section 504 service plan in place that specifically recognizes that a child with limited social skills and other disabilities may be especially vulnerable to teasing and bullying and that addresses how bullying and teasing will be handled.
- Be aware of where and when bullying is most likely to occur. Make sure that there is proper supervision during recess, lunch, before and after school, between classes, and in areas such as hallways, playgrounds, restrooms, locker rooms, and on the bus.
- Document incidents of bullying and report them to school officials. Remind your school district personnel—orally and in writing— that an atmosphere of harassment constitutes a violation of your child's right to a free appropriate public education and make it clear the first time you contact them that you will pursue the matter as far as necessary.
- If your school district is unresponsive or unable to protect your child, report incidents to local law enforcement officials. Several OASIS families discovered that the harassment did not stop until they involved the police. This may not be the best first response, but if your child is in danger you may have no choice.
- Call a lawyer who specializes in special education law. Your child is being teased and harassed because of his disability, and the school's failure to protect your child may constitute a form of discrimination.
- Supply your school with a copy of *Gray's Guide to Bullying* by Carol Gray.[2] In this guide she discusses bullying and how it impacts children with ASDs. She points out that the definitions of bullying that are currently being used by most school districts are clearly not inclusive of children with Asperger Syndrome. As a result, the usual types of interventions may not be as effective.

- Be aware that bullying may be happening to siblings of your AS child. They may be too frightened or embarrassed to tell you. Be very clear with all of your children: Teasing and bullying are not acceptable and you can and will protect them.
- Carefully weigh what you teach your child about how to handle teasing and bullying. There are a number of books on the market that outline how to "bully-proof" your child, but these tactics may be ineffective for our children, who may not have the skills to carry them off. Social skills training often addresses this very issue, teaching skills such as the right "comeback," how to find help, and ways to behave that may discourage bullying. Be aware that among certain groups, ignoring—something some bullying programs and well-meaning advisors promote—can be interpreted as the ultimate sign of disrespect and a provocation.

THE BASIC SOCIAL SKILLS

Different authorities have different opinions of what constitutes a basic social skills repertoire. Unfortunately, there are few widely available, basic resources that outline a comprehensive step-by-step program for teaching social skills. (See "Recommended Resources," page 393.) You'll doubtless devise a program using a number of different interventions. You can help your child most, however, by looking through "Asperger eyes" at every conceivable social opportunity and finding a way to make the world make sense to her and, equally, help her to be better understood by the world.

A good place to start is assessing your child's current level of social ability. Dr. Tony Attwood and Carol Gray list the following behaviors as crucial components of effective social interaction or, as they term them, "friendship skills."

Friendship Skills
1. Entry skills
2. Assistance
3. Compliments
4. Criticism
5. Accepting suggestions

6. Reciprocity and sharing
7. Conflict resolution
8. Monitoring and listening
9. Empathy
10. Avoiding and ending

Learning How to Join In

When it comes to approaching other children, or responding to another child's approach, many children with AS literally don't know where to begin. You can see their discomfort as they remain on the sidelines of the action, fail to pick up on the invitations (verbal and nonverbal) to join, or seem to ignore a peer who expresses an interest in them or what they're doing. This inability to connect stops the action before it even has a chance to start. A child who doesn't respond to social overtures may be viewed as rude or uninterested.

How parents can help. Chances are, there are situations in which your child joins in or invites others to join him. For many children with AS, that may occur only at home, with family. If that's the case, talk with your child, perhaps using a Social Story or a Comic Strip Conversation, about what he's doing right. For example, "I notice that when you see your little sister Jasmine doing something you want to do, you first get her attention by saying 'Hi, Jasmine,' or 'Excuse me, Jasmine,' and then you ask her if you can color, too. That's a friendly thing to do. You can also say those same things to your cousins, and kids at school, no matter what they're doing."

Sometimes persons with AS simply miss the social cues, partly because they don't recognize them and they pass by quickly. For children who are more literal-minded, hearing someone say "Do you play ball?" "Are you a good catcher?" "We're short a few guys today," or "I haven't seen you here before" doesn't sound anything like "Would you like to join our game?" Be sure that when you consider the social situations your child may encounter, you cover other possible verbal cues. For some kids with AS, "Cake?" "Are you hungry?" "Got room in that tummy for dessert?" or "Do you like cake?" don't automatically translate into "Would you like a piece of cake?"

Through looking at pictures, watching videos, or drawing a Comic Strip Conversation, you can stop time, so to speak, and spend minutes pointing out and explaining the dozens of ways in which a few seconds' communication said, "Welcome. Would you like to play?" With the help of friends and family members, you can "stage" situations, so that your child can practice his skills.

Learning How to Ask for and Offer Help

Children with AS aren't always aware that someone else may know or be able to do something that they do not. This may prevent them from seeking assistance from others. Because a child with AS may not be able to read the "signs" that someone else needs help—an expression of confusion, frustration, sadness, crying, and so on—he also misses opportunities to offer help. Seeking and providing help is a basic social exchange that we use to do everything from finding out directions from strangers to starting a conversation that sparks a friendship.

How parents can help. Remind your child when he can or should ask others for help. Identify for him the types of people in different situations who may be helpful: in the doctor's office, the nurse; in the store, the clerk; at the movies, the cashier, the usher, the ticket taker, or the snack bar attendant. Teach a number of possible "opening lines"—"Excuse me. I was wondering if you could help me," "Can you help me, please?"—as well as the appropriate tone of voice, posture, gestures, and so on. Some persons with AS worry that they will "look stupid" to others. Remind your child that asking for help is a smart thing to do.

As for teaching your child how to offer assistance, focus on the "signals" that indicate another needs help. Using various visual media—photographs, videos, mirror, video recording—point out to your child the signs that someone might like assistance, everything from the polite "Excuse me" to a scream for help. Teach your child to respond appropriately and talk about what constitutes a friendly, helpful response. Talk about those situations in which he should seek out help in turn (a playmate getting hurt, an emergency) and how he would go about that (shouting, finding and telling an adult).

Unfortunately, peers and adults who seek to take advantage often initiate their contact with a request for help. Studies have shown that even typical older children who have been well trained to recognize "stranger danger" will respond to a child molester's plea to help him, for example, find his lost puppy. Teaching any child how to distinguish a legitimate, friendly request from a dangerous one is difficult. You might begin by teaching your child that while it's good to help certain people in certain situations (classmates in school or at play, an adult you know, for instance), there are other times when "helping" isn't appropriate. It's easy enough to tell your child never to help anyone do anything that is dangerous or wrong, yet it may be impossible for her, in the moment, to recognize the potential danger. Using a Social Story format, a list, or a chart, you might outline the types of help different people might ask them for, how they would show it, and what it's okay to help with: sister putting on her skates, the postman asking you to carry in the family's mail, your friend asking you to help him finish his Lego castle. Then you might talk about the types of people and requests for help that are never okay: anyone asking you to keep a secret, anyone asking you to go someplace with them, anyone asking to let them touch you or asking you to touch them. Obviously, it gets tricky, because statistically children are taken advantage of and abused by persons they know far more commonly than by strangers. And how do you make it clear that it's a good thing to keep the secret about Mom's birthday party but not to keep the one about the beer the school bully tried to coax him to drink? Unfortunately, there are no hard-and-fast rules. Just keep talking about, teaching, and demonstrating it whenever you can.

Learning How to Offer and Accept Compliments

The inability to offer and gracefully receive compliments shuts down another bridge to initiating and maintaining social relationships. A child who doesn't acknowledge compliments may appear snobbish, aloof, cold, or simply mean. We may wonder why it's so difficult for our children to give (and sometimes receive) compliments when it seems, on the surface at least, to be such a simple act. However, in her *Gray's Guide to Compliments* (a special issue of *The Morning News*; see "Recommended Resources," page 393) Carol Gray explains that there are three types of compliments—on appearance; on skills, talents, and efforts; and on personality. The basic compliment involves two people (the Sender and the Recipient) and three parts, Noticing, Paying a Compliment, and the Response.

Breaking a compliment down into steps is a good way to help our children learn how to make them. Compliments serve many social functions beyond the obvious. We usually think of a compliment as a means of showing someone that we like or care about them, but a compliment can also be a means of acknowledging someone's efforts, shoring up their confidence, cheering them up, taking the edge off a disagreement, or repairing a social faux pas.

Persons with AS may not automatically recognize situations that call for compliments, or they may not understand the point of telling someone something they "already know." As one eight-year-old observed, "My dad knows I like his cinnamon toast because I eat it. Why do I have to tell him again?" By the same token, they may not recognize the true intention, the unspoken communication, behind a compliment they receive. "I know this is a cool shirt," one young teenager said, "so why is she telling me?" It has been noted that persons with AS may respond to compliments by ignoring them, giving too little acknowledgment, or appearing visibly uncomfortable.

How parents can help. Be generous and specific in compliments you pay to your child; express your appreciation through your gestures as well as your words. You may even want to tell your child why you are complimenting him while you're at it, since for some persons with AS the "why" of compliments is not always clear. "Good job not shouting in the car" is just not as good as "I really like the way you sat quietly during the car ride. I know it's not always easy for you and I know you tried very hard. I appreciate the extra effort you put into that. It made it a pleasant ride for everyone."

In their important article "The Discovery of 'Aspie' Criteria," Carol Gray and Tony Attwood remind us that when we compliment our kids, it's best to note those qualities and accomplishments they value. A child who values his intelligence may very well appreciate a compliment on how smart he is over a compliment on how well he sat down during the test, even though the good behavior may be what you feel is the greater accomplishment. They suggest mentioning the talent itself when you acknowledge social achievements; for example, "How smart of you to remember to raise your hand when you needed to ask a question."[3]

The types of compliments that may be more meaningful for your child may change over time. For quite some time, Patty has gotten a lot of mileage out of telling Justin how his socially appropriate behaviors are "cool" and "like what a teenager would do." This works because he has a small circle of friendly preteen and teenage family friends, sitters, and acquaintances (camp counselors, social skills group helpers, and so on) he admires.

Talk to your child about compliments, explaining that they do seem illogical sometimes, but they are a way to let others know that we care about and appreciate them. Stress that paying and receiving compliments is a friendly and smart thing to do, because most people like to receive and give compliments. Remind your child that even if something is "obvious" to a person with AS, those of us who do not have AS have a "problem"—we often need to be told certain things we already know (that my dress is pretty) or that may or may not be entirely true (that it looks great on me) in this particular, illogical, redundant way. And then point out occasions to compliment, and prompt your child, if necessary, to practice the art.

Use the *Gray's Guide to Compliments* workbook (which appeared in *The Morning News*; see "Recommended Resources," page 393) as an aid to help your child understand the types of compliments and to practice giving and receiving them.

Learning How to Understand and Respond to Criticism

This is a difficult issue for children with AS for many reasons. Due to a lack of social understanding, a person with AS may criticize another person unintentionally, usually as a result of being blatantly honest. A child with AS may tell his chess-playing friend, "That was a dumb move," where a typical child might suggest, "Are you sure that's the move you want to make?" or "Did you see this move?" As discussed previously, children with AS usually have not built up an arsenal of social "sweeteners" (asking questions, making suggestions, using less highly charged words) with which to blunt or disguise a critical remark. Nor can they always know what *not* to say. For those who like rules, old saws like "If you can't say something nice about someone, don't say anything" can be helpful.

As objects of criticism—or what they perceive to be criticism— persons with AS can be extremely sensitive. Some have a lot of difficulty interpreting a difference of opinion as anything but criticism of them personally. The supposed esteem-saving value of such parental standbys as "I'm not upset with you; I'm upset with your behavior," may not be as clear or as effective as you'd think. As parents, we feel that part of this is due to the fact that most children with AS are the recipients of so much help, intervention, correction, reminding, prompting, and discussion about what they say and do that they reach a point of overload. Although it may seem obvious that we and others are just trying to help, most children past a certain age understand that no one "helps" or tries to "fix" what isn't wrong, broken, or could stand improvement. Problems with pragmatics and reading social cues may also cause a child with AS to see criticism in innocuous comments. Ten-year-old Peter became furious when his friend said, "Bet you can't beat me at Crash Team Racing today." Instead of interpreting it as a friendly invitation to play a video game, Peter took it literally and as an insult.

Parents have frequently mentioned that in addition to having difficulty telling the difference between a friendly suggestion and criticism, their children often seem to misinterpret the volume of the speaker's voice. We both remember numerous times when we were speaking to our sons in a completely calm voice only to be told, "Quit yelling at me!"

How parents can help. First, monitor how much criticism your child receives and over what. Criticism laced with hyperbole, sarcasm, anger, and coldness is never appropriate. If you don't do so already, get in the habit of offering necessary criticism in a caring, constructive way that protects your child's self-esteem. Model accepting criticism, too: "You know, Dad's right. I should have put the garbage out last night after dinner. I said that I would, so I can understand why he's a little annoyed."

Explain to your child and model what constitutes acceptable criticism and what does not. Help her to distinguish between criticism of something someone does or thinks and criticism of who they are (which is a very sensitive point for many with AS). Rather than saying, "Don't tell your friend Greg you think *Star Trek* is stupid!" expand the concept and offer alternatives. "It's okay not to like what Greg likes. Everybody likes different things. Friends just have to like each other; they don't have to like everything the other friend likes. One way to be a good friend is to tell Greg that *Star Trek* isn't your favorite program and that you'd rather watch something you both like. Or you can take turns watching the programs you each like."

Pay attention to the role of pragmatics in "misinterpretations" and work on making your child aware of the many ways in which people say the same things. Also teach them to recognize criticism that is unacceptable, personal, and intended to hurt.

Avoid the tendency to overexplain or repeat yourself. Give your child time to absorb the suggestion before you start talking again. Keep your suggestions clear, short, and to the point.

Learning How to Offer and Accept Suggestions

Being able to listen to, consider, and adopt other ways of doing things is a crucial skill, from the playground to the boardroom. Children with AS may have two different challenges in learning how to accept suggestions. One is that they may be interested only in doing things "their way." Those who are particularly locked into strict, ritualistic patterns of play may become upset at any suggestion that something be done differently. The second problem arises when a child interprets a suggestion of an alternate activity or way of doing things as a personal criticism. Either way, this can easily become ground zero for an emotional outburst.

How parents can help. Model flexibility by soliciting suggestions from your child (but only if you are prepared to follow them)—"Hmm, do you think we should drive home the long way or take the highway?"—and compliment him when you accept one. You might say, "I really like to take the highway because it's faster, but your idea to take the long way home is a good one. Look at all the great trees and gardens we get to see. I'm glad I listened to you. That was a great suggestion. Thank you." If your child has problems accepting suggestions from others, make a point of practicing them in low-stakes situations that you know he isn't sensitive about or that can be fun (dessert-first dinners, extra TV or video time, for instance). The point is to show your child that suggestions can have good outcomes. When you think about it, many things that don't appear to be suggestions can be dressed up to look like them for the sake of practice. Instead of saying "You can have an extra cookie," try, "May I make a suggestion? How about another cookie?"

Prior to play dates and other social occasions, remind your child that we can do only what we want to do when we are alone but that being with friends and others means we have to take turns. If you can anticipate a friend's interests, talk with your child about some of the possibilities ahead: "You know, Dan really likes your toy robot. He may ask to play with it," or "If you want to play with trains and Dan wants to build a tent in the den, we could make the train run in and out of the tent and pretend it's a secret cave. What do you think of that?"

When your child does accept suggestions and demonstrate flexibility in play, praise her specifically and generously, pointing out how much fun both she and her friend had. Also focus on teaching your child how to rephrase his requests and demands in the form of a suggestion, as well as how to adopt the appropriate tone of voice. Remind him that just like him, people prefer to be told something in a nice, friendly way.

Learning to Share and to Reciprocate

Most people would name sharing—of time, ideas, activities, objects, interests—as the essential foundation of friendship or membership. However, children with AS experience the social world differently, so they're limited in their ability to derive the full emotional, social, and cognitive benefit of what they do experience. Among the AS-related problems that may affect a child's ability to interact with others are one-sided conversational style (usually related to the special interest); lack of spontaneous curiosity about or interest in the thoughts, feelings, and behavior of others; aversion to new or novel situations and activities; insistence on sameness and routine; and difficulty understanding the purpose of "small talk" and other social exchanges that do not seem "logical."

How parents can help. Using Social Stories, pre–social event prompting, and postevent review and encouragement, explicitly explain to your child what constitutes appropriate behavior. If there is a behavior that you consider inappropriate, discuss why (in terms of how it would make the other person feel if, for example, "you sat alone in the corner and read your *Titanic* books"), and in what situations that behavior would be appropriate ("in your room before bedtime"). Point out to your child any and every time someone shares something with him—be it a joke, a smile, or a cupcake—and don't forget about yourself, family members, teachers, friends, and others.

You might consider substituting words such as *share, trade, exchange,* and *cooperate* for some of the less descriptive terms we usually use. For example, rather than "I'm going to tell you what happened when I took Sparky to the vet today," say "I'm going to share with you what happened with Sparky at the vet today. I know you care about Sparky and would like to know." Or instead of "I see you're reading a book about the Beatles. What do you think?" try posing questions that will lead to others (not "yes," "no," or "I don't know") and giving answers in which you model an appropriate response (e.g., answers with "because" clauses). You might say, "I like the Beatles, too. Let's trade thoughts. I'll ask you a question, then you ask me one. What's your favorite Beatles song?"

" 'Ticket to Ride.' What's your favorite song?" (Prompting may be required for some children to ask the question: "It's your turn to ask me a question," "I want to share my thoughts with you, but I can't if you don't ask me.")

"It makes me feel good that you asked [smile]. Thank you for asking. I like 'Ticket to Ride,' and I also like 'Daytripper' because of the guitar sound. Why do you like 'Ticket to Ride'?"

"I like 'Ticket to Ride' because it makes me feel happy and it could be about a train."

One way parents can help their children is by gently imposing limitations on common AS conversational styles that make reciprocity impossible. Setting rules for special interest talk and activity is an important one. It would be unfair, however, to limit talk among those who share the special interest. Even then, though, your child should learn the socially appropriate way to discuss the special interest and any other topic.

Try to restrict special interest talk to two times a day, for no more than five to ten minutes each time, and only after the completion of specific chores (e.g., being ready for school in the morning, setting the dinner table). You can expand this time as a reward for good behavior or other accomplishments, though you should never reduce or take it away as punishment. One family has also built into the special interest exchange other social skills practice: asking a listener if it's a good time to talk about it (and handling delays and refusals appropriately) as opposed to simply launching in; pausing to answer the listener's questions and responding to the listener's comments, which greatly reduces the run-on, one-sided nature of the talk; noticing and observing the listener's cues that it's time to wind it up (the listener breaking eye contact, humming, crossing his arms in front of his chest, distractedly saying, "uh-huh"). When the child fails to pick up on the cues, the parents verbally draw his attention to them: "I'm looking away and humming. That's how I'm letting you know that I would like to talk about something else." In this case, long-winded, seemingly endless monologues have gotten shorter as the parents give their most enthusiastic praise for "a good ending."

When it comes to sharing objects, time, or a third party's attention, children with AS may act immature for their age. Here again, the solution is making your child aware of the value of sharing in terms of how it makes others feel, and reassuring him that he isn't "losing" anything. This is sometimes a difficult concept because some children with AS see things in black-and-white terms and may be limited by certain play and behavior "rituals." Tony Attwood has identified this as the "Frank Sinatra syndrome" because everything has to be "my way."

Eight-year-old Eddie was extremely possessive of his favorite toys (a toy airport, airplanes, and related things) and was distressed when anyone interfered with his play. After a series of play dates in his home that ended in full-blown tantrums over his friend's playing with "his" toys, his mother wisely arranged for play dates in other children's homes (with her present). After each, she would remind her son that someone had shared with him and talk to him about how good it felt. She also realized that Eddie was worried that his play guest would abscond with his toys, so she reminded him many times that while he did get to play with Joey's Nintendo, he didn't take it home with him; Joey still had it. When Eddie was ready to have guests at his home, his mother removed the toys he was most possessive of, leaving him and his friend a large selection of "neutral" toys. If Eddie asked about his airplanes, she would offer him two—one for him and one for his friend—on the condition that they take turns sharing. Once Eddie's guest left, his mother reminded him that no one had taken his toys and that he also had fun playing with other things. As Eddie got older and began to treasure his play dates, his mother would include him in the planning and ask, "Tell me which toys you think you will have a hard time sharing. I don't want them to spoil your great play date with Jordan." Eventually Eddie felt secure enough that he could share his favorite toys and even play with them in different ways.

One mother found that "formalizing" her daughter's role in the play date has been helpful. She is officially "the hostess" and now very much enjoys being told she was "an excellent hostess" and specifically why. Another unexpected benefit is that it has paved the way for discussions about the role of a host and that of a guest, and how they are different (e.g., the rules of the house you are in prevail).

Learning to Avoid, Recognize, and Resolve Conflicts

A skill that rarely comes naturally to anyone, conflict resolution is essential for persons with AS. Their social deficits place them at increased risk for misunderstandings while at the same time leaving them with few, if any, effective strategies for avoiding conflict or resolving it appropriately. Every one of the "Friendship Skills" listed on page 374 should be considered an essential component of a conflict resolution "program."

Two of the more socially stigmatizing aspects of AS are the inability to consider different opinions or ways of doing things and the inability to express disagreement in a socially appropriate manner. Unfortunately, these deficits are too often read by others as stubbornness, arrogance, hostility, or worse. Persons with AS sometimes perceive personal criticism or rejection where none is intended. They may have difficulty seeing the difference between a disagreement with their idea and a dislike of them personally. One mother recalled her daughter Caroline becoming angry when a playmate declined to share in her daughter's favorite snack. Even though her friend said she just wasn't hungry, Caroline felt rejected and hurt. Another mom discovered her twelve-year-old son, Tom, screaming at his younger brother, Carl, because Carl wanted to watch a favorite television program. Even though Tom had no intentions of watching television himself, he was angry because he felt his brother's choice was "stupid," which he continued repeating long after he had made his point. When his mother suggested he go watch what he wanted in a different room, he refused. The argument was not about who had control of the TV but Tom's intense response to someone having a difference of opinion.

How parents can help. First, realize that your child isn't trying to be difficult, argumentative, or unlikable. Whenever possible, even when unacceptable behavior is involved, try to keep your focus on resolving the conflict and modeling behavior conducive to achieving that goal. The moment when your child feels most misunderstood and under attack isn't the best time to forcefully impose your own views. Also remember that most persons with AS consider their intelligence one of their greatest strengths and, like all of us, may use their opinions to demonstrate how smart they are. We find it revealing that one child we know automatically assumes that anyone who disagrees with him "thinks" or "is saying" that he is "stupid."

Whenever possible, point out when you or others disagree appropriately. Discuss in clear, explicit detail why one person might disagree and what that does ("different people think different things") and does not mean ("that someone dislikes you personally"). Reassure your child that you can disagree with someone else and still like them, that even people who love each other very much disagree. Most marriages and partnerships offer a treasure trove of compromise examples: Dad likes chicken and Mom likes fish; Dad watches science fiction and Mom is into sports; Dad rides his motorcycle and Mom thinks it's dangerous. When your child or someone else reaches a compromise, point it out, label it, and talk about the consequences. "Dad wanted us to go see *The Matrix,* and I wanted to see a love story. But instead of arguing or being upset with each other, we made a compromise: Dad gets to pick the movie this week, and I get to pick the movie next week. Even though I probably won't like Dad's movie, and he probably won't like mine, we'll have a good time, because we're together."

If your child is younger or socially immature, you might consider reducing or eliminating videos, music, television programs, movies, or video games that promote inappropriate conflict resolution styles or in which characters express disagreement with personal attacks on others, rage, or violence. Point out when people do the right thing, and encourage your child by praising even the smallest compromises in a way that the disagreement is not forgotten. Rather than just saying "That was very fair and friendly of you to compromise and let your sister watch *Beauty and the Beast,*" you might add, "even though I know you don't like that video."

If your child tends to respond to conflict inappropriately, don't deny his feelings but teach him better ways of expressing them. These can range from basic rules, such as "no shouting, throwing things, or hitting," to a structured program geared toward teaching him to monitor and control his emotions through relaxation techniques, cognitive behavior therapy, and so on.

Learning to Notice the Behaviors of Others and Oneself

For various reasons, some children with AS just don't seem to be paying attention to what goes on around them; nor are they aware of the message they send to others through their behavior, words, and body language.

How parents can help. Gently and sensitively draw your child's attention to what other people are doing and saying. Help him become, as Dr. Temple Grandin, a woman with autism, describes herself, "an anthropologist from Mars." One of the first professionals who spoke to Barb about her son and his AS pointed out the need for her to begin explaining everything to her son. For example, he recommended that she point out instances in which a boy and girl were walking down the street together chatting and suggest that by their body language and the way they were walking that they might be "friends" or even "brother and sister." If she and her son later passed by a girl and boy who were holding hands, she should explain to her son that these two had a different relationship than the other couple.

The idea behind this was not only to get her son to see what social skills look like from the outside, but also to get into the habit of being aware of his surroundings. It is not an easy lesson to learn and, as Barb's son has reminded her many times over the years, "Mom, you should know by now that I just don't notice those kinds of things." However, in many situations he has learned to take a step back and observe—very much the anthropologist. The key seems to be to teach our kids to "stop, look, and listen"—and, we would add, "think" or "analyze"—before reacting. Generally, this is more easily accomplished by older children and adults than by younger children. Even so, it takes a great deal of constant practice and gentle reminding by parents and other "cultural guides."

Learning to Respond to Others in an Appropriate Way

It may seem that the rules are fairly clear-cut: You comfort someone who is crying, you smile back when a stranger smiles at you. But if you begin to look closely at just a handful of common situations, you appreciate how much more complex the rules really are. You may put your arms around someone who is crying if you know them well, but that response would be inappropriate for a stranger. Since the ability to empathize depends so much on having theory of mind, "teaching" empathy is one of the harder challenges parents face. How do you teach someone to "care"? How do you teach a person with AS how to "decide" the appropriate course of action?

How parents can help. Use techniques such as Social Stories and explicit teaching for what types of behavior are acceptable and expected in different situations. Look at the world through your child's eyes and try to break down for him the unspoken rules of social behavior. Always bear in mind your child's penchant for taking things literally, and be sure that you teach in such a way that allows for exceptions. It is important to teach your child not only what is expected in a given situation but why, what it means, how it makes another feel, and so on. Eight-year-old Chrissie's best friend's grandmother passed away a few weeks earlier, so before their next play date, Chrissie's mother said, "Lisa's grandmother died, and she feels very sad about it. When you see her, remember to say 'I'm sorry to hear that your grandmother passed away.' "

Chrissie looked perplexed, then asked, "Why am I saying I'm sorry? I didn't do anything wrong. I didn't do anything to make her grandmother die."

Realizing her mistake, Chrissie's mother considered for a moment and then said, "Sometimes we tell someone we care about 'I'm sorry' when something happens that makes them sad or unhappy. You're right: sometimes you say 'I'm sorry' to apologize for something you did. But there are other times, like when someone passes away or somebody gets hurt, when we say 'I'm sorry' as another way of saying 'I wish this bad thing didn't happen to you, because you are my friend.' This tells Lisa that you care about her and hope that she feels better. When you say that to Lisa, it will make her feel glad that you care."

Narrate your own socially appropriate empathetic behavior and that of others, in real life, as well as in movies, books, and so on. This is particularly important if your child seems to miss or misunderstand the "point" of doing favors, being courteous, or saying or doing things (as in the case of Chrissie) that at first blush seem "illogical." After a major snowstorm, a thirteen-year-old boy was confused as to why his father was shoveling the walk of an elderly neighbor, because "Dad said shoveling snow is a big pain in the neck and he hates it." His mother explained what it meant to be a good neighbor and reminded her son of the many ways in which the neighbors had helped him in the past (by feeding his fish when the family was on vacation and bringing over cake on his birthday). When Dad got back in the house, Mom made a point of prompting him to explain that even though he didn't care for shoveling, it made him feel good when the neighbors said thank you.

When discussing a past mistake (and Comic Strip Conversations can come in handy here), try to be understanding and gentle. Rather than criticize, walk your child through understanding not so much "what was wrong" as how his behavior made others think, feel, or act. Help him to understand the possible alternatives in a given situation and recognize when to ask for help. Until your child can be reasonably expected to respond appropriately, prompt him and prepare him ahead of time, especially when it comes to "high-stakes" situations such as weddings, funerals, social events, and any situation where the rules of "behavior" and/or the other persons involved may be less flexible and forgiving of mistakes. If your child does commit an embarrassing faux pas, remind him that everyone makes mistakes sometimes (be sure to tell him about a few of your own), and be supportive. Also try to have in place a good backup plan so that he is not put at social risk unnecessarily. If, for example, you must attend the big family reunion, have a baby-sitter on call or a friend or relative who has agreed beforehand to take him to a quiet place for a short time while you fulfill your social obligation. Allow him to bring his Game Boy (sound off) or a book, keep a snack or two in your purse, and ignore anyone who feels you are coddling him.

Learning How to Avoid and End Social Interaction

Just as children with AS must be taught explicitly how to join or initiate a social exchange, they also need instruction on how to "leave the scene" appropriately. Another, related skill is knowing how to let others know that you prefer to be left alone without coming off as rude. We all know the value of first impressions, but last impressions can be equally lasting.

How parents can help. Respect your child's feelings about the people with whom he wishes to interact. Teach him the verbal and the nonverbal ways to let another person know that it's time for him to go, he's finished with the conversation, or he has no interest in an exchange. Model and practice spotting the other person's cues, finding the correct opening, making eye contact, and using the right words. Left to their own devices, children with AS sometimes appear to give short shrift to leave-takings and declining conversation. More than a few parents have noticed that even the beloved grandparents who may not be seen again for another year get the same perfunctory " 'bye" as the mailman.

Excusing oneself, saying good-bye, or telling someone you cannot talk to her right now are all occasions that have special rules. When we follow these rules and say these things in a polite and friendly way, we remind people that we care about them even though we're going to do something else or prefer to be alone. Teach your child appropriate expressions to use—"I'm sorry, but I have to go home now," "Excuse me, but I'm going to spend some time in my room," and so on—especially if your child is one to question why he just can't get up and leave. Barb remembers a New Year's Eve party at which her son (age nine at the time) quietly pulled the hostess aside and said very politely, "I sometimes get overwhelmed at large parties. Is there a room where I can read my book?" The hostess was charmed and delighted at the boy's request, offered a bedroom, and asked him if he would mind her joining him if she got "overwhelmed." While some would criticize this kind of behavior as being antisocial, look closely and you can see that her son demonstrated a number of great and necessary skills. He realized when he was in danger of becoming overwhelmed and figured out how he could avoid that. He took the initiative of approaching the hostess politely, explained his problem (self-advocacy), and asked for help.

Model the right behavior, and talk about it with your child. Help your child develop a repertoire of exit lines for a wide range of situations.

SOCIAL SITUATIONS: SIX BASIC RULES FOR SETTING YOUR CHILD UP FOR SUCCESS

1. Put your child in situations that show off his strengths, not those that expose his weaknesses. For virtually every social activity, there is an alternative. It would be unwise, perhaps even cruel, to send a boy with motor skills deficits to try out for the basketball team or demand that your sensorily challenged daughter attend her sister's birthday pool party "just like everyone else" at the noisy indoor public pool. In fact, that boy would probably do well and derive great benefit from one-on-one activities such as weight training, private or small-group lessons in martial arts, bowling, or other "individual" sports. Your daughter can celebrate her sister's birthday in a way that is more comfortable for her. Perhaps she can skip the pool portion of the program and arrive in time for snacks and cake.

2. Understand and respect your child's social limitations. For some kids with AS, a social situation with fewer social demands is ideal. For some kids, a movie and pizza afterward provides a chance for companionship without them constantly having to listen to, look at, and respond to someone else. Seeing the movie together gives them a shared experience both probably will be eager to talk about afterward. If your child can handle an hour-long play date, but invariably melts down after that, then make sure the play date runs only about an hour. Better yet, resolve beforehand that the play date will end *immediately* at the first sign that your child (or another) is unable to maintain control. That may mean accompanying him to his room while his guest gets ready to go without the standard long, polite good-byes at the door or, if you are at someone else's house, leaving carrying your child's jacket in your hands. Don't let the fact that things are going so well undermine your good judgment. Many parents can tell you from experience that those last extra ten minutes can spell the difference between social success and social disaster.

3. Go out of your way to create a social setting in your home. Creating social opportunities for a child with AS can be time-consuming, frustrating, and difficult. The reality is that you'll probably spend far more time hosting other children than your guests' parents do. However, creating a "controlled" social environment for your child has the potential to be very rewarding, with benefits that could pay off over his lifetime. As much as possible, try to make your home the place where other children will feel welcome and come to play. If you can, offer to have other children over after school (a self-limiting, short, and usually manageable type of play date) regularly. Both of us have seen our sons grow socially because we offered to baby-sit good "friend candidates" on a regular basis, which allowed both our sons and their guests a chance to get to know one another. Don't forget to involve children who are a little bit older as well as those who are a little younger. Sometimes a child with AS is more comfortable with someone not exactly his own age. Try to keep expanding your pool of potential playmates. So-called rent-a-friends are a good idea for younger children. However, they may not be as easy to come by once children grow old enough to choose their own playmates. Depending on one "friend" who suddenly stops coming over can be heartbreaking. One caveat: Be sure other parents don't abuse your hospitality and that drop-off and pickup times are observed, for your child's sake and your own.

4. Accept your child's friendship on his or her own terms, not your—or anyone else's—idea of what friendship "should be." Your child's special interest may provide the foundation for a relationship with another who shares that interest. In fact, their social interaction may appear to be about nothing but the special interest. Some parents find this distressing; however, remember that even if your daughter and her friend talk of nothing but horses, they're still experiencing companionship and acceptance. Many parents find that special interest relationships often do grow to encompass other activities. To someone not familiar with AS, our children's friendships may seem "different," and their interaction may appear atypical (which it is), but that doesn't mean it isn't valuable or meaningful to your child.

5. The play's the thing—in more ways than one. Play and social practice are perhaps the most valuable experiences you can give your child. Rehearse, practice, prompt, discuss, and review to teach your child systematically the unspoken social rules. Then provide him every possible opportunity to practice, generalize, and expand on his skills. That can include everything from having your daughter telephone her friend to invite her over to corresponding with pen pals who share her interests.

6. Acknowledge and reward every attempt at social sufficiency—even if it results in "failure." Don't forget that even when everything seems to go wrong, your child did do one brave, smart, and admirable thing: he tried.

Recommended Resources

See pages 218 and 223 for resources specifically designed to teach social skills.

BOOKS

Sabrina Freeman and Lorelei Dake, foreword by Shelley Davis, *Teach Me Language: A Language Manual for Children with Autism, Asperger's Syndrome, and Related Developmental Disorders* (Langley, B.C., Canada: SKF Books, 1996).

Rebekah Heinrichs, foreword by Brenda Myles, *Perfect Targets: Asperger Syndrome and Bullying: Practical Solutions for Surviving the Social World* (Shawnee Mission, KS: Autism Asperger Publishing Co., 2003).

Ami Klin and Fred R. Volkmar, "Treatment and Intervention Guidelines for Individuals with Asperger Syndrome," in Ami Klin, Fred R. Volkmar, and Sara S. Sparrow, eds., *Asperger Syndrome* (New York: Guilford Press, 2000), pp. 340–66.

Michelle Garcia Winner, *Inside Out: What Makes the Person with Social Cognitive Deficits Tick?* (SLP, 2000). This book is designed primarily for children of junior high school age and older. Order through www.socialthinking.com.

JOURNALS

Autism Spectrum Quarterly, P.O. Box 799, Higganum, CT 06442, (860) 345-2155. Online at www.asquarterly.com. (Formerly *The Morning News*; order back issues at www.thegraycenter.org.)

VIDEOS

Social Language Groups, by Michael Thompson Productions. In this video, Sally Bligh, a speech and language pathologist, demonstrates the use of social language groups to facilitate peer communication. For more information go to: www.aspergersyndrome.org/as_videos.html or phone (630) 357-0696.

Last One Picked . . . First One Picked On: Learning Disabilities and Social Skills, by Richard Lavoie, a leading authority on the social, emotional, and psychological aspects of learning disorders and disabilities. With grace, insight, and humor, he offers practical solutions. This is one in the Learning Project series of acclaimed videos; all of them are worth seeing. Order through PBS (800) 344-3337 or online, through LD OnLine, at www.ldonline.org.

Chapter 11

YOUR CHILD IN SCHOOL

THE strengths and weaknesses of many children with Asperger Syndrome seem to converge most glaringly in school. Those who are academically gifted or have developed special interests that are validated in school may get their chance to shine. Unfortunately, the social, sensory, and organizational challenges of school also provide ample opportunities for even these children to crash and burn. Students with AS who also contend with learning disabilities, comorbid disorders, emotional difficulties, or other issues may find each school day a struggle.

In previous chapters, we have addressed the issue of diagnosis and evaluation and the basics of special education law. This chapter is devoted to ensuring that the student with AS is understood and accommodated.

WHAT CAN BE GOOD ABOUT SCHOOL?

Your school district is obligated to provide an appropriate curriculum for children who are identified as gifted, talented, or exceptional, which many children with AS are.[1] School allows your child the chance to learn to interact with a range of personality types, to practice flexibility, and to grow toward greater independence. Finally, as a major ground for socialization of all children, school provides "practice" for simply learning to live among and get along with others.

— • • • —

AS and Giftedness

To most people *gifted* merely means exceptionally intelligent (usually an above-average measurable IQ) and/or talented. Contemporary definitions of these students also recognize other traits, including creativity, leadership, or a specific talent in practically any field of endeavor. Giftedness is also evidenced in abilities to manipulate abstract symbol systems (dance or music notation, mathematics, etc.); acquire, retain, and discern associations among quantities of information; solve problems in novel ways; and exercise sound judgment. For the *highly gifted* (IQ at or above 145), researchers have identified other qualities: intense curiosity, perfectionism, difficulty conforming to the way others think, and precocious concern with moral and existential matters, among them.[2]

The challenges and the joys of being gifted or raising a gifted child are quite complex and not always well understood by educators and other professionals. You might be surprised to learn, for example, that between 10 percent and 20 percent of high school dropouts are intellectually gifted, and 40 percent of those who graduate in the top 5 percent of their high school class do not complete college.[3] One possible explanation for these statistics is that learning disabilities are as common among the gifted as other students. Studies have demonstrated that gifted students with conditions such as ADHD are often underdiagnosed and, because of their giftedness, fail to qualify for extra help, special education, or related services.[4] Another is that the psychological and emotional experience of giftedness brings its own challenges.

Stephanie S. Tolan's 1994 essay "Giftedness as Asynchronous Development"[5] is deservedly one of the most reprinted explanations of giftedness. She quotes a widely accepted 1991 description of giftedness, attributed to the Columbus Group: "Giftedness is asynchronous development in which advanced cognitive abilities and heightened intensity combine to create inner experiences and awareness that are qualitatively different from the norm. This asynchrony increases with higher intellectual capacity. The uniqueness of the gifted renders them particularly vulnerable and requires modifications in parenting, teaching, and counseling in order for them to develop optimally." Because of the asynchrony of giftedness, these children can "appear to be many ages at once," according to Tolan—eight (his chronological age) on his bicycle, but fifteen in algebra class and two when sharing a cookie with a sibling. Further, gifted children experience an internal reality that is very different from that of their peers. The brilliance, the creativity, the achievement that we see are only the external products of an "internal reality" we probably cannot imagine, and which without the proper understanding and support can foster emotional and social problems.

We all seem to "know" or suspect that gifted children have emotional difficulties. But why? Tolan writes, "Often the products of gifted children's special mental capacities are valued while the traits that come with those capacities are not. For example, winning an essay contest on the dangers of global warming may get a student lots of attention and praise while her intense emotional reaction to the threat technology poses to the planet . . . may be considered excessive, overly dramatic, even neurotic. . . . Writing a winning essay is deemed not only okay, but admirable; being the sort of person she had to be to write it may not be considered okay."

Remember that so far we are discussing neurotypical gifted individuals. When you add AS (and other comorbid conditions) to the gifted mix, certain strengths (intensity, concentration, focus, tendency toward nonconformity, highly developed moral sense) and weaknesses (disparities between chronological age and social and emotional maturity) can increase exponentially. A child who is twice (or thrice or four or five times) exceptional needs the benefit of specialized attention, individualized educational programs, and emotional support to reach his or her potential. There is no federal law protecting the rights of gifted students, despite their clearly different and urgent needs. Most, but not all, states have mandates requiring special services for gifted and talented children. Unfortunately, in absence of a federal mandate like IDEA, when education funding gets tight or school districts find themselves meeting the requirements of other mandates for other types of students (or all students, as is the case for No Child Left Behind), gifted programs often suffer. After all, some would say—wrongly—gifted students "don't really need help."

Despite research that demonstrates gifted students' need to be educated with their academic peers,[6] many of them are being pulled back into mainstream classrooms, like too many students, swept away in the tide of inclusion. There they may be "assigned" to helping less able students instead of using the time to pursue a curriculum that challenges them. Current research dispels many of the myths about gifted children: their parents are not more aggressive about pushing them, they benefit from accelerated placement in "ability-grouped" classrooms, they do not report having lower social self-perception than others their age.

If your child with AS has been identified as gifted, learn all that you can about the issues surrounding this exceptionality. Contact national and local advocacy groups for the gifted; there are wonderful resources online. Most important, however, do not allow your child's intellectual abilities to exempt him from any special education, services, or supports he may need. Giftedness does not "cancel out" your child's preexisting needs because of AS, learning disability, emotional issues, or social challenges. It only complicates them. If anything, your child will need more individualized attention and support to reach his potential, not less.

WHAT IS TOO OFTEN WRONG WITH SCHOOL?

If asked to design an environment specifically geared to stress a person with AS, you would probably come up with something that looked a lot like a school. You would want an overwhelming number of peers; periods of tightly structured time alternating with periods lacking any structure; regular helpings of irritating noise from bells, schoolmates, band practice, alarms, and crowded, cavernous spaces; countless distractions; a dozen or so daily transitions with a few surprises thrown in now and then; and finally, the pièce de résistance: regularly scheduled detours into what can only be described as socialization hell (aka recess, lunch, gym, and the bus ride to and from school). It's a wonder that so many children with AS manage to do so well. That's not to say, however, that most of our children couldn't be doing a lot better and experiencing more pleasant, less stressful days. This chapter is designed to help you encourage, cajole, demand, or threaten your child's teachers and your school district to meet their obligations and become adept at applying the many techniques and accommodations that we know can be effective.

• • •

Zero Tolerance Policies in Schools

In the past few years, there has been an increase in violent acts in schools throughout the United States. The movement toward so-called zero tolerance of violence and aggression gained force in spring 1999, after two students opened fire on their classmates, killing twelve students and one teacher and wounding twenty-one before committing suicide at Columbine High School in Littleton, Colorado. Although it is imperative that all children be safe in school, indiscriminate application of zero tolerance policies have placed children with AS and other neurological differences at risk for being labeled or "profiled" as a danger to others. In some places, this has fostered a witch-hunt environment, in which hearsay and isolated incidents carry far more weight. For example, a straight-A student with Tourette's syndrome, few friends, and a limited social life was suspended from his school a day after Columbine because a fellow student told a teacher that she "could imagine that he might commit such a crime."[7] This teen and many other students throughout the country have been subjected to interview, review, suspension, and expulsion for exhibiting behaviors that fall well within the diagnostic criteria of AS and other disorders.

We mourn the loss and the pain of students victimized by school violence. The fact remains, however, that our children are far more likely to be victims of such actions than perpetrators. We must protect our children from becoming, in a very different way, victims of these tragedies. Persons with AS may respond with aggression or violence when threatened, bullied, rejected, frustrated, or otherwise provoked. They may voice the thoughts and feelings most other children would know better than to share: "I hate you," "I'm going to blow up this school," "I hate everybody," "I'd like to kill the kid who knocked me into the locker," and so on. While these behaviors are likely related to AS, and the person is someone who responds like this under stress, they may make your child a target for zero tolerance enforcement.

There are other things about persons with AS and ASDs that add to what some would call a "suspicious" profile. They may choose to wear loose clothing or wear the same clothing every day. Because of sensory issues, they may hold their bodies in such a way that they appear to be hiding something. If this same child lacks friends or has formed relationships with other children who are perceived as outside the mainstream, he could be perceived as being "antisocial," a "loner."

It is very important that your child's school district be made aware of his diagnosis and that he have an IEP (and thus the disciplinary protections under IDEA) in place before something happens. (There are no special provisions regarding discipline for disability-related behaviors under Section 504.) In addition to taking the actions mentioned throughout this book to increase your child's social skills and create a positive environment in school, establish your own zero tolerance policy for bullying and teasing of your child as well as inappropriate responses from teachers, administrators, and staff.

If your child does experience outbursts, be sure that their occurrence and the circumstances surrounding them are documented. Be sure that your child's doctor, therapist, or another professional familiar with him addresses the nature of his behavior in a letter to your child's teachers and principal, with copies sent to the superintendent and your board of education. If necessary, obtain written backup from an advocacy or mental health official or organization documenting the fact that your child's behavior is a direct result of his disability. Let everyone know—in writing—that in the event he is threatened with disciplinary action, you will vigorously defend your child's legal rights.

Finally, the wisest course is preventing such incidents from occurring. Again, helping your child develop social skills and emotional control, coupled with a supportive and understanding educational environment, can go a long way toward preventing misunderstandings and undesirable behavior.

THE EXPERT PARENT

Your primary responsibility as a parent of a student with AS is determining how much the professionals in your child's school know about the disorder and then filling in the blanks however you can. "Code" statements that betray a clear misunderstanding of your child and AS that you might hear include "If only he applied himself," "He's so smart, why can't he . . ." "Her inappropriate behaviors get in the way of her learning," "He uses his sensitivity to noise to avoid work," "His outbursts are nothing more than attention-seeking; the more attention we give them, the worse they will get," and, our personal all-time favorite, "She simply has to get used to the noisy lunchroom/teasing/remembering to bring home her books/[you name it]."

Few educators can expect to fully understand the ramifications of autism spectrum disorders without some training. Don't wait for your school district to provide this special training (although, legally, it is obligated to) or allow well-intentioned but unprepared staff to try to figure it all out on their own. Don't assume that simply by having an IEP, a 504 service plan, or other education program in place that your child's teacher will fully understand either him or AS. Take the initiative. Create a notebook for your child's teacher (and consider making a second copy to go in your child's file for others to see) that includes information about AS and the specific behaviors and issues he faces. You might use colored divider tabs and organize information under such sections as "Sensitivity to Noise," "Play Skills," "Dysgraphia," and so on. Rather than fill the notebook to the brim with every piece of information you find, try to pick the one or two most comprehensive and authoritative pieces you can find. Lend educators videos and books, provide print material, and let everyone know that you are always available to talk about AS. However, try always to do so with tact and understanding. The sudden rise in autism spectrum disorders caught most educators by surprise. In many instances, your child may be among the first in the school district correctly diagnosed with AS.

It's important to establish a good relationship with your child's teacher. You can be cooperative and friendly in the classroom without undermining your effectiveness as an advocate at the IEP table. Even when you feel strongly about a matter or wish to share information, be tactful above all else. Educators may feel self-conscious because they lack, through no fault of their own, adequate training or experience in dealing with children like ours. Try to be sensitive in how you present your ideas and suggestions. Even if you are, for now, the resident "expert," be sure everyone knows that you are first and foremost a team player who is interested in helping create an environment at school that works not only for your child but for everyone: teachers and other students alike.

THE OASIS ASPERGER SYNDROME GUIDE FOR TEACHERS

There's a lot more to your child than what his teacher might read in his records or his IEP. Rather than leave your child's teacher to develop a relationship with him based on trial and error, introduce your child through a letter that you can copy and distribute to anyone who may need it. Be sure to send a copy to your school district and ask that it be included as part of your child's permanent records.

This letter is based on the work of OASIS forum members. In 1999, OASIS forum member Elly Tucker invited other members to contribute suggestions for a "letter of introduction" for teachers about Asperger Syndrome and how it affects a particular child. The result was a thorough, detailed, but succinct overview of AS. (You can see it in its original form at the OASIS Web site under "Education.") Because we have covered elsewhere in the book many of the points in her original guide, we are not reprinting it here verbatim but offer this suggested format based on her work. The material in italics is the type of thing you might add. Feel free to add or delete sections to fit your child. You can download this form letter from OASIS ("Education") and tailor it to your needs. Since we first published it in late 2001, it has been downloaded thousands of times.

— • • • —

Letter of Introduction

Dear _____,

We are the parents of _____. Our child has been diagnosed with Asperger Syndrome, a neurological disorder that is related
to autism. He also has the following comorbid conditions [list] and
learning disabilities [list]. While AS affects many aspects of behavior, it
shares with autism the "core" deficits in social understanding and language. Simply put, our child sees and experiences the world differently from people who do not have AS. He may seem to "overreact at
nothing" or become very emotional "for no reason." We have learned
that in most instances, there is a reason for why our child responds
the way he does. And it is a reason that "makes sense" once you
understand AS. We have also learned that there are things we can do
to help him. The first and most important is accepting that many of his
behaviors are not under his control.

If you have not heard of AS, it is because it is a fairly new diagnosis
here in the United States, although it has been recognized elsewhere
in the world since the 1940s. People with AS often have a unique and
at times unusual mixture of abilities and deficits. They may appear to
be more capable than they actually are. AS is a pervasive developmental disorder, and it can affect virtually every facet of a child's academic, social, and emotional life, sometimes in ways that may be
unfamiliar to you. There is no "cure" for AS, but research on the disorder and new interventions and therapies are moving ahead quickly.
We will be happy to share with you whatever information we find that
may be helpful to you in helping _____ have a positive,
productive experience in school. Please feel free to call us anytime at
[phone number] or e-mail us at _____.

Every child with AS is unique. No two have the same pattern of
behaviors, skills, or deficits. A technique or approach that worked
for one child may not necessarily work for the next. Or what worked
last month may not work today. In the _____ years
since our child was diagnosed, he has received the following therapies and interventions: [list]. We found [list the most effective ones]
the most helpful. He is currently receiving [list other interventions].

[Add if relevant] He is taking [name of medication(s)] to address [list the behavior(s)].

- Our child's main strengths are: [list strengths]
- The praise he values most is: [list: *being told that he is bright, wise, fun to be around*].
- The most effective rewards would be: [list].
- The strongest disincentive would be: [list].

Like many people with AS, our child has special interests: [list special interests]. You may find it helpful to allow him to indulge his special interest by talking about it for a limited period of time as a reward. You may also use his interest as an instructional tool (e.g., write math story problems about trains, allow book report on interest-related book).

AS affects numerous areas. Below is a list of the difficulties _____ faces and what we and his other teachers and therapists have discovered works and does not work.

General Personality and Behavior

_____ is [list the positives: *warm, loving, has a great sense of humor, etc.*].

The areas in which he is most seriously challenged are: [list challenges]. We believe that these can be most effectively addressed by [list interventions and tactics that have proved successful].

Some other approaches such as [list what does not work for your child] do not work for our child and tend to make him feel [describe adverse or undesirable behavior]. When that occurs, we find that it helps to [describe action].

Social Skills with Adults

_____ is [list the positives: *warm, loving, polite, etc.*].

The areas in which he is most seriously challenged are: [list challenges: *has difficulties following multistep directions, a tendency to ask for help with things when he does not necessarily need it, etc.*]. We believe that these can be most effectively addressed by [list interventions and tactics that have proved successful: *breaking all oral* directions down into short, simple steps; gently encouraging him to do those things you know he can do].

Some other approaches such as [list what does not work for your child: repeating complex instructions several times; forcing him to do things he feels inept at] do not work for our child and tend to make him feel [describe adverse or undesirable behavior: anxious, dumb]. When that occurs, we find that it helps to [describe action: calm and comfort him to regain control].

Social Skills with Peers

_____ is [list the positives: interested in other children and anxious to make friends].

The areas in which he is most seriously challenged are: [list challenges: his inability to join in appropriately, participate in conversations, and understand how to reciprocate]. We believe that these can be most effectively addressed by [list interventions and tactics that have proved successful: using Social Stories to cue and remind him of appropriate behavior; setting up situations where he can practice these new skills with other children]. Some other approaches such as [list what does not work for your child: simply leaving him in a group of children on the playground to "find his way"] do not work for our child and tend to make him feel [describe adverse or undesirable behavior: stressed, anxious, and sad]. When that occurs, we find that it helps to [describe action: gently remove him from the situation and set up another experience that is "rigged" for success].

Expressive and Receptive Language

_____ is [list the positives: has a large vocabulary, tells interesting make-believe stories].

The areas in which he is most seriously challenged are: [list challenges]. We believe that these can be most effectively addressed by [list interventions and tactics that have proved successful]. Some other approaches such as [list what does not work for your child] do not work for our child and tend to make him feel [describe adverse or undesirable behavior]. When that occurs, we find that it helps to [describe action].

Auditory Processing

_____ is [list the positives: *can completely recall songs or poems he has heard only once or twice*].

The areas in which he is most seriously challenged are: [list challenges]. We believe that these can be most effectively addressed by [list interventions and tactics that have proved successful]. Some other approaches such as [list what does not work for your child] do not work for our child and tend to make him feel [describe adverse or undesirable behavior]. When that occurs, we find that it helps to [describe action].

Sensory Issues

_____ is [list the positives].

The areas in which he is most seriously challenged are: [list challenges]. We believe that these can be most effectively addressed by [list interventions and tactics that have proved successful]. Some other approaches such as [list what does not work for your child] do not work for our child and tend to make him feel [describe adverse or undesirable behavior]. When that occurs, we find that it helps to [describe action].

Fine- and Gross-Motor Skills

_____ is [list the positives: *almost at age-level with basic living skills; he can tie his shoes, zip his jacket*].

The areas in which he is most seriously challenged are: [list challenges]. We believe that these can be most effectively addressed by [list interventions and tactics that have proved successful]. Some other approaches such as [list what does not work for your child] do not work for our child and tend to make him feel [describe adverse or undesirable behavior]. When that occurs, we find that it helps to [describe action].

Organizational Skills

_____ is [list the positives: *able to pack his book bag at the end of the day if prompted; sometimes able to work at his desk without prompting*].

The areas in which he is most seriously challenged are: [list challenges]. We believe that these can be most effectively addressed by [list interventions and tactics that have proved successful]. Some other approaches such as [list what does not work for your child] do not work for our child and tend to make him feel [describe adverse or undesirable behavior]. When that occurs, we find that it helps to [describe action].

Perseverations

_____ is [list the positives: *engaging in perseverative behaviors less this year than he did last year, and is becoming aware that they are stigmatizing*].

The areas in which he is most seriously challenged are: [list challenges]. We believe that these can be most effectively addressed by [list interventions and tactics that have proved successful]. Some other approaches such as [list what does not work for your child] do not work for our child and tend to make him feel [describe adverse or undesirable behavior]. When that occurs, we find that it helps to [describe action].

Transitions

_____ is [list the positives: *managing to handle transitions, provided he is given clear, detailed explanations of what is expected*].

The areas in which he is most seriously challenged are: [list challenges]. We believe that these can be most effectively addressed by [list interventions and tactics that have proved successful]. Some other approaches such as [list what does not work for your child] do not work for our child and tend to make him feel [describe adverse or undesirable behavior]. When that occurs, we find that it helps to [describe action].

Changes in Routine, Surprises

_____ is [list the positives: *still uncomfortable with surprises but less likely to scream when they occur than he was a few months ago*].

The areas in which he is most seriously challenged are: [list challenges]. We believe that these can be most effectively addressed by [list interventions and tactics that have proved successful]. Some other approaches such as [list what does not work for your child] do not work for our child and tend to make him feel [describe adverse or undesirable behavior]. When that occurs, we find that it helps to [describe action].

Eye Contact, Gaze Modulation
_____ is [list the positives: *making as much eye contact as he comfortably can right now*].

The areas in which he is most seriously challenged are: [list challenges]. We believe that these can be most effectively addressed by [list interventions and tactics that have proved successful]. Some other approaches such as [list what does not work for your child] do not work for our child and tend to make him feel [describe adverse or undesirable behavior]. When that occurs, we find that it helps to [describe action].

[Add any other information you feel is important.]

Sincerely,

[your name]

CLASSROOM STRATEGIES FOR DEALING WITH AS

In addition to your letter, you may also want to provide the teacher with this simple, easy-to-read table. It was adapted from "Educating the Student with Asperger Syndrome" from *Teaching Students with Autism: A Guide for Educators* (1998), a document prepared by the Special Education Unit of the Government of Saskatchewan, and is based on the work of several recognized experts in AS and autism.

Suggested Solutions for Common AS-Related School Problems[8]

DIFFICULTIES WITH EXPRESSIVE LANGUAGE	STRATEGIES
• Makes irrelevant comments • Interrupts others • Talks about one or a few topics excessively • Talks over the speech of others	• Use Comic Strip Conversations. • Use Social Stories. • Provide explicit instruction in conversational skills. • Provide small-group speech and language instruction for conversation skills.
• Has difficulty sustaining a reciprocal conversation • Has difficulty beginning, maintaining, and ending conversations appropriately	• Teach turn-taking: board games, card games, tossing a ball, using a talking stick. • Teach cues for when to reply, interrupt, listen, change the topic, or end the conversation. • Teach introductory remarks ("Can I tell you something interesting about Grand Central Station?") and then give *one* interesting factoid, not a dissertation.
• Speaks without giving listeners information necessary for their comprehension	• Practice theory-of-mind exercises to improve student's ability to understand what listeners may or may not know about his topic. • Teach the difference between general information most people can relate to ("I go on trips with my family to see old steam engines") and information that is overly detailed, arcane, or of interest to aficionados only ("The Big Boy had a 4-8-8-4 wheel arrangement").
• Seems to take "too much time" to answer questions or respond	• If student's response seems slow, pause before restating the question, commenting, or orally prompting; avoid derailing the student's train of thought. He may be actively processing what you have said.

DIFFICULTIES WITH EXPRESSIVE LANGUAGE	STRATEGIES
	• Teach the student "holding" phrases (e.g., "Let me see," "I'm thinking," "That's interesting," and so on).
	• Pause between oral instructions and check for understanding.
	• Make the same point several different ways, using different words for the same thing (appositives) (e.g., "In the story, Frodo defeated Gollum," "How did the hero vanquish the villain and destroy the ring?" "Why did Frodo have to destroy Smeagol?").

DIFFICULTIES WITH RECEPTIVE LANGUAGE	STRATEGIES
• Complex language	• Limit oral questions or restrict to a number the student can handle comfortably.
	• Consider providing oral material in written form as well (e.g., a list of tasks to be completed within the period; instructions for filling out a form or test paper).
	• Allow the student to tape-record lessons given orally so that he may review them later.
• Words with multiple meanings (*drive, heart, snow, dog*)	• Using books, videos, role-playing, and examples from real life, draw the student's attention to use of homonyms, idioms, figures of speech, metaphors, similes, sarcasm, irony, and hyperbole.
• Words that sound the same but have different meanings (homonyms: *here/hear, phase/faze*)	
• Idioms or figures of speech ('barking up the wrong tree," "skating on thin ice")	• Explain and point out the signals and cues—facial expressions; body language; tone, volume, rhythm, and the cadence of speech—that indicate when someone is using sarcasm, irony, or hyperbole.
• Metaphors ("my head was spinning," "on the road to freedom," "the apple of my eye")	
• Similes ("as white as snow," "cried like a baby")	• Use the Mind Reading software program to illustrate the cues and signals.
• Symbolism (the whale in *Moby-Dick,* the owls in the Harry Potter	

books, "the road" in innumerable books, movies, songs, poems)
- Sarcasm ("yeah, right" meaning "no"; "you think?")
- Irony (the shoemaker's children have no shoes)
- Hyperbole ("His hair was on fire," "I died!")

- When a student correctly identifies the use of these types of expression, ask him to explain how he knows what they are "saying."
- Point out examples of symbolism and metaphor.

INSISTENCE ON SAMENESS AND ROUTINE, PROBLEMS WITH TRANSITIONS, CHANGE, AND THE UNEXPECTED	STRATEGIES

Remember: For children with AS, sameness and routine provide much-needed structure to an often unpredictable world. Work to improve flexibility, not to extinguish rigidity. In addition, children sometimes cling to the familiar because of a lack of ability to generalize, or to "carry over" knowledge and experience gained in one situation to another. When possible, point out the similarities between different situations and remind the student of specific skills he has that can help or past experiences in which he was successful.

- Consider the student's resistance to change as possible indication of stress.
- Wherever possible, prepare the student for potential change by explaining fully what will happen.
- Use pictures, schedules, and Social Stories to explain or illustrate an upcoming change in routine.
- Help the student to recognize when skills learned in one situation can be applied to another (e.g., "Going on the bus for the field trip is a lot like taking the bus to school, and you do great on the bus every day").
- Once the student is comfortable in the classroom, deliberately change some small detail from day to day to help him practice flexibility using a "low-stakes" issue (i.e., an object or routine he is not obsessed with).

INSISTENCE ON SAMENESS AND ROUTINE, PROBLEMS WITH TRANSITIONS, CHANGE, AND THE UNEXPECTED	STRATEGIES
	• Count down to upcoming transitions and emphasize with visuals (clock, timer, pictures, schedule): "We have ten minutes until we go back to class," followed by "We have five minutes before we leave," then "Let's start getting ready to return to class," and so on. When possible, make your prompts nonverbal (point, tap the student lightly on the shoulder, place a card with the words *check time* on his desk). Oral prompts are the most difficult to fade and most likely to increase prompt dependence.

IMPAIRED SOCIAL INTERACTION	STRATEGIES

Note: Students must be protected from teasing and bullying at all costs. Failure to do so is a violation of a student's right to a free appropriate public education (FAPE).

• Has difficulty understanding the rules of social interaction and the so-called hidden curriculum (the rules of life we know but were never explicitly taught)	• Provide clear expectations and rules for behavior. • Explicitly teach rules of social conduct through Social Stories, modeling, and role-playing.
• May appear naive, tactless, or lacking in common sense • May not be able to distinguish good-natured, playful teasing from serious threats • May interpret what is said literally as if unaware of social context, the speaker's tone of voice, body language, or other signals	• Teach the student to look at other children for cues as to what to do. • Teach the student how to start, maintain, and end play appropriately. • Teach flexibility, cooperation, and sharing. • Develop structured social skills groups.
• May apply rules rigidly, regardless of mitigating circumstances	• Be on the lookout for situations where an exception to the rule you know the student knows may come into play and prepare the student for that possibility ("Usually we don't jump up and scream during assembly, but because today is

	graduation, most students will probably do that when the ceremony is over. It's okay. It's a way of expressing happiness, and you can do it, too, if you'd like").
• May have problems maintaining the correct, socially appropriate physical distance between himself and others • May touch inappropriately (e.g., hugging every child he sees, kissing adults on the lips, touching other people's hair or clothing)	• If necessary, develop a behavioral plan and intermittently reinforce the student for appropriate social behavior. • Create a diagram that visually depicts the appropriate distance we keep and levels and types of acceptable touching for different groups of people (family, friends, teachers, classmates, adult friends, strangers, etc.).
• May become the target of covert teasing and bullying because typical peers are more skilled at "hiding their tracks" and lying convincingly. This leaves the student with AS to"react," often with inappropriate behavior	• Educate peers about how to respond to the student's disability in social interaction in a way that does not stigmatize the student. • Encourage class participation in cooperative games and endeavors, particularly the type in which the student with AS can be seen as a valuable member of the class team. • Provide the necessary level of supervision and support for the student at breaks, recess, lunch, and traveling to and from school. • If necessary, provide alternate arrangements for breaks, recess, lunch, and transportation. • Assign a high-status, sympathetic peer as a "buddy" to assist the student through nonstructured times. If possible, try to rotate the buddy duty among two or more students.
• May become emotionally overwhelmed by the social strain	• Teach relaxation techniques. • Impose no penalties for those times the student needs a break from the classroom or other activity. • Teach the student how to monitor his emotional responses and behavior. Where possible, use visual and written devices.

IMPAIRED SOCIAL INTERACTION	STRATEGIES
	• Strongly reinforce the student's attempts to communicate his feelings and needs *before* he hits the crisis point.

EXCESSIVE FOCUS ON A RESTRICTED RANGE OF INTERESTS	STRATEGIES

Remember: A student's behavior concerning his special interest is often a source of comfort and joy, as well as a hedge against stress and an opportunity to excel or shine. Focus on "appropriating" the special interest and channeling it toward more socially appropriate expressions rather than completely extinguishing it (which would probably prove impossible and ultimately undesirable anyway).

	• Establish clear rules to limit perseverative discussions and questions (e.g., limit time, place, circumstances of the discussion). • Provide an acceptable outlet for the interests (e.g., allow child to give a presentation or report, incorporate interests in activities and assignments). • Use the special interests to teach other skills and information. • Use permission to talk about the special interests as an incentive or reward.

POOR CONCENTRATION	STRATEGIES

Note: Many students with AS also have an attention deficit disorder (ADHD, ADD). While there is a lot of good information on handling attention deficits in the classroom, teachers should keep in mind that some commonly used strategies for students with ADHD (e.g., maintaining a brisk pace of instruction, use of novel, visually or aurally stimulating materials) may make things harder, not easier, for the student who has AS as well.

• Is often off-task • Is distractible • May be disorganized • Has difficulty sustaining attention	• Provide frequent teacher feedback and redirection, preferably nonverbally. • Break down assignments into manageable portions. • Allow student to work in shorter sessions with frequent breaks.

• Reduce or eliminate homework assignments.
• Seat the student at the front of the class or in the area with the least number of distractions.
• Use nonverbal—as opposed to oral—cues to get attention to reduce prompt dependency.

POOR ORGANIZATIONAL SKILLS	STRATEGIES

Note: Poor organizational skills are usually the result of several neurologically based deficits, namely in executive planning. Consider setting up a data sheet that travels between school and home; reinforce student for displaying organizational skills.

• Often forgets to take home materials necessary for completing homework and/or forgets to bring them back to school • Loses or misplaces notes, books, and other necessary items	• Provide duplicate sets of necessary books and materials for home and for school. • If the student frequently forgets to pack his books and materials, assign an aide or classmate to prompt him (but not do the job for him); fade the prompting as quickly as possible while maintaining the desired behavior. • Help the student establish "one place for everything" at home and at school to help reduce "lost" items.
• Seems "paralyzed" when faced with a task that requires organization or planning	• Place visual supports that guide daily activities (e.g., how to get ready to do work, what to take to lunch, etc.) inside locker, in notebook, or inside or on the desk. Also consider creating a small, wallet-sized laminated card for each task the student needs help with that he can refer to throughout the day. • Provide verbal, nonverbal, and visual prompts; systematically fade prompts as the student learns the skill.
• Seems unable to organize thoughts or materials	• Use schedules, calendars, to-do lists, checklists, planners, and other visual and/or written reminders.

POOR ORGANIZATIONAL SKILLS	STRATEGIES
	• Maintain lists of assignments and their due dates; consider including notes about what is required at each stage of a lengthier project or in preparation for a test (e.g., "Monday: define words for Friday's spelling test," "Thursday: review spelling words; write each five times; check your work"). • Be sure that parents are aware of homework, upcoming tests, projects, and other assignments, as well as upcoming special events at school, such as assemblies, that may require the student bring something to school or dress in a special way. • If the student seems to have difficulty locating materials, place small photographs showing the contents on the outside of bins, closet and cabinet doors, book-shelves, and so on.

POOR MOTOR COORDINATION	STRATEGIES
• Has difficulty with handwriting and other fine-motor skills (e.g., using scissors, manipulating art supplies appropriately)	• Take slower writing speed into account when giving assignments, oral instructions, tests, or when presenting material orally on which students must take notes. • Provide extra time for tests and other work. • Support the student's access to a computer, scribe, or other assistive technology for written assignments. • Consider using a massed-trial approach to teaching skills such as cutting paper. This might involve ten daily trials of cutting increasingly complex shapes—1 line, then an L, then a square or rectangle, etc.—using graduated guidance, errorless teaching, and immediate reinforcement.

416

	• Consider teaching skills like cutting or applying glue through graduated guidance, fading from hand to hand, to hand on wrist, then elbow, at shoulder, and then faded completely as the student gains mastery. • "Reteach" handwriting systematically, using an established program such as Sensible Pencil or Handwriting Without Tears. • Try using different types of writing instruments and modifying them with different pencil grips, etc. • Provide the student with a slightly slanted writing surface. • Set reasonable standards for acceptance of that student's handwriting. • Consult with school physical therapist or occupational therapist (if the student has those services) on how best to coordinate your respective efforts to address this problem.
• Has difficulty maintaining a comfortable posture at his desk without slumping or leaning against things or nearby persons	• Provide an ergonomically correct work area and a chair that supports and/or encourages better muscle coordination of the upper torso. • Consult with school physical therapist or occupational therapist (if the student has those services) on how best to coordinate your respective efforts to address this problem.
• Has difficulty with gross-motor skills	• Encourage participation in physical activity, bearing in mind that persons with AS tend to fare better at noncompetitive, nonteam activities.

ACADEMIC DIFFICULTIES	STRATEGIES
• Has poor problem-solving skills • Has problems with comprehension, oral and/or written • Has problems with processing • Has difficulty with abstract concepts, which may include time • Is often strong in word recognition and decoding; may learn to read very early (hyperlexia, see page 81), but have difficulty with comprehension • May do well at mathematical computations but have trouble with more complex problem solving (e.g., story problems, computations that require multiple steps and/or operations) and more abstract mathematical concepts (algebra, trigonometry, geometry, calculus)	• Do not assume that the student understands the material or what is expected of him simply because he can restate the information or the question. • Be as concrete as possible in presenting new concepts and abstract material. • Use activity-based, experiential, or hands-on learning strategies whenever possible. • Use outlines and graphic organizers such as semantic maps. Focus the student's attention on the different categories you can place different facts in, or the different cues that signal to you which operation is called for in a mathematical problem. • Break down all tasks into smaller steps. • Provide direct instruction as well as modeling. • Show examples of what is required to do the work and of the finished product. For example, if a three-paragraph essay is required, provide an example or write out the specific requirements. ("The book report should be between two and three pages long with at least three paragraphs: one that introduces the book, one that briefly discusses the characters and storyline, one that reflects your thoughts about the book.") • Avoid verbal overload: give student time to process what you have said, answer questions, ask questions, etc. • If necessary, provide all instructions given orally in writing, too. • Become familiar with and consider using interventions and strategies designed for students with non-

verbal learning disability (see page 79).
- Look into Lindamood-Bell Learning Processes programs, particularly Visualizing and Verbalizing for Language Comprehension and Thinking.

EMOTIONAL VULNERABILITY	STRATEGIES
• May have difficulties coping with the social and emotional demands of school • May be easily stressed • May have low self-esteem • May have difficulty tolerating mistakes or failure, even the most innocent and minor • May be prone to depression and anxiety • May have rage reactions and temper outbursts	• Remember, a student with AS is actually working on two separate "curricula" at school: the academic and the social. • Provide positive, explicit, and specific praise (e.g., "You were very smart to use colored folders to organize your notes for the paper" is more effective than "Good job"). • Word your praise using terms that are meaningful to him and that acknowledge those qualities he values in himself: "wise," "clever," "smart," "creative," "thorough," "neat," "detailed," "comprehensive," "brilliant," "sharp," "bright," "original," "unique," "different," "novel," etc. • Teach the student to recognize when he has exhausted his own problem-solving options and to ask for help. • Teach techniques for coping with difficult situations and dealing with stress. • Set up situations that allow the student to make choices. • Help the student to understand his behaviors and the reactions of others. • Educate other students without stigmatizing the student. • Use peer supports such as a buddy system or peer support network.

Remember that for some individuals with central auditory processing difficulties or sensitive hearing, there is no "getting used to it." Exposure to troublesome sounds can be a physically painful, emotionally terrifying experience not unlike a panic attack. Do not try to "reason" a student through a bad reaction once it's taken hold and he shows signs of distress. Get him out of the situation as soon as possible. This is especially true if the problem is a noise that has come on suddenly, like a fire alarm.

- Types of noises that may be perceived as extremely intense may be anything, including sounds most people do not hear (such as the hum of fluorescent lights). Typically troublesome sounds include sudden, unexpected noises; high-pitched continuous noise; confusing, complex, or multiple sounds such as what one would hear in a classroom, playground, hallway, gym, assembly, sports event, or concert.
- May have an extreme reaction to particular sounds (e.g., a certain individual's voice, the school bell in the east hallway but not the west hallway)
- Such extreme reactions can result in stress, anxiety, and even phobias and difficulties over the mere possibility that the sound could occur.
- May be averse to or avoid sounds most young children delight in: music, videos, recordings aimed at younger children; electronic toys and figures that "talk" or make sounds (e.g., musical toys; toys that make "realistic" motor, weapons, crowd, and other sounds)

- It may be necessary to entirely avoid some sounds.
- Minimize background noise.
- Allow the use of earplugs that block volume or specific frequencies without distorting sound.
- Teach and model relaxation strategies and diversions to reduce anxiety.
- If the student is to participate in an "aurally challenging" situation (e.g., assembly, school concert, sports event), be sure you have provided an alternate plan and the student is aware of his ability to escape the situation if he begins to feel overwhelmed. Sometimes
- just having that degree of control over the situation can help him cope.

SENSORY SENSITIVITIES	STRATEGIES
• May have extreme or unusual responses to sound, touch, taste, smell, sight • May also have difficulties with vestibular system (which regulates balance) and proprioception (which essentially lets the student know where his body is in space) • May demonstrate an aversion to certain activities that seems "inexplicable" or "extreme" but in fact has an underlying sensory cause (e.g., a refusal to go to art class may be about an aversion to the smell or texture of a material such as clay, paper, paint, the scent of markers, the feel of crayons on the fingertips)	• Suspect sensory difficulties when the student's avoidant behaviors seem "illogical" or "out of proportion"; specifically ask the student if an item, activity, or environment bothers him (e.g., "Does the feel/smell of the clay make you uncomfortable or feel funny?"). • Be sure that any child who appears to have sensory difficulties is screened for them; consult an OT. • Be aware that normal levels of auditory and visual input can be perceived by the student as too much or too little. • Keep the level of sensory stimulation within the student's ability to cope.

DIFFICULTIES WITH SCHOOL-RELATED PHYSICAL ACTIVITES AND SPORTS	STRATEGIES
• Has poor coordination • Lacks basic sports-related skills (catching, throwing, etc.)	• Work with occupational and/or physical therapist to help student develop skills needed for school-related physical activities. • Consider using massed-trial and graduated guidance techniques for teaching skills like catching and throwing. Remember that for some students with AS, imitating motor movements is difficult, especially when they are presented mirror-image style (teacher facing student to teach throwing, for instance). More effective may be standing behind the student and using twenty consecutive daily throws with hand-over-hand prompting, for instance, gradually fading the level of prompting to independence.

DIFFICULTIES WITH SCHOOL-RELATED PHYSICAL ACTIVITES AND SPORTS	*STRATEGIES*
• Has sensory difficulties in gym or on a field • Is highly distractible or inattentive during team play • Has aversion to activities in which physical contact is routine or may occur • Has aversion to gym class and physical activity	• Become familiar with the basic philosophy and techniques of adapted physical education (APE). • Focus on providing opportunities for individual as opposed to team activities. • Focus on activities that have no winners or losers and that are cooperative and without "leaders." • Consider developing alternate opportunities for students with AS to exercise individually or with a partner or smaller group than the full phys ed class.

● ● ●

Selected Resources for Teachers

Despite growing awareness of autism spectrum disorders, they have yet to warrant the amount of attention they deserve in teacher education programs. Most of the handful of graduate programs that concentrate on autism are concerned with teaching students more likely diagnosed with autistic disorder or PDD-NOS and may promote the use of ABA over most other approaches. We consider this list the "AS library" we wish every school serving our kids had (and every educator read). Because most of these books are written especially for and by educators, they are invaluable as backup for sticky situations and IEP tussles. See also "Recommended Resources" throughout this book for other topics.

Tony Attwood, *Asperger's Syndrome: A Guide for Parents and Professionals* (London and Philadelphia: Jessica Kingsley Publishers, 1998).

Val Cumine, Julia Leach, and Gill Stevenson, *Asperger Syndrome: A Practical Guide for Teachers* (London: David Fulton, 1998).

Catherine Faherty, *Asperger's: What Does It Mean to Me?* (Arlington, TX: Future Horizons, 2000). Note: If your child's teacher is using this

book, make it clear that you do not want anyone at school informing your child of his diagnosis (this is the first exercise in the book).

Beth Fouse, *Creating a "Win-Win IEP" for Students with Autism: A
How-to Manual for Parents and Educators* (Arlington, TX: Future
Horizons, 1999).

Deirdre V. Lovecky, *Different Minds: Gifted Children with AD/HD,
Asperger Syndrome, and Other Learning Deficits* (London and New
York: Jessica Kingsley Publishers, 2004).

Jennifer L. Savner and Brenda Smith Myles, *Making Visual Supports
Work in the Home and Community: Strategies for Individuals with
Autism and Asperger Syndrome* (Shawnee Mission, KS: Autism
Asperger Publishing, 2000).

Pamela B. Tanguay, *Nonverbal Learning Disabilities at Home: A Parent's
Guide* (London and Philadelphia: Jessica Kingsley Publishers, 2001).

Sue Thompson, *The Source for Nonverbal Learning Disorders* (East
Moline, IL: LinguiSystems, 1997).

Diane Twachtman-Cullen, *How to Be a Para Pro: A Comprehensive
Training Manual for Paraprofessionals* (Higganum, CT: Starfish Specialty Press, 2000). Though ostensibly designed to train paraprofessionals and aides, this 200-page spiral-bound book is indispensable
for teachers.

Journals

Autism Spectrum Quarterly, edited by Diane Twachtman-Cullen, Ph.D.
In 2004, Carol Gray's *Jenison Autism Journal* (formerly *The Morning
News*) evolved into a new format. It provides ideas and examples for
teachers and parents on ASD-related topics. For information go to
www.asquarterly.com. To order back issues, see www.thegraycenter.org.

Web Sites on Adapted Physical Education (APE)

Here are two excellent Web sites devoted to Adapted Physical
Education.

Project I.N.S.P.I.R.E. APE Web page from Texas Women's University:
www7.twu.edu/~f_huettig/index.htm.

PELINKS4U
www.pelinks4u.org/sections/adapted/adapted.htm.

THE SCHOOL-HOME CONNECTION: KEEPING THE LINES OF COMMUNICATION OPEN

Consistency is crucial to a child with AS. While it's unreasonable to expect that you and your child's teacher will handle every situation exactly the same way, your child will benefit greatly if you and those at school agree on key issues. How to manage "high stakes" situations such as emotional meltdowns, misbehavior, and social issues top that list. A teacher who persists in trying to stop a rage attack, for instance, or forces a child out on the playground every day despite obvious signs of stress must be persuaded to adopt strategies that are effective.

The key is, obviously, communication. Make it your first priority to see that your child's teacher understands AS and how it affects your child. Next, propose (and insist, if necessary) that you and the teacher exchange a notebook, checklist, or some other written update of your child's school day. Checklists are often preferred, since for many teachers, time is at a premium and they have other children to teach.

It is impossible to track every behavior of the day. To make the data you or your child's teacher collect and analyze meaningful, follow these guidelines:

1. Be specific: Target behaviors (tantruming, pushing in line, greeting teacher and peers each morning, hitting other students, bringing in homework) that you can observe and count, not states of mind, moods, or attitudes you cannot.

2. If you are concerned with a mood, attitude, or state of mind, identify behaviors that might be indicative of it and document the behavior. For instance, rather than "rate" Neil's anxiety on a scale of 1 to 5, if you know that higher anxiety tends to result in more tantruming, count the tantrums.

3. Define your terms so that you and your child's teacher are talking about the same thing. Let's take the tantrum. What will define the tantrum? Your child raising his voice, complaining or whining or crying loudly, hitting objects or persons, getting out of his chair, falling to the floor, running out of the classroom—these could all be parts of tantrum behavior. Specify what defines a tantrum, or an appropriate greeting, and agree with your child's teacher to count only that. So,

for example, a tantrum has to include loud complaining, or whining, or crying *and* refusal to return to his seat; your child should not be scored as tantruming if he's annoyed and muttering under his breath while he sits in his seat. A greeting would have to include your child initiating the greeting and saying audibly while making at least a second of eye contact, "Good morning," "Hi," "Good day," "Hello," or whatever and the person's name. A silent wave won't cut it.

4. Choose behaviors that have a clear beginning and an end.

5. Pinpoint specific times to observe the behavior. It would be impossible for Tali's teacher to chase behind her and count up every time she greets anyone over the course of a school day. But her teacher or an aide can watch Tali for the first three minutes after she's entered the classroom and track whom she greets and how.

6. How much data do you need? If Tali's just learning to greet others, every day for a week or two would establish whether or not Tali's mastered the skill. After that, you might want her teacher to observe her once a week until it's clear she's got it.

7. What will you do with it? Make a simple chart, like the one shown on page 426. (Or, if you are handy with a spreadsheet program such as Excel, you can create something a bit fancier.) What does it tell you? We can see that for Neil, tantrums are significantly more common on Monday than on any other day. This suggests you might look at ways to help him make the transition back into the school routine.

• • •

Tracking Neil's Tantrums

A tantrum: Neil cries or complains loudly for more than 30 seconds *and* gets out of his seat *and* refuses two or more requests to return to his seat; scores a plus (+). Any other behavior or lack of tantruming scores a minus (-). Data will be taken during first period, fourth period, and eighth period (the last of the day). [Note that we are not concerned with what goes on in the other periods of the day; these three periods have been identified as the three during which Neil has the most difficulty so we are focusing on them.] Here is Neil's data for the first week of the month. Note: + indicates tantruming occurred; – indicates absence of tantruming.)

Period	Monday	Tuesday	Wednesday	Thursday	Friday	Weekly total
1st	+	+	−	+	−	3
4th	+	−	−	−	−	1
8th	+	−	−	−	−	1
daily total	3	1	0	1	0	5

You could keep a graph that charts data from week to week to help you spot trends. Here's Neil's data for the month by daily totals. Connecting the dots will give you a clearer picture of the data. Parents and teachers who know their way around Microsoft Excel or other spreadsheet programs can produce graphs like the one pictured opposite. This one had date and day in the "A" column, number of tantrums in "B." Charting on regular graph paper works just as well.

Clearly, having real numbers is more useful than comparing statements like "Neil had a terrible day today," "Neil seemed a little happier," "Neil did not seem so anxious." If Neil is improving, we can see that. We can also measure how much he has improved and specifically when. This month's chart tells us that while Neil is tantruming less frequently, Mondays are consistently the day on which he tantrums the most. You might want to explore with his teacher, What is it about Mondays? Don't forget to ask Neil. You might find out that on seven of the last nine Mondays, there has been a fire drill, and Neil has very sensitive hearing. But maybe that's not it. So you might explore what it is about the other days that may be contributing to his tantruming less. Perhaps Monday is the only day he is not pulled out of the classroom for OT or speech therapy. Could it be that spending the whole day in the classroom is difficult for him? Collecting and charting data will not yield these answers, but it will help you narrow your search and give you concrete evidence of improvement (or lack of it).

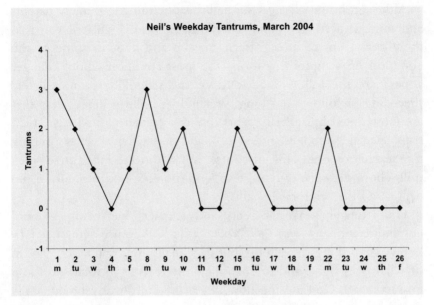

Because the source of our children's difficulties and behaviors can be so mysterious, always keep your child's teacher posted on changes at home, changes in schedule, or anything that may be upsetting to your child. This includes the obvious ones (changes in medication, illness, family crisis) and seemingly less important things (an unsuccessful weekend play date, an after-school dental appointment, concern over the fact that music class has been moved to right before lunch instead of right after). Children with AS can become troubled over things most people wouldn't even notice.

Keeping specific data over a period of time can help you see where your child is making progress and where he needs some extra help. We've heard from too many parents who learned their child was having a problem only after it had reached crisis proportions. This lack of communication not only deprives the student of the chance to benefit from effective, timely intervention, it threatens the openness and trust parents and teachers need in order to work together. Often we become so fixated on the "biggies" that we often lose sight of the real and important accomplishments that accrue slowly, over time. It can be encouraging, for both you and your child, to look back and see that his ability to tolerate transitions has improved. On the other hand, keeping track can also help you pinpoint patterns of behavior.

Although no one has yet studied this phenomenon, many parents and some experts, including Dr. Tony Attwood, will tell you that there does seem to be a pattern, an ebb and flow, to some of the common AS symptoms. Among the most common school "danger zones" are the following: Mondays; the school days immediately preceding or following a long weekend or holiday break; days that are interrupted by special events (holiday concerts, field days, field trips, special assemblies, and so on); and days when there is a substitute teacher or aide. This, of course, is in addition to the run-of-the-mill school stressors: quizzes, tests, and projects, not to mention fire drills and other sensory "assaults."

Unfortunately, many parents and teachers view home-school communication as *The Bad News Daily*. Of course, you need to know when things go wrong, but it's equally important to be aware of what goes right, and to encourage the teacher to focus on those positives, too. Considering how much difficulty many of our children have with telling us what they did in school, saying, "I see that you've been asking for help instead of getting upset. That's the smart thing to do. You're doing a wonderful job," might be a good opener. Besides, our children can never receive enough specific praise for their accomplishments and their efforts.

You need to know what goes on in school, particularly if it's been a rough day. For many children with AS, school-related stress and anxiety don't end when the bell rings. If your child hasn't had the best day, you should know and plan accordingly, perhaps postponing the dreaded haircut, reducing the homework load (talk with your child's teacher about doing this), or rescheduling a play date.

HOW MUCH HELP?

As we've said, it's impossible to generalize about the "best" educational placement for a child with AS. Different children need different things, and some children with AS need the help of a one-on-one paraprofessional, or aide. Unfortunately, in some school districts, aides function merely as in-class baby-sitters. There are so many ways in which a well-trained "para pro," as autism and education expert Diane Twachtman-Cullen terms them, can help a student with AS not only develop academically, emotionally, and socially but learn to do so with a degree of independence. Para pros who are not well trained may actually be more of a hindrance than a help, and school districts are quick to point out the "ineffectiveness" of previous aides as an excuse not to provide them. There are resources for training staff, including paraprofessionals, to work with students with ASDs properly. The "ineffectiveness" lies with school districts that fail to meet their obligations under IDEA to provide the appropriate staff training.

If your child needs a para pro, required reading for you, your child's teacher, and your child's para is Twachtman-Cullen's *How to Be a Para Pro: A Comprehensive Training Manual for Paraprofessionals* (see page 423). Frankly, we strongly believe that as long as there is a copy of this book available, no school district has an excuse for undertraining staff—and that includes teachers, principals, and administrators—in autism spectrum disorders generally and the theory and application of appropriate, effective, and practical strategies. In fact, we recommend that you read the book even if your child does not have a paraprofessional, because as one OASIS parent commented, "Parents *are* paraprofessionals when it comes to our children."

It's in your child's interest for you to initiate and maintain a relationship with his para pro. If your child requires such support, you can assume that it may not be the easiest job. Anything that you can do to help your child's para to better understand your child will probably be appreciated. (If it's not, you should talk with his teacher and consider requesting another para.) When things go well, be sure that you let your child's para know that you appreciate her work, and let others—your child's teacher, special education administration, and even your school superintendent and board of education—know it, too. Remember, many school district policies are created out of default, or a lack of positive input. If your child's para has helped facilitate his progress, write a letter outlining specifically what has improved and the para's role in making that happen. You may be doing other parents whose children require the same level of help a big favor by offering evidence that one-on-one intervention for children with AS is not only appropriate but effective.

If your school district doesn't routinely include para pros in meetings related to IEP and 504 service plan development, encourage it to do so. (One problem is that such meetings usually occur during school hours, and since your child's teacher must attend, also insisting the para pro do so may create a gap in classroom coverage.) If she cannot attend, ask that she write up a report of her observations of your child, including challenges, progress, strategies (effective and ineffective), and so on.

LUNCH AND RECESS: WELCOME TO THE JUNGLE

For many students with Asperger Syndrome, some parts of the school day are easier to negotiate than others. The most common areas of difficulty are the "unstructured" activities—namely, recess, lunch, and the school bus ride—when sensory overload, social confusion, and anxiety can become overwhelming. Depending on how your child's school handles things, these may be prime settings for tantrums, meltdowns, and other inappropriate behavior, the social ramifications of which are only magnified by it being witnessed by the student's peers. If your child indicates that these activities are difficult for him, or if his behavior—before, during, and after—suggests that this may be the case, work with his teacher to create alternatives. Quiet free time inside spent reading, playing, or working on the computer can take the place of recess. Lunch can be spent with a small, supervised group. It may be very informal or an opportunity to provide a structured social skills experience.

PHYSICAL EDUCATION CLASSES

While most neurotypical children find gym class a welcome release from the academics and look forward to the games, activities, and the social aspects of physical education, children with Asperger Syndrome often find the opposite to be true. In most schools, gym class is an environment that showcases his weaknesses rather than his strengths. From a sensory perspective, the noisy atmosphere of the gym and the piercing sound of the coach's whistle can be painful to a child who experiences auditory difficulties. The smell of the locker room and the sensation of changing clothing and showering can easily overwhelm a child with AS. A child who struggles with shoelaces and buttons will take longer to change into gym clothes than his peers and may find himself late for class.

While there are exceptions, most children with Asperger Syndrome are to some extent clumsy and have difficulty with both small- and large-motor planning issues. They may not run fast, catch, or throw well. They may struggle with playing as part of a team, and often find games such as basketball, baseball, and dodge ball extremely difficult. We often forget that what many of us loved about physical education and team sports is exactly what makes them so challenging for kids with AS: the social component. Think back to your own days on the court, in the field, or staring down your tetherball or foursquare opponent on the blacktop. What did you say to one another? Little or nothing; you communicated nonverbally for the most part using everything from simple glances and gestures to elaborate play-calling gestures. In addition, many children with Asperger Syndrome do not do well with competition and have difficulty with winning and losing. Because of problems with making realistic attributions they may blame themselves or others for things that happen in a game that are beyond their control. And unless your child's teammates—and their opponents—are exceptionally sensitive, mature, and well versed in sportsmanship, any player's errors will not go unnoticed. For some would-be team players with AS, these factors combine to make even the prospect of team sports unappealing, to put it mildly.

Off the field and the court, probably the most challenging aspect of a PE class for an AS child is the social aspect. Although educators almost automatically mainstream children with AS for gym, even if most of their other classes are in special education or related services, this may not be the best idea. Unlike, say, a science class, phys ed has its own social rules. Children who are not athletically inclined easily become the objects of teasing and taunting by other children and, unfortunately, sometimes by the gym teachers themselves. The combination of sensory overload, lack of athletic ability, and all too often being the object of teasing can have a devastating effect on the self-esteem of a child with Asperger Syndrome. Adapted physical education (APE) can help address many of these issues. For suggestions on what can be done, see the chart "Suggested Solutions for Common AS-Related School Problems" on page 421.

Some parents have persuaded their school districts to grant their child credit for regular, documented participation in health or fitness activities outside of school. If your child is having a particularly difficult time with physical education in school, or your school just doesn't seem to get it, find out if your child could substitute a couple of weekly sessions working out, swimming, or taking exercise classes at your local Y, community center, college, or private health club. Some of these places offer special programs for individuals with disabilities. You might also find local instructors in martial arts, dance, archery, bowling, or other nonteam activities your child might enjoy. Don't give up on finding a Little League or other team that would welcome and work with your child.

THE SCHOOL BUS

If the problem is the school bus, look carefully at what factors might be changed to make the trip more pleasant. One solution is using a smaller bus, which, theoretically at least, might result in a quieter, shorter, and better supervised trip. You might request that your child be given special seating (at the front of the bus rather than in the back) or an aide, or that the bus route be altered so that he spends the least possible amount of time in transit. Arranging a small car pool with children your child feels comfortable with may be another option. It's quicker and quieter and provides a low-stress opportunity for informal socialization. Other parents drive their child to and from school. One mother feels that the ride to school provides her child with a more gradual transition between home and school. "I learn a lot in those fifteen minutes about how he feels, what may be bothering him," one mother told us. "It gives me a chance to get in a little pep talk or correct some misconception he has about the day ahead. If necessary, I can also give his teacher a heads-up. I like to think of the ride home as 'the decompression zone.' If he had a problem, he gets it all off his chest before we pull into the driveway, and we can start the afternoon on a fresh page."

THE HOMEWORK QUESTION

In the spring of 2000, Dr. Tony Attwood posted a paper on his Web site posing the question many parents and teachers were asking themselves: "Should children with autistic spectrum disorder be exempted from doing homework?" As Dr. Attwood points out, for many children with AS, the "stress and mental exhaustion" of coping through the school day, as well as cognitive difficulties, may render homework an exercise counterproductive to both the student's emotional well-being and his academic progress. Emotionally, some children with AS need to separate school from home. They need the school day to have a clear and precise ending. If the child has other challenges that affect his cognitive abilities, the prospect of tackling additional schoolwork when tired may prompt refusal, defiance, tantrums, and other unpleasant avoidant behaviors. Parents may also find homework a difficult, frustrating experience. "The worst feeling in the world for me," one mother told us, "is sitting there and watching him struggle to write, and erase, and write, and erase, and write the same letter over and over. I want to grab the pencil myself and break it, or do the work for him, or throw it all out the window. Rather than be upset when he melts down, I find myself marveling that he stuck with it as long as he did."

With the ever-increasing emphasis on academic achievement, most parents, particularly those whose children have other learning disabilities, may be reluctant to forgo this opportunity to get in a little more learning. Dr. Attwood suggests that parents do all they can to create a pleasant homework environment. It should be quiet, free of distractions, and follow, to the extent possible, strategies that have been successful in class, such as the use of a timer, frequent breaks, incentives, praise, and ample, undistracted supervision. Many parents find it best to make homework part of a strict routine, so that children know what to expect.

Teachers can help by providing explicit instructions for both the student and the parent regarding what is expected. If you're unsure about some aspect of your child's homework, contact his teacher as soon as possible. If your child's teacher won't respond to phone calls or e-mails off-hours, arrange for your child to have extended deadlines so that he can stop working on an assignment he does not understand. If homework is difficult for your child, ask your teacher to use it for reviewing rather than teaching new material.

If you and your child's teacher have tried everything and your child is still having problems, you must then consider if the negative repercussions may be outweighing any potential benefit. We say "potential" because several studies have questioned the academic value of homework, particularly for children in elementary school.

For children who are chronically frustrated by learning disabilities, it isn't unreasonable to wonder what is gained from insisting he engage in an exercise that undermines his self-esteem and creates negative feelings about school and learning. Be honest with your child's teacher. What is the point of a specific homework assignment? Is he learning something new (as when he reads a book for a class book report) or is he just practicing an acquired skill? Perhaps you can reach some agreement about what types of homework must be done and which are optional. If Kate can answer the first twenty of fifty algebra problems correctly, does she really need to do the other thirty? If it's possible, you might also ask if your child could work on the homework he must do during recess times (unless he would prefer to join his classmates and take a break).

WHEN SCHOOL IS JUST TOO MUCH

With the appropriate accommodations and interventions, most children will find a school placement that works for them. Even then, however, it's not unusual for some students with AS to need a break from school. During periods of particularly intense stress or difficulty, some children benefit from an extra day away from school. (Of course, you should get your child's work in advance so she can complete it at home, if possible.) Discuss this issue with your child's teacher.

For a small minority of students with AS, school is nothing short of torture. Even with the seemingly appropriate programs, services, and interventions in place, there are students who simply cannot cope comfortably with the stress of school. And by "cope comfortably," we don't mean just "holding it together" until they can fall apart after school. Sometimes the stress in combination with other conditions, such as depression, anxiety, and obsessive-compulsive disorder, creates serious problems. Or the stress can even cause anxiety, depression, OCD, and other psychiatric disorders. For this small group of persons with AS, the esteem-shattering experience of school—whether the result of emotional stress, social failure, teasing or bullying, academic difficulties, or anything else—is not unlike war, and the experience may profoundly affect them for years hence.

In fact, some adults with AS do suffer a form of posttraumatic stress syndrome as a result of their school experiences.

You must learn to recognize when enough is enough, when your child has reached a point at which his current academic placement poses a threat to his current and future well-being. Alternate school placement—to a smaller classroom, a smaller school, or a school that specializes in autism-related disabilities, the gifted and talented, or children with specific behavioral and emotional issues—may be appropriate. We've heard from a number of parents who, often in the wake of their child's emotional crisis, opt for home schooling, with good results. If your child is emotionally or psychologically unable to attend school, he should be provided with a home tutor. Fortunately, relatively few parents face these options. Because there are matters of law involved, consult with a local advocacy group or a special education advocate or attorney if you're considering these courses. Protect your child. Know and exercise your rights. Be especially careful if you are contemplating voluntarily removing your child from his current placement and enrolling him in a school or home-schooling program for which you will seek reimbursement from your school district. Speak with a special education attorney before you act.

— • • • —

Home Schooling

You may decide that the best and most appropriate educational environment for your child is home schooling. Perhaps the situation at school is so desperate that the child cannot function in the school environment, or perhaps you're an advocate of home schooling to begin with.

One great concern is whether a child with AS will have access to social opportunities if removed from the school environment. As one mother stated, the "social interactions that my son was involved in were so detrimental to his self-esteem that no contact with other children would be better than continued contact with bullies." The quantity and quality of this boy's social interactions actually increased because the mother was able to protect him from the bullying at school and he was able to interact with other children in her home-schooling network. In many ways she felt she was much more able to help her son learn appropriate social behavior due to her involvement and support.

Most home schoolers belong to networks in which they have contact with other children of a variety of ages. They may meet a couple times a week for gym or other activities. Home schooling provides opportunities for a child who has sensory issues or gets tired or overwhelmed easily to work in a quiet environment. Those who struggle with OCD, attention difficulties, or other issues and may not be able to succeed in a classroom situation can learn at their own pace. Home schooling takes a tremendous amount of time and dedication, and it is not for all families and children. But those who have used this method feel that it offers their children the best opportunities for successful learning and socialization. Again, if your child is eligible for or receiving special education or related services, be sure you are fully aware of your rights and responsibilities *before* you withdraw your child from his current placement. We strongly suggest consulting an attorney or advocate.

Resources for Home Schoolers

Homeschooling Children Who "Aut" to Be Home is the title
   of the Aut-2-B-Home Support list. It can be accessed at
   http://home.earthlink.net/~tammyglaser798/authome.html.
Tony Attwood, Ph.D., "Appropriate Educational Placements for
   Children with Asperger's Syndrome," January 2000, online at
   http://www.tonyattwood.com.au.

THE OLDER STUDENT

As students enter their teens, most parents' thoughts turn to life after high school. Whether that means college, special job training, or employment depends on numerous factors. Most students with AS will require special support through the years when most other students require significantly less.

Plan ahead, bearing in mind that the special education, related services, and supports your child has received in school under IDEA will end when he either graduates from high school or turns twenty-two. IDEA requires that IEP meetings and IEPs written when a student is fourteen years of age or older provide specific information on transition services. If you believe that your child may need extra time to prepare for life after high school, IDEA provides that transition can be discussed and planned for earlier, "if determined appropriate."[9] Transition services are defined in IDEA as a coordinated set of activities for a student with a disability that: "(A) is designed within an outcome-oriented process, which promotes movement from school to post-school activities, including post-secondary education, vocational training, integrated employment (including supported employment), continuing and adult education, adult services, independent living, or community participation; (B) is based on the individual student's needs, taking into account the student's preferences and interests; and (C) includes instruction, related services, community experiences, the development of employment and other post-school adult living objectives, and, when appropriate, acquisition of daily living skills and functional vocational evaluation."[10]

Note that the purpose of transition is to help prepare the student for a wide range of postschool activities, including college. Don't let your school district persuade you that your college-bound child is "too smart" to benefit from transition services. Among special education experts and advocates, transition services often get low marks because they're not always sufficiently individualized, intensive, or creative. If you can locate a public or private organization that specializes in providing such training in your area, make an appointment. It may be the best way to learn what really can be done, as opposed to what your school district usually does. Persons with AS may require very specialized training and preparation for independence. Insist that your school district call in outside professionals, if you feel it's necessary.

If college is an option, be prepared to do a lot of research. Just as there is no one school placement appropriate for every student with AS, there are no "guidelines" for finding the right college beyond the by now obvious: support, understanding, and accommodations. We've heard from many parents of adults with AS who look back and regret that their child did not receive the training in social skills, emotional self-management, and daily living skills that would have supported success in higher education or a job. One development we are very pleased to see is the slow but steady growth in post-secondary programs that recognize and support the student with ASDs.

While the needs of an elementary school student may be radically different from those of the high school student, the primary goal for all students with AS is that their educational environment allows for both academic and social development. Even if your child was diagnosed late or didn't require services in previous years, it's never too late to initiate supports at school or to make changes in the educational environment.

Chapter 12

GROWING UP

As children with Asperger Syndrome grow, they face new and different challenges. As they enter the teen years, parents find themselves looking forward in a way that they may have subconsciously avoided until now. Before we look ahead, however, it's a good idea to stop for a moment, look back, and consider how far your child (and you) have come. Take an objective look at the problems and challenges facing your teen, but also remember what has been overcome and remind him and yourself of his wonderful qualities, talents, and skills.

THE CHALLENGES OF ADOLESCENCE

If this time of life is difficult for most children, it is understandably more trying or challenging for those with AS. The early teenage years are typically a time when children strive to seek a measure of independence from their parents. Gradually, the opinions and approval of peers become paramount, as they find their place in a new social realm separate from their family. Most teens want desperately to fit in with their peers. Typical teens begin to explore dating and express an interest, at the very least, in sexual relationships. Adolescence can be trying for anyone. For the teen with AS, the problems can be more complex, especially since he may lack peer support and shared social experiences.

PARENTS GROW UP, TOO

One day you realize that the boy who learned to ride a two-wheeler at age eleven and still has difficulty holding his fork properly is starting to grow facial hair. Suddenly the term *milk mustache* takes on an entirely new meaning. Or you notice boys at the mall looking at your daughter, who still faces challenges in reading nonverbal communications, in a very different way.

Your child's adolescence may also bring with it a heightened sense of your own not fitting in with parents of neurotypical kids. As children grow up and away, parents face an important rite of passage as well. Typically, they experience the bittersweetness of seeing a child grow into a life of his own. At the same time, many parents are also looking ahead at changes in their own lives, wrought by added responsibility for their own parents, retirement, career changes, and so on. Here is yet another generational journey on which we as parents may feel left behind or entirely left out. The one thing that parents of children with AS may not be able to foresee is a time when there will be an empty nest or they will not be needed to the extent they were when their children were much younger.

While our peers are worried about their children staying out too late, drinking and driving, or experimenting with sex and drugs after a school dance, parents of AS teenagers may feel out of the loop. Friends may tell us that we are "lucky" to find our son happily involved in his special interest and totally unaware that the school dance was even scheduled. Be prepared for the totally ridiculous moments when you find yourself thinking, *I wish she would sneak out to see her boyfriend,* or *I wish he did complain when he couldn't have the keys to the car.* It's not because you want to place your child in danger, or because you advocate premarital sex, or because you wouldn't worry while your son was behind the wheel. It's something else. After all, that's the growing up most of us have lived ourselves, that we can teach from and that we know signals the presence of important emergent abilities and drives. At the very least, we know where to go for help with those types of situations. We could commiserate with friends; we could one day look back on it and, hopefully, even smile.

Instead, the quickly passing years of adolescence tend to make parents of an AS child anxious and worried. If your child has received special education and/or related services, you may feel that the clock is running out. As one mother put it, "There is so much left to do, and so little time."

WHAT WE KNOW ABOUT AS AND ADOLESCENCE

Unfortunately, there isn't yet a great deal of information available to assist parents in raising an adolescent with AS. Parents and, most important, the teens themselves are again blazing a grassroots trail. Fortunately, parents of children who were diagnosed at the time the diagnostic criteria appeared and parents of newly diagnosed teens and young adults are banding together via both local and online support groups to share information on ways to best help teens and young adults reach their potential. One such online support group is the OASIS Raising Teens and Young Adults Forum, which can be accessed through OASIS. Parents also look to the wisdom of other parents who are willing to share their experiences raising "difficult" children who were diagnosed with AS in adulthood.

VOICES OF EXPERIENCE

Perhaps most important—and encouraging—are the contributions from adults who have been recently diagnosed with AS and HFA. Their stories are often painful, and their courage in sharing both the good and the bad is to be commended. In most cases, no matter how difficult their lives were, they are intent on making sure that things are better for children and teens now being diagnosed. Some local support groups have set up programs in which adults with Asperger Syndrome mentor children and young adults, and quite a few online relationships have developed after parents corresponded with adults with AS who participate in online support groups.

There are adults with AS willing to offer suggestions as to how we as parents can make things better for our children and the AS community at large. However, parents and others should understand the context of their comments. In many cases, these adults were misdiagnosed or not diagnosed at all, misunderstood, and, too often, horribly mistreated. In addition to the unfortunately "usual" teasing, bullying, and loneliness, some persons were subjected to emotional, physical, and sexual abuse at the hands of parents, professionals, and strangers; misdiagnosis and resulting treatment that was traumatic (institutionalization, electroconvulsive therapy—previously known as shock treatment—over- and mismedication), or attempts to "self-medicate" through alcohol and drug abuse. Because of experiences like these, some adults with AS have a profound (and understandable) distrust of parents, professionals, and the community in general. In some cases, their anger is truly justified. It may be unrealistic to expect them ever to understand and forgive. And, to be honest, in some situations, there can be no forgiveness. As advocates for persons with AS and related disorders, we have a moral obligation to raise awareness about their plight, to respect their point of view, and to refrain from imposing upon them our opinions regarding appropriate interventions and treatments for them.

Parents of children with AS are often understandably curious to learn from adults with AS. For the most part, those who make themselves available to answer questions or serve as mentors do so because they feel a sense of community with the child with AS. Some parents, however, have been taken aback and surprised when the AS advisor expresses an opinion that does not agree with theirs. A typical flash point is the subject of medication. Some adults with AS have had such horrific experiences that their only advice to parents considering medication is simply "don't." Parents and persons with AS may not always agree, but it is disrespectful of those of us who do not have AS to presume to tell those who do that their views are somehow wrong. Particularly when seeking input from persons with AS on matters of parenting, realize and accept the terms of engagement. Be prepared to receive input about your views; don't ask expecting endorsement or validation for them. And you need not "correct" views that don't dovetail with your own.

Persons with AS, particularly those who are older, more confident, and have found a place for themselves in the world, are extremely proud of their independence and their differences. Some have an almost reflexive aversion to anything and anyone that seems to place a higher value on conformity to social norms than on the happiness and the acceptance of the individual. Given that we neurotypicals have the ability to adopt different perspectives, should it not be we who bend to accommodate those who cannot rather than to force those with AS to be what they naturally are not?

SOME TRUE PIONEERS

We parents should never overlook the fact that well-known persons with autism spectrum disorders, such as Liane Holliday Willey, credit their positive outcomes to their parents' courage to follow their hearts and do what they felt best for them. Holliday Willey, who is an author, a frequent speaker, a parent of a child with AS, and by most standards a great success story, admits to the tremendous struggles she faces every single day as an adult with Asperger Syndrome:

> I, like many on the light end of Asperger Syndrome, am an inbetweener. After years and years of hard work, solid intervention, constant support, and much trial and error, I have found I am close enough to normal to touch it, if I want to. If I have the energy to. The sheer effort it takes to maintain neurotypical standards of normal is overwhelming and, at times, brutal to the "real me" few people ever get to know. Sometimes I dream people with Asperger Syndrome have purple tongues. If we did, there would be no doubting our struggles and our twists and turns. We could open our mouth, pop out our purple tongue, and never again have to explain the reality behind who we are. People would know, they would understand, they would accept that what they perceive as our shortcomings were really just manifestations of our Asperger Syndrome and not a shortcoming at all. And maybe, just maybe, they would stop calling us names like rude, ungrateful, obnoxious, weird, and strange. In my dreams I live in a world where I don't have to become anyone else to make my goals come true. In that pretend place, I am respected for my humanity and never turned away because of my differences. I am forever happy there.

TEENS AND YOUNG ADULTS SPEAKING OUT

It has been more common lately to hear from teens with Asperger Syndrome who are speaking out and sharing their insights through Web pages, message boards, and participation on conference panels. In some areas, local support groups are now beginning to focus on the needs of the adolescent, young adult, and adult with ASD.

Online support groups for college students are available, and there are safe chat rooms and message boards available for teens where they can discuss their Asperger Syndrome or find persons who share common interests. (No matter where your child is chatting, you should be vigilant. AS teens have been taken advantage of online. In two cases we know of, naive AS teens gave out personal information that resulted in sexual assault. It is important to note that this did not occur as a result of participation in autism-related forums. Talk with your teens about Internet safety. Don't assume that your son or daughter will "know" how to respond to inappropriate advances.)

WHEN DIAGNOSIS COMES LATE

If your child wasn't diagnosed until his teens or later, you may feel you've lost so much time that it's too late to help. We would like to stress what we feel is one of the most important messages of this book: It is *never* too late for a child or parent to seek assistance. Through the years, Barb has heard from countless adults who have been diagnosed with Asperger Syndrome, and with very few exceptions, they have felt that finding out about their AS was a positive thing.

Even if years have passed in which your child's AS behaviors were incorrectly viewed as discipline problems or something else, you, teachers, friends, and, most important, your child himself can benefit from understanding and intervention. For example, we know of one therapist who runs social skills groups for people with AS well into their fifties and beyond.

If your child has been diagnosed at an older age, you may be more inclined to see behaviors and attitudes as "set" or inextricable from "who he really is." We urge you to try viewing it in a different light.

What you see today may be "who he is," but it is who he is without intervention, support, awareness of more effective strategies, and help. Although we cannot possibly change everything about a person with AS, nor would we wish to do so, some of the changes that can occur have the power to make a world of difference in that person's future well-being and happiness. For many older adolescents and adults the relief of finally knowing that there is a explanation for what they have felt and experienced is welcome.

LATER DISCLOSURE

Late diagnosis also raises another important issue: disclosure. Several experts we asked agreed that adolescence is probably not the optimal time to tell a child she has a lifelong disability. Certainly by that point, most adolescents will be aware that something is wrong. Still, to be told that you are different at a time in life when it is so important to be the same can be a devastating blow. (See page 116 for more on telling your child about the diagnosis.) Unfortunately, parents of children who are adolescents at diagnosis probably have no choice but to tell their children and, possibly, their school district. If your older child is planning to pursue employment or college after high school, he needs to know because there may be types of support, training, and accommodations that are available to him. The question then arises, Who else needs to know?

When your child is younger, you may tell whomever you choose. Once a child reaches a certain age, however, he has the right to decide who knows. You may not always agree with his choices, but you should certainly give them serious consideration and err on the side of protecting him to the extent possible. After all, he's the one who has to go out into the world "known as" a person with AS. Parents often ask whether it is a good idea to tell classmates and friends about a child's AS. There are compelling arguments supporting either decision. Those who are for informing peers take the position that understanding encourages tolerance and acceptance. One expert told us a heartwarming story about a class of elementary school students who took a substitute teacher to task for not understanding the behavior of their classmate with AS. Even though every student may not become more supportive, and you do run the risk that teasing may actually increase, we have heard from many parents whose experience was positive.

The argument against informing a group of classmates or peers is equally compelling. For one thing, it's risky. No one can predict how peers will respond, and the presence of one or two domineering troublemakers may outweigh the goodwill of other students. There is also the question of whether telling simply stops harassment or truly fosters inclusion. If your child is being teased and bullied, and the school has failed to secure the environment against such antisocial behavior, revealing that he has AS may not necessarily solve the problem. If the school has created a climate in which such behavior is accepted, you should consider whether news of your child's AS might not simply become another weapon against him. Demand that your school district meet its obligation to protect your child from harassment, teasing, and bullying first. (See box on "Bullying and Teasing," page 371.) Understanding does not always equal acceptance, and your child may feel exposed by everyone knowing something so personal.

If your child is an adolescent, we believe that he should be involved in the decision-making process concerning telling his peers. Discuss the situation with him openly, and consider the unique variables of your situation: your child; the attitudes of classmates, teachers, and school administration; and the individual personalities of his classmates. While we as parents may want to shout to the world that Asperger Syndrome is nothing to be ashamed of and feel that it is important for her peers to know and understand what it means, she may not yet be ready to share her diagnosis with others.

PRACTICAL SUGGESTIONS FOR COMMON PROBLEMS

Many parents report that their teens find high school more comfortable than junior high. Greater emotional maturity in both the AS child and his peers can have a positive effect on everyone's behavior. Some of the issues that are problematic for children and teens do get easier just by virtue of being a young adult. People are less likely to comment on a teenager wanting to spend time in her room or refusing to eat everything on her plate than they did when she was eight years old.

The one thing that doesn't change with age is how persons with AS learn the skills they need. They still need more "show and tell" and more practice. Expecting them to grow out of AS or become "typical" can only be frustrating for everyone involved. As parents, our goal should be supporting and protecting our child, as the situation warrants. Throughout the book, we have discussed the various social, emotional, and educational challenges parents and children face. The advice offered there applies to adolescents as well. What follows are some of the common problems and difficulties faced by adolescents with Asperger Syndrome, along with some suggestions.

Fitting In

Children with AS enter puberty and adolescence at the same time as the typical child. However, developmentally and emotionally, they may still be lagging behind well into adulthood. Some adults with AS have remarked that they sometimes feel that they never totally grow up in the way others do. Once a person with AS reaches early adulthood, perhaps in the midtwenties, he or she may well have "caught up," so that some differences aren't as glaring. On a humorous note, one father observed that since his son with AS probably wouldn't consider seriously dating until his midtwenties, all he would be missing is the first bad marriage and divorce so many of his neurotypical peers would have experienced.

Due to economic changes and other factors, it's not unusual for a young neurotypical (NT) adult to try several different educational or vocational possibilities, to delay serious romantic involvement or marriage until the midtwenties or beyond, or even to live at home past college age. As parents, we can really help our children by not buying into the idea that "everybody"—NTs included—makes a smooth leap into adulthood. The fact is, not "everybody" does.

For typically developing kids, adolescence is a time of conformity and nonconformity, of slavish devotion to certain social demands (usually their peers') and absolute disregard for others (their parents'). The key, for all teens, is exploring which values, mores, and attitudes they will ultimately adopt as their own. Children with AS are less prepared than typical adolescents to do personal and social exploring. They may be less aware of or interested in the trends and fads through which adolescents claim their membership in their social group. A teenage boy who is still wearing sweatpants for every occasion or a teenage girl who insists on wearing only pink may be inviting ridicule. Persons with AS are not alone in feeling that appearance should not matter and that those who judge them by it are "shallow." That is certainly a valid viewpoint, but peers of any age, though particularly adolescents—who may be hyperconscious about fitting in themselves—can be cruel. There are good reasons for teaching a child with AS to blend in as much as possible by, for example, encouraging him to dress in an age-appropriate manner or have a reasonably stylish haircut. Though you may not be able to persuade your daughter to adopt a "special interest" in current fashion, it will accrue to her social benefit if you can teach her to save talking about her special interest in the literary history of unicorns for a more "receptive" audience.

Most parents worry about their children fitting in, and it's easy to forget that plenty of NT children, for various reasons, choose not to join the crowd. It may well be that your child will find her niche among those kids rather than with the "in" crowd. While there may be a social toll to pay for nonconformity, there is nothing inherently wrong with it.

On the other hand, you may have the type of child who is so lonely and desperate for friendship that he's likely to go along with anything just to feel a part of the group. Often AS teens find themselves in trouble because they have been led astray by more socially adept peers who have no problem allowing the teen with AS to be the scapegoat.

BEHAVIORAL ISSUES

The problem behaviors children with AS may have don't always fade easily with maturity. In fact, hormonal changes, social pressures, and other forces may exacerbate your child's current difficulties or foster new ones. Adolescents generally resist parental hovering and intrusion. It may have been necessary for you to help your child at seven or nine or eleven with taking his shower, for example, or quietly coaching him through placing a telephone call. By the teen years, however, you should strive to be out of the picture. If you are involved in your child's daily life on this level because he is dependent on you to help him do things he should be doing himself, teach him—or find someone to teach him—the skills to be self-sufficient *before* he faces life after high school.

Anger and Aggression

Dealing with frustration and anger can be difficult. For teens with AS who may have other issues, learning difficulties, and awareness of their differences, adolescence may be a time in which tantrums appear, reappear, or increase. However, many parents report that with the onset of puberty, their children are much calmer and more in control. For those who do have problems with acting out, recovery time may be longer, and in the heat of the moment, teens with AS may not be able to exercise the best judgment. The kindergartner who punches a playmate in frustration is viewed far differently than a sixteen-year-old who, caught in a rage cycle, takes a swing at the principal or a stranger.

In terms of controlling behavior, teens with AS are hit from both sides. On the one hand, legally, socially, and emotionally, the stakes are higher. On the other, the external supports and controls many of them depended on in the past and may still need are reduced or eliminated. Suddenly, instead of one teacher having to recognize the signs of impending meltdown and intervene, in middle and high school there are five or six different teachers who may or may not be interested or able to help. Children who had one-on-one aides and other obvious supports and services may be reluctant as they grow older to appear to need help. In addition, we parents as well as educators may feel that it is time to wean the adolescent from the types of support he cannot realistically expect once he's out in "the real world." As a result, full responsibility often lands squarely on the shoulders of the teen himself, who may or may not be able to recognize that he is approaching the end of his rope.

As in the younger years, teens with AS may "hold it together" throughout the school day and then fall apart at home. That this is a "natural" occurrence is something you may hear from teachers and other parents, who repeat it unquestioningly. However, some experts vehemently disagree with the "accepted wisdom" that after-school meltdowns are inevitable. Look at it from a different perspective: What's happening at school that's giving the student so much "to hold in" to start with? Some common culprits: classroom environments, inadequate support, stress during unstructured and loosely supervised parts of the day (break, lunch, gym, bus ride), and so on. Though your teen may be less than forthcoming, do all you can to discover what's happening during his school day that may be adding to his stress.

Don't overlook how the prospect of coming home may be making him anxious. Because both parents may work, many teens will come home to empty houses. Though many are responsible enough to get themselves organized, it may be difficult for some to get started on their homework, for example.

How Parents Can Help

- Make sure your teen has time to wind down after school.
- Unless your teen is exceptionally responsible, don't expect him or her to provide child care for siblings after school.
- If you think your teen is missing lunch, pack a snack in her backpack.
- If you work, make sure that you arrange for a check-in, be it by phone call or by e-mail.
- If your teen is home alone after school, go over the basic rules of safety. Post them prominently and review them often. Assume nothing. Make sure there is a contact available for emergency situations.
- If you are at home when your teen arrives, try not to bombard him with questions the moment he walks in the door. Just as parents need time to wind down after work, AS teens may need time to readjust after a hard day at school. One mother reported that her son goes directly to his room after school for a twenty-minute rest during which he is not to be disturbed. He emerges later, rested, relaxed, and ready to talk.
- If there are siblings, help them understand that their brother or sister needs this time. It's good for everyone.

We stress again the importance of securing an IEP for children whose behavior may likely be misinterpreted. All who will encounter the teen need to be made aware of AS and its implications. It is far too easy for an AS teen who is reacting with frustration, be it over an academic problem or a social difficulty, to react in a way that might be incorrectly viewed as dangerous. The research on AS does not support the idea that persons with the disorder are inherently more dangerous or violent than anyone else. One unfortunate result of the education system's lack of understanding about AS is that children with it are sometimes removed from their usual school environment and placed among children who do have serious emotional disturbances. Every expert on AS will tell you that this inadvertently produces a perfect match between the perfect victim (the child with AS) and the perfect victimizer (the emotionally disturbed, antisocial, or violent student). You should protect your child from such placements at all costs.

What parents can do. In addition to the suggestions offered throughout this book, you can:

- Remember that tantrums and outbursts are likely tied to frustration. If at all possible, try to discover the source of the problem.
- Make sure your teen knows where he can go if he becomes overloaded, confused, or stressed. At home, that might be his room. At school, it could be the resource room, school psychologist's office, nurse's office, or guidance counselor's office. Wherever it is, make sure that someone knows how to handle the situation and that your child will not be punished for being late for class if she takes a break before something happens.
- Everyone dealing with your child in school should have information about him, AS, and how AS may affect his behavior. Don't wait for a major incident, such as a suspension or arrest, before you avail yourself of professionals, such as psychologists and psychiatrists, who can help your child *and* provide your school district with the correct information about the disorder.

DEPRESSION AND ANXIETY

For various reasons, adolescents are at increased risk for anxiety, depression, and other disorders. Some psychiatric disorders make their first appearance in the teen years. For persons with AS, simply the fact of being an adolescent can exacerbate existing problems or create new ones. One of the main differences between a depressed or anxious teen and a depressed or anxious ten-year-old is that the teen is in some ways at greater risk. More time spent with less adult supervision, coupled with access to alcohol, illicit drugs, cars, and sex make any psychiatric disorders arguably more risky because the opportunities for and risks of acting out are so much higher.

Know the signs of anxiety and depression (see pages 69 and 71). If you have any question about your child's behavior or mood, see a qualified professional. If your teen has never taken medication and finds that she is having increasing difficulties that cannot be managed by other methods (such as support, environmental changes, relaxation exercises), you may want to discuss the possibility of medication. If your teen is suffering from depression, something that is not at all uncommon for typical teens and very common for teens with AS, please discuss it with your teen's physician.

If your teen with AS is currently taking psychotropic prescription medicine but is still experiencing increased anxiety, depression, or behavioral problems, see your doctor. Adolescence brings hormonal changes and growth spurts that may require adjustments in medication.

HYGIENE AND PERSONAL APPEARANCE

Though many teens with AS are meticulous in their grooming and love adopting the latest trends, others display a near-total lack of interest in personal hygiene and general appearance. In the same way that a young child with AS may forget to bring home his math book, an older child with AS may forget to use soap, shampoo, or deodorant, put on the same dirty clothes day after day, and neglect to change her underwear. It's not at all uncommon to hear stories of teens who need to be reminded on a daily basis to take a shower or wash their hair.

Why should this be so? In some cases, a child simply forgets or is distracted by other concerns. For children who have difficulty staying focused or who are prone to obsess over things, the mere thought of an upcoming test or yesterday's unpleasant bus ride home can overwhelm everything else. Another possibility is that there are sensory issues that even the child cannot totally identify, such as the smell of a particular brand of soap or shampoo. Many individuals with AS don't like the sensation of water hitting their skin, the feel of the soap or washcloth, or the texture of deodorant. One child we know literally cringes at the feel of baby powder on his skin; another simply cannot stand for her face to be wet.

While others their age may be very focused on the "impression" they make, particularly on peers and members of the opposite sex, teens with AS may seem quite unconcerned. The idea of agonizing for hours over the right skirt or shirt may strike them as irrational and even silly. They may find it difficult to imagine that anyone would notice what they wear because chances are they don't notice what anyone else wears. At the same time, they may develop certain strong feelings about what they wear and how they look. One girl we know, for example, goes through periods where she absolutely refuses to wear anything red, although there are times when it has been her second-favorite color. In addition, tactile sensitivities may cause some teens to prefer worn, soft, unstructured clothing to new, stiffer, and more structured or tight-fitting clothes. Some teen trends—such as the loose or baggy grunge, surfer, or hip-hop styles—are far more easily adopted by teens with AS than anything that's figure-hugging, overly tailored, or just plain tight. They also may prefer the same haircut they have been wearing since they were younger. This may be due to a preference for sameness, a sensory aversion to the experience of having hair cut or styled (the sound of the blow dryer, the smell of hair gel), or simple lack of interest. The difficulty recognizing faces may also apply to one's own reflection. In other words, for persons with AS who have a degree of prosopagnosia, too much change in their own image may be disturbing.

How parents can help. For better or worse, in our culture, and particularly among adolescents, style is a form of communication. Shallow, market-driven, and sometimes ridiculous, style is nonetheless here to stay. While you can rest assured your teen probably will not become a local trendsetter, there is much you can do to help him or her sidestep the more grievous fashion faux pas.

- Casually mention or point out styles and colors that you think would be attractive on your teen. Encourage her to notice what others are wearing.
- Elicit the help of a friend or sibling near the same age as your teen to help her pick out clothing.
- At the child's first hint that he or she wants what the other kids are wearing, run, don't walk, and do your best to provide it. This is not "caving in" to teenage whims, but supporting your child's burgeoning awareness of his own image.
- Remind your child when it's time for a haircut. If possible, try to encourage your child to try subtle changes in his style: a little shorter on top, for example, a little more closely cut at the side. Approaching it like this means it may take you a few months to leave your son's Beatle cut or your daughter's wild mane of curls behind. However, it's better to go at it gradually than to traumatize your teen with a dramatically different 'do.
- Post a list in the bathroom of things to do: brush teeth, comb hair, wash (using soap), shave. If necessary, prepare visual supports and other prompts and reminders. When your child does practice good hygiene and grooming, compliment her generously and specifically.

SCHOOL-RELATED PROBLEMS

Ensuring Services and Protections

Teens diagnosed as children with AS or some other disability covered under IDEA should have an IEP that includes plans for transition by age fourteen (see pages 281 and 303). However, teens who were diagnosed late have probably been struggling without any assistance and understanding. Those students who don't have academic or learning difficulties probably have no supports in place. If you don't have an IEP (or if appropriate, Section 504 services plan) currently in place, we strongly suggest you consider initiating one now. You may meet resistance from your school district, which may take the position that your child has been doing "well enough" thus far without services or accommodations. The fact is, a number of children with AS manage without help only to find that, upon entering middle school or high school, they cannot cope. Services and accommodations are based on *current* need. The fact that a student didn't seem to need special education, services, or accommodations yesterday has no bearing whatsoever on what he needs—and is entitled to receive—today.

In addition, if your child is college bound and may require accommodations (e.g., extra time, use of laptop) for SAT, AP, and ACT testing, plan well ahead. These accommodations must be the same accommodations offered to your child at school, and medical documentation must be current and up-to-date. Universities also require current documentation of disability and accommodations if those same accommodations are to be provided in college. Even if your child managed without accommodations through high school, carefully consider the possibility that he may need them when faced with a more demanding curriculum, less parental supervision (if he goes away to school), and other new academic, emotional, and social challenges. If your child qualifies for accommodations, he can always opt not to use them. At least if you have put them in place for him, he has a choice.

Fortunately, there is no age limit on when a student can be evaluated and provided special education, related services, or accommodations, provided he has not graduated from high school or reached the age of twenty-two. Either of those two events terminates eligibility under IDEA.

Unfortunately, it may be up to you and, we hope, with the help and support of professionals, to educate the educators. (See chapter 8.) Because your child is so close to the end of his public school years, and therefore his eligibility to receive FAPE (free appropriate public education), time is of the essence. If you must call upon professional help to expedite the process, do so by all means.

Self-Advocacy

School is the ideal environment for teaching your child to advocate for herself. Once she leaves the shelter of school and possibly the IEP or 504 services plan, no one else in the world will have "advance warning" of her limitations and areas in which she needs help. Many special education experts encourage you to include your child in IEP and other school-related meetings as soon as she's old enough to understand her disabilities and the type of assistance she needs. They also suggest that you teach your child to speak up for herself and learn to say "I need more time to complete this test," or "I didn't catch everything you said. Could you please repeat the question?"

Teaching self-advocacy is teaching independence. Starting early allows your child time to get used to expressing her need for assistance without embarrassment or shame. It also allows her to better understand her limitations and her skills, which in itself can be empowering.

When School Problems Cannot Be Solved

Despite everyone's best efforts, some persons with AS find school, particularly high school, simply unbearable. The pressure to perform and conform, the rejection, the harassment and abuse from peers can be so psychologically damaging that some never recover.

If your child is showing signs of anxiety, depression, suicidal ideation, or any other dramatic change in behavior, seek help immediately. Demand that your school protect your child from harassment and abuse, and be prepared to act if it does not. Though it may pay to stand your ground and fight on principle in some areas, if your child is being hurt by remaining in school, it may be wisest to find another school, home-school, or have the child provided with instruction (at the school district's expense) at home. Again, consult a special education advocate or attorney *before* unilaterally changing your child's current educational placement.

WORK EXPERIENCE

We've heard from dozens of parents whose children had brilliant academic careers yet are virtually unemployable due to lack of previous work experience and adequate social skills. Not surprisingly, the first after-school or summer job is one rite of passage many parents sidestep, for several reasons. Many of the jobs available to teens are in the service industries (fast-food worker, movie usher, camp counselor) and demand a lot of personal interaction. It's challenging to place an AS child in a new environment where his success depends on understanding people he may not know.

It may not be easy to find the "perfect" job, but AS teens can really benefit from a summer or part-time job during the school year that doesn't detract from their schoolwork or time needed to wind down from school. Although many NT teens can juggle school and work, AS teens may find this extra responsibility stressful. In addition to exposing teens with AS to the real world, being employed in some capacity during the summer or school vacations can also help eliminate the "what to do in the summer" problem faced by teens with AS. By the time they reach age thirteen or fourteen, most summer camp programs are no longer appropriate. By this age many NT kids are becoming camp counselors or attending advanced skill- and sports-oriented camps. Many AS parents express their dismay at summer, and in all too many instances, summers are spent at home with the teen involved in few activities other than their particular special interests. Math and science summer camps or music camps appeal to a certain percentage of teens with AS. Others may participate in camps for special-needs children.

Contact your school district to discover counselors and organizations that specialize in placing persons with disabilities in jobs. If possible, try to find a job for your child that will capitalize on his abilities (say, an interest in computers or music) while avoiding his disabilities (by, for example, working directly under one or two people, having limited contact with strangers). Roger Meyer, an adult with AS, wrote *Asperger Syndrome Employment Workbook: An Employment Workbook for Adults with Asperger Syndrome.* If all else fails, he suggests that you or someone in your family who works in a field of interest to your child consider asking that he be allowed to spend a day or two "on the job." When you're out with your child, point out the different kinds of jobs other people have and encourage him to find out more about occupations that may be of interest to him.

FRIENDS AND EXTRACURRICULAR ACTIVITIES

As an AS child enters her teen years, it becomes harder for parents to actively facilitate friendships by arranging play dates and birthday parties. There are fewer opportunities to get to know other parents as well. The parents at the middle school or the high school level are the ones who are boosting the athletic teams, cheering from the bleachers, helping decorate for the prom, or chaperoning the Spanish Club trip. If your child isn't involved in such activities, you probably will never meet these parents, either. Even those AS children who are athletically gifted and do participate in sports often have difficulty once they leave the playing fields. And, even if you could, it's unlikely that you would be able to do much to facilitate a friendship.

Still, it's not hopeless. There are probably others in your child's school, community, or religious group who share common interests. Many high schools do offer math league, computer clubs, chess club, and band, orchestra, or chorus. Several adults with AS have mentioned that they have success in drama. If your child is interested in history, there are reenactment groups in most states, for example. Contact your local disability-related organizations for information on dance, martial arts, swimming, crafts, art, photography, and other classes either especially designed for or that welcome persons with differences. Also check out volunteer positions your child might enjoy. Depending on the type of work, the people supervising your child may be very open to and patient with a person with disabilities.

You can help your teen find a group that shares his or her particular interest. Or you can volunteer to help run such a group, which will also keep you on hand to help your child with any difficulties. In addition, we feel that it's never too late for a child to participate in social skills training. Many high schools have social facilitation groups and peer mentor systems in place. However, it's *essential* that those who facilitate these programs understand the unique needs of adolescents with AS.

Of course, you can continue to make your home a welcome environment where your child's friends will feel comfortable.

DATING

The teen years are a time when most young adults become interested in forming intimate relationships. For those with AS, such relationships are not easily formed. Those interested in dating may find that they lack the skills to play the dating game. Knowing whether or not someone likes you, knowing how to approach someone in a way that lets her know that you like her, finding the courage to ask someone out, and handling rejection if she says no—these have the power to prompt anxiety, fear, embarrassment, and pure mortification in even the most socially adept. For people with AS, they can be an emotional and social minefield.

In relationships, it's important to learn to read signals and pay attention to the other person's likes and dislikes. Perhaps there are a few who sail through this gracefully, but for the majority of teens, it is definitely a learning process. Teens with Asperger Syndrome may feel particularly lonely as they see their peers become involved in dating relationships. They may make awkward attempts and develop crushes, only to be disappointed.

How parents can help. If your son or daughter wants to have a relationship and it isn't working out, try to be as understanding as possible. Encourage your teen to participate in activities where he's likely to meet other teens who share similar interests. Remind your teen that not everyone dates in high school, and that most people are interested in many other people before they find the "right one." Reassure your teen that there is no time limit on when people begin dating, and that while it may not seem so right now, most people don't find a true, serious relationship until they're in their twenties or older.

If your son or daughter does begin dating, you and your child may have to consider whether to tell the boyfriend or girlfriend about the AS diagnosis. This decision can be particularly difficult if peers at school are unaware of it. The boy or girl your child is dating may well realize that something is different but may blame themselves or your child for behaviors that are a result of AS. Although many teenage dating relationships are short-lived and some end dramatically, it may be wise to limit the information shared until you're sure where the relationship is going.

You'll probably want to assure your child that someday he or she may find someone special who will love and care for them and appreciate them as they are. Yet at the same time, you may secretly wonder if this is true. You may waver between wanting to encourage your child to take the initiative and ask someone out and wanting to protect him or her from rejection and disappointment. Perhaps the best approach is to gently offer suggestions and always be there, no matter what the outcome.

SEXUALITY

Long before the issue of dating arises, it is imperative that both boys and girls with AS are educated about issues concerning sexuality (including sexual abuse, contraception, safer sex [to prevent transmission of HIV and other sexually transmitted diseases], and date or acquaintance rape). Remember, children with Asperger Syndrome reach puberty at the same age as typical children, but they may be more confused and unprepared for the changes occurring in their bodies. Parents wonder if their children, who have a tendency to take things literally, will misinterpret sex education information. Considering that schools are introducing discussion of these matters at increasingly younger ages, you would do well to start talking about sexuality early and often, in terms that your child understands.

Most high school health classes cover many of these topics, but there has been some discussion as to whether this is the best environment for a student with AS to learn about and discuss these issues. Classes taught using a social skill/group discussion format may create awkward situations for a teen with AS. Some adolescents with AS can be literal and ask or answer questions in a way that might elicit teasing. Students harassed one AS teen after he told the members of his health class that he was "not interested in girls" and thought dating was "a waste of time." He was simply telling the truth as he saw it, not making a statement about sexual orientation.

Contact your local autism or Asperger Syndrome organization, university or university hospital, or therapy practice that specializes in treating persons with AS. There is an increasing need for sex education for persons all across the spectrum, and programs are cropping up. For example, on Long Island, the Cody Center for Autism at the State University of New York at Stony Brook offers programs on sexuality designed for individuals on the spectrum as young as nine.

A pervasive lack of social skills can result in difficult situations for both young men and women who don't engage in the full complement of culturally accepted gender-specific behaviors. Young women who dress for comfort and take a casual approach to grooming, and young men who aren't into sports or avidly pursuing girls may be labeled "gay." Of course, individuals with AS, as in the general population, can be gay or straight. However, the teasing and harassment that usually happen to both boys and girls is generally based not on true sexual orientation but on how teens with AS are perceived by their peers.

The lack of social skills can place teens and adults with AS at risk because they may not understand the intentions of others or be able to express their own intentions clearly. Women with AS are at higher than normal risk for sexual harassment, date rape or attempted date rape, and sexual assault. Men with AS, who may lack subtlety in their approach to women, are sometimes perceived as overly insistent and forward. Men with AS are also sometimes presumed to welcome homosexual advances because they lack the social sophistication to "read" the signals correctly.

How parents can help. With little expert advice at hand, we can only suggest that you include issues related to sexuality in your on-going conversation with your teen. Individual cognitive behavior therapy, social skills training that addresses these issues and situations particularly, and frank discussion about the "rules" of social-sexual behavior may all be necessary. Remember how long it took our teens to learn other social skills; dating and sexuality are no different. You must provide clear information when you discuss these topics with your teen and, perhaps more important, make sure that he or she knows you will always listen and welcome questions.

DRUGS AND ALCOHOL

Illicit use of drugs and alcohol pose problems and risks for all kids. However, for persons with AS, these risks are multiplied. The social disability makes our kids easy marks for those who would take advantage of them—by asking them to "hold" or sell drugs or steal beer from a store, for example. Peer groups that are heavily involved in such illicit activities tend not to be as picky as some groups you might prefer your child associate with. Our children with AS may be more readily accepted by them. We are all well aware of the role of peer pressure in teenage drinking and drugging. However, peer pressure takes on a whole new meaning and a lot more force when directed at a young person with AS who may be even more desperate to fit in and lack the social savvy to fully appreciate all aspects of a situation.

Our teens will be exposed to drugs and underage drinking just as all other teens are, so it's important to discuss these issues early and often. What do you say? Once again, the research is not yet in, but common sense tells us that we can do several things to help our kids steer clear of problems.

- Exploit the AS tendency to see moral issues in terms of black and white. Tell your child that drugs and underage drinking are illegal (resulting in possible arrest, going to jail) and dangerous (resulting in addiction, overdose, alcohol poisoning, etc.). Explain that drugs and underage drinking are not good for anyone and that a real friend is someone who would never ask you to place yourself at risk.
- Although the typical teenager may scoff at the idea that drinking or doing drugs is "stupid" or makes people "look dumb" and do embarrassing things, a teen with AS may accept those as compelling reasons to abstain.
- Explain how drugs and underage drinking can hurt people by impairing their judgment, making them attractive prey to bullies and others who would take advantage of them sexually or otherwise, and making it all too easy for them to be caught in bad situations.
- Establish and reiterate rules of behavior such as not visiting anyone's home or "hanging out" where there is no adult supervision; immediately leaving any situation in which drugs or alcohol are used; telling you or another adult of drug or alcohol use; never holding or transporting drugs or alcohol, no matter who asks you to do it.
- Build a network of friends and activities to counter the boredom, lack of supervision, and peer pressure that often precede alcohol and drug use.
- Make sure that your teen knows how to respond if he is offered alcohol or drugs and that he knows to leave any situation where they're being used.
- Be sure that your teen knows how to respond to law enforcement officials and other authority figures, particularly if alcohol or drugs are present.

A special note for parents who may have experimented with drugs in the past or who use alcohol or drugs now: Whether or not you personally agree with a hard-line, "just say no" approach, that may be the only sound advice to give your child. A "do as I say, not as I do" position may be confusing, and recounting your own past experiences (though arguably helpful with typical kids in helping them relate to Mom and Dad) may simply complicate and cloud the issue for the teen with AS.

Some parents of AS children worry that the use of prescription psychotropic medication will lead to drug abuse. In fact, children whose serious emotional and psychological problems are not addressed are at the highest risk for underage drinking and illicit drug use. (See pages 237 and 257.) The fact that drinking and illicit drug use serve the function of "self-medicating" is well established among both pediatric and adult populations. If anything, prescription psychotropic medication, when used correctly, may actually reduce your child's risk of experimenting with alcohol and street drugs.

Warning: *If your child is currently taking any prescription psychotropic medication, she should understand that alcohol or other drugs may cause adverse reactions, including sudden death. If you suspect that your child who is taking medication may be experimenting with alcohol or drugs, or is at high risk of doing so, speak with your child's prescribing doctor immediately.*

DRIVING AND GETTING AROUND

One of the most talked-about topics on the OASIS Raising Teens and Young Adults forum is driving. Can a young person with AS learn to drive? Get a license? Become a safe driver? The good news is that all of that is possible, but like anything else it may take a little bit longer (just like it probably took a bit longer to learn to tie shoes or ride a bike). We have heard from parents whose children have failed their driver's tests, sometimes several times. The first concern for most parents is not whether or not their child will ever drive, but how safe a driver she will be once she does.

The most obvious obstacle to safe driving is the trouble many persons with AS have in doing more than one thing at a time and quickly shifting focus from one second to the next. Teens and young adults who do not have their temper under control, who are prone to rages or aggression, who are extremely easily distracted, or who become easily flustered or frustrated by circumstances beyond anyone's control should delay getting behind the wheel. On the positive side, most AS individuals are fairly rule-oriented and do abide by the law. They are also probably less likely to drink and drive, blast loud music, or show off for their friends. That said, driving can be very challenging (there are plenty of neurotypicals who simply cannot or will not drive), and your child may not receive his license until years after his peers.

For those who do drive, here are some tips. First, practice, practice, and more practice is essential. Driving is all about looking for and dealing with the unexpected. Be sure your child has massive amounts of supervised practice so that the act of driving comes more naturally and he can focus his attention on the road. To reduce distractions, opt for an automatic as opposed to a manual transmission, be sure the car is in good repair, and be sure your child always has a cell phone (with every conceivably important phone number he may need preprogrammed in). One mother we both know very well has her eighteen-year-old son call when he arrives at school or work and call home before he leaves school or work in the afternoon. If you can afford it, the OnStar navigation and tracking system is a good idea. Needless to say, talking on the cell while driving—even with a headset that makes it hands-free—is not allowed. Studies have shown that drivers engaged in conversation perform on the road no better than someone who is legally intoxicated. Set some rules for driving: Change radio stations and CDs only when the car is stopped; no friends in the car without your prior permission.

Make sure your teen knows the most basic rules of car safety: how to get off the road and park safely in the event of mechanical trouble, whom to call, where to wait until help arrives, and so on. Also drill him on what to do if he's involved in an accident. He should know who to call immediately and be able to produce all the required insurance documents and see those of the other driver, too. He should not admit to any wrongdoing and know how to talk appropriately to the police. (See below.)

ENCOUNTERS WITH LAW ENFORCEMENT
AND OTHER AUTHORITIES

Because of their Asperger Syndrome, children and adults may run into unforeseen misunderstandings and difficulties when dealing with law enforcement officers and other authorities. There is no research indicating that persons with AS are more likely to be involved in illegal activity. However, parents should take seriously the risk that having such a pervasive social disability poses. Persons with AS are at greater risk for being victims of any kind of crime, for being "misled" into situations they cannot foresee or understand (including illegal or suspicious activity), for being coerced or forced to take part in illegal activity, and so on. Despite the fact that many persons with AS are rule-abiding to a T, they often lack the social sophistication to fully appreciate the possible implications of a particular action or to fully foresee how certain types of behavior (for example, standing outside the public restroom in a park at night or following a woman walking down the street too closely) may look to others.

We have heard of cases from around the country where a person with AS was left holding the bag, so to speak, after being involved by more savvy companions who then convincingly denied any involvement. In these cases, peer pressure, a need to feel accepted, and a lack of social understanding conspired to create the setup. In other cases, a person with AS reacted aggressively or violently after being attacked, provoked, or overwhelmed. Here again, the real perpetrators could stage it in such a way that their claims of innocence were believed.

Sometimes a person with AS finds himself in trouble based solely on the way he responds to a police officer or other authority. By their very nature, persons with AS can sometimes "look suspicious" even when innocent. A teenage boy who walks through a store wearing an oversized coat (because of sensory issues) and holding his arms close to his body (because of unusual posture) could appear to be shoplifting. He may not know how to respond to the store manager or security guard's "Hey, what have you got in there?" in the expected way. Rather than assume a friendly demeanor, make eye contact, volunteer to open his coat, and apologize for any misunderstanding, he may reply "My arms," start walking or running away, or panic—each of which may exacerbate the situation. Under stress, he may begin having tics, become echolalic, start talking to himself, scream, or behave in other ways that give the impression he is unstable, dangerous, or under the influence of drugs or alcohol. If approached, touched, or restrained, he may become more agitated and even violent out of panic and fear. Consequently, this misinterpreted behavior may incur the use of force.

Persons with AS can seem uncooperative or threatening by virtue of their body language or how they respond to routine questions. Dr. Brenda Smith Myles gave the example of a man stopped for speeding. When the police officer asked, "Do you know how fast you were going?" the man replied simply, "Yes." The fact is, he did know how fast he was going, so he was telling the truth and answering the officer's question. However, most of us recognize that in dealing with police officers and other authorities, the "right" answer is not always the literal truth. Instead of using his answer to demonstrate the expected degree of respect, the man with AS communicated defiance and lack of respect.

If a person with AS is the victim of or witness to a crime, he or she may not be a good witness. The trauma of the incident coupled with difficulties in recognizing faces or noticing details may make him unable to describe perpetrators—what they looked like, what they did, or what they said. Sometimes law enforcement officials mistakenly assume that no crime was committed or that the person may be "covering up" for someone else.

Finally, most persons with AS—even those with average IQs and above—don't understand their legal rights. They may interpret what is said to them literally or not understand the ramifications of what they say or do. In one case we know of, a man with autism confessed to a crime he did not commit because he wanted the interview to end. He believed that if he "did what the police wanted," they would let him go home.

Dennis Debbaudt, creator of the Web site Avoiding Unfortunate Situations (http://policeandautism.cjb.net), believes that law enforcement personnel need to be educated about the behaviors and needs of persons with ASDs. For example, he says, there are ways to interview individuals with autism that will make it possible for them to provide the right information if stopped by police. Debbaudt recommends the Maryland Autism Police Curriculum.

How parents can help

- Take the first steps to make your local police, fire, emergency, and other helping personnel aware of autism and AS. Present them with information about the Maryland Autism Police Curriculum and urge them to obtain it. Get your local and national AS-related organizations to press this issue.
- Educate your child about police and fire safety. Many communities sponsor programs such as Safety Town or school visits from firefighters and police officers who talk about how to respond in emergencies. Ask your school district to work with your local police department and fire department to develop a program designed for children with disabilities. If that isn't possible, consider setting up one through your local support group. Invite police officers, firefighters, and EMT personnel to meet your children and give a presentation about the issues facing persons with ASDs. Be sure to offer print material as well.
- Design a wallet-sized card, which you can have laminated, that identifies your child as a person with Asperger Syndrome (see page 352).
- Teach your child the proper way to respond to police, fire, and EMT personnel. Keep in mind that these encounters may include sirens and other troubling noises.

COLLEGE AND EMPLOYMENT

Many children who were among the first diagnosed back in 1994 are now approaching adulthood, and parents are blazing yet another new trail. Long before your son or daughter begins considering life after high school, you need to have an individualized plan for transition up and running (see chapter 8). No matter how bright, gifted, talented, or diligent your child is, chances are good that he or she will require a great deal of support for a much longer time than the typical teen. Begin the process early.

If college is the direction you're headed, visit possible schools early and discuss with admissions officers the accommodations your child will require. Once your child is accepted, visit the campus frequently with your child (if possible) so she can become familiar with where things are and what is available. Coulter Video has put together a College Prep Portfolio, which is an organizer that can help students and parents begin to prepare for college and work. This organizer or something like it can be very helpful in compiling and organizing resources for work or college. In addition, consider putting together a binder or organizer that will help your child once he or she is in college. Consider and discuss the what-ifs. What if you have a toothache? What if you oversleep? What if you run out of deodorant? What if you get lost on campus? What if you find yourself falling behind in your work? Now is the time to have another discussion about sexuality, safe sexual practices, and date rape. Again, discuss all possibilities (including walking in on a roommate, or your roommate walking in on you). And don't forget to talk about managing money, alcohol and drugs, (relatively) healthy eating, and so on.

If your child is living on campus, make sure you come up with ways to stay in touch. Be aware that unless specific arrangements are made, universities will not contact you if there is a problem.

Some children with Asperger Syndrome will not attend a traditional college, for any number of reasons. The rise in universities offering online courses and degrees may be an option for some. Others may prefer to pursue an interest or begin work in a field for which a college education is not necessary, though training may be involved. Contact your state department of education and find out what is available in terms of vocational training, which has come to encompass everything from culinary arts and computer programming to health care and jet engine repair. Inquire in your community about businesses or corporations that have made a commitment to hiring and supporting individuals with disabilities. Such organizations may be a good place for your child to get his or her first job experience.

THE FUTURE WITHOUT YOU

This is perhaps the hardest thing to consider for most of us: the day when we will no longer be able to be involved in our children's lives the way we are now. As much as we all wish for a long, healthy life, the fact is that that dreaded day could come at any time. What can you do today to help your child tomorrow?

• Be prepared for the unthinkable and the inevitable. None of us enjoys planning for tragedy, but our children need these arrangements made on their behalf. If you find it difficult to make the proper arrangements, simply picture your child in the temporary custody of social services personnel or other strangers who know nothing about him, or AS, for the weeks or months it may take to establish legal custody or find him a new home. Then get to work.

• Working with an attorney who specializes in estate planning for families with children who have disabilities, write your will and set up a special-needs trust. Choose your child's guardian wisely, and be sure you have discussed it thoroughly and the person you have chosen has agreed to assume responsibility for raising your child. Because of your child's disability, you may consider setting up a trust or other arrangement through which your child's financial needs will be met without him inheriting the money directly. Laws concerning inheritance vary from state to state, so consult with a knowledgeable attorney who specializes in this area. (*Note:* Will-writing software and "form" wills will not suffice. You need a specialist to write a will that will provide for and protect a disabled child.)

• Be sure that family members and friends you can count on have copies of critical information about you and your child: the location of his school and how to get there; any medication he may be taking, the schedule, where to find it in the house, and the name of the prescribing physician as well as the pharmacy where it is filled; the names and numbers of all of your child's doctors; where to find important papers, keys to safe-deposit boxes, and other items that may be needed in the event you are incapacitated or deceased.

• If your child is old enough and you believe the disclosure would not provoke anxiety, discuss the arrangements you have made and what will occur in the event that you can no longer care for him.

LETTING GO WHILE STILL HOLDING ON

Parents of teens and young adults with Asperger Syndrome are often criticized by those who don't understand their need to remain deeply involved in their children's lives. Some of us also question when to loosen the strings, by how much, and how. Just as many of us were judged for "hovering" over our three-year-olds and "babying" our nine-year-olds, so we may be seen as "smothering" or "coddling" our teens. The fact remains that our children may need more support, more care, and more assistance than others their age, perhaps even for the rest of their lives. As a parent of a child with AS, you have probably weathered other criticism by now. Our advice: Take it on the chin, ignore it, then go on doing what you believe is best for your child today, while you are still here and have this opportunity. As difficult as it may have been to imagine for so many years, your child with AS will become an adult with AS. What does that mean? And what is the best thing you can do?

Our job as parents is not to change our children into who we would like them to be, but rather to help guide them to be the best they can be. Liane Holliday Willey writes in her book: "I know the real me, the one that truly matters, was nurtured and shaped by the lessons my mother and father taught me. The heart and soul of their parenting was simply that I take pride in my individuality, idiosyncrasies and all."[1]

Kalen Molton, an adult on the spectrum, once said, "I try to remind myself that I am a high-functioning autistic, not a low-functioning normal person, as others would have me believe."

We must light the way for others to understand our children in terms of what they are rather than what they are not and perhaps never can be. Those who choose to enumerate the many ways in which the rare lavender rose "fails" to be a classic red rose not only miss the point, they miss the beauty. Learning to see, to understand, and to appreciate every rose is an opportunity to learn something new, not only about that flower but about themselves. As we help our children to better adapt to a world that is not very good at accepting people with differences, we should remember Kalen's words. Simply in persisting through a life that is neither predictable nor easy, our children exhibit courage, resilience, and an unusual strain of hope.

How parents can help

• Help your child form a network of support. This network could consist of family members, friends, community members, medical professionals, and others. For example, a friend who is an accountant might be willing to keep an eye on taxes, or a member of your church or synagogue might be willing to include your child in holiday celebrations. Just as we made sure our children knew where the safe places were when they were younger, they should also know this as adults. Most of us know on whom we can count in an emergency. Make sure your young adult knows who's available for support.

• Introduce your child to the community; including law enforcement, fire, and ambulance personnel, if you feel this may be useful in the future.

FINALLY

We both truly believe that by offering to individuals with Asperger Syndrome help in areas such as social skills training, behavior management, independence, and understanding, we are not attempting to "cure" Asperger Syndrome, but rather to give the children with AS the necessary tools to make choices in their lives. Everyone with Asperger Syndrome should be respected and celebrated for their differences.

Recommended Resources

Asperger Syndrome: Transition to College and Work (With College Preparation Checklist), Coulter Video, 2002, www.coultervideo.com.

Tony Attwood and Carol Gray, "The Discovery of 'Aspie' Criteria," originally published in *The Morning News*; also on Attwood's Web site (http://www.tonyattwood.com.au/paper4.htm) and at the Gray Center for Social Learning and Understanding (www.thegray center.org/discovery_of.htm.).

Teresa Bolick, *Asperger Syndrome and Adolescence: Helping Preteens and Teens Get Ready for the Real World* (Gloucester, MA: Fair Winds Press, 2001).

College Prep Portfolio: Preparing and Organizing the Paperwork That Will Give You an Edge in Applying to the College or Job of Your Choice. Coulter Video, 2004, www.coultervideo.com.

Yvona Fast, *Employment for Individuals with Asperger Syndrome or Non-Verbal Learning Disabilities: Stories and Strategies* (London and New York: Jessica Kingsley Publishing, 2004).

John Harpur, Maria Lawlor, and Michael Fitzgerald, *Succeeding in College with Asperger Syndrome* (London and New York: Jessica Kingsley Publishing, 2004).

Gail Hawkins, *How to Find Work That Works for People with Asperger Syndrome: The Ultimate Guide for Getting People with Asperger Syndrome into the Workplace* (London and New York: Jessica Kingsley Publishing, 2004).

Patricia Howlin, *Autism: Preparing for Adulthood* (London and New York: Routledge, 1997).

Roger N. Meyer, *Asperger Syndrome Employment Workbook: An Employment Workbook for Adults with Asperger Syndrome* (London and Philadelphia: Jessica Kingsley Publishers, 2001).

Brenda Smith Myles and Diane Adreon, *Asperger Syndrome and Adolescence: Practical Solutions for School Success* (Shawnee Mission, KS: Autism Asperger Publishing, 2001).

Jerry Newport, *Your Life Is Not a Label* (Arlington, Tex.: Future Horizons, 2001).

Jerry Newport and Mary Newport, *Autism-Asperger's and Sexuality: Puberty and Beyond* (Arlington, Tex.: Future Horizons, 2002).

Digby Tantum, "Adolescence and Adulthood of Individuals with Asperger Syndrome," in Ami Klin, Fred R. Volkmar, and Sara S. Sparrow, eds., *Asperger Syndrome* (New York: Guilford Press, 2000), pp. 367–402.

Liane Holliday Willey, ed., *Asperger Syndrome in Adolescence: Living with the Ups, the Downs and Things in Between* (London and New York: Jessica Kingsley Publishing, 2003).

NOTES

Chapter 1. What Is Asperger Syndrome?

1. Lorna Wing, "The History of Asperger Syndrome," in Eric Schopler, Gary B. Mesibov, Linda J. Kunce, eds., *Asperger Syndrome or High-Functioning Autism?* Current Issues in Autism series (New York: Plenum, 1998), pp. 11–27.
2. Peter Tanguay, "Pervasive Developmental Disorders: A 10-Year Review," *Journal of the American Academy of Child and Adolescent Psychiatry* 39 (9) (September 2000), pp. 1079–95.
3. Christopher Gillberg and Mary Coleman, *The Biology of Autistic Syndromes,* 2nd ed. (London: MacKeith Press, 1992), p. 44.
4. Sue Thompson, *The Source for Nonverbal Learning Disorders* (East Moline, IL: LinguiSystems, 1997).
5. Dr. Ami Klin and Dr. Fred R. Volkmar, handout to conference "Asperger Syndrome: Diagnosis, Assessment, and Treatment," New York City, May 3, 2000.
6. Peter Tanguay, "Pervasive Developmental Disorders: A 10-Year Review," *Journal of the American Academy of Child and Adolescent Psychiatry* 39 (9) (September 2000), pp. 1079–95.
7. Klin and Volkmar, "Asperger Syndrome" conference handout.
8. For our purposes, we will not be referring to Rett's disorder and childhood disintegrative disorder when we use the term PDD.
9. "Autism Facts," Autism Society of America, online at www.autism-society.org/site/PageServer?pagename=autism_Facts; "Fact Sheet: How Many People Have Autistic Spectrum Disorders?" the National Autistic Society (U.K.), online at www.nas.org.uk/nas/jsp/polopoly.jsp?d= 108&a=3527; U.S. Census, online at www.census.gov.; United Kingdom census figures, online at www.statistics.gov.uk. All accessed May 22, 2004.
10. Dr. Eric London, National Alliance for Autism Research (NAAR), speech at the David Center, Uniondale, NY, December 2000.
11. Eric Frombonne, "The Prevalence of Autism," *Journal of the American Medical Association* 289 (1) (January 1, 2003), pp. 87–89.

12. "Autism A.L.A.R.M.," January 2004, online at medicalhomeinfo.org/screening/Autism%20downloads/AlarmFinal1.jpg.
13. Statistics from Fighting Autism, based on data from the U.S. Department of Special Education. "Autism Incidence: U.S. School Years, 1992–2002" and "Autism Incidence Cumulative Growth: U.S. School Years 1992–2002," online at www.fightingautism.org/idea/autism.php.
14. Ibid. "Incidence Annual Growth: U.S. School Years 1992–2002," online at www.fightingautism.org/idea/autism.php.
15. Frombonne, "Prevalence of Autism."
16. Byrna Siegel, *The World of the Autistic Child* (New York and Oxford: Oxford University Press, 1996), p. 55.
17. For more information on the savantism, visit Dr. Darold A. Treffert's pages on the Wisconsin Medical Society Web site at www.wisconsin/medicalsociety.org/savant/default.cfm.

Chapter 3. How Asperger Syndrome Is Diagnosed

1. CHADD Facts. "The Disorder Named AD/HD," online at www.chadd.org.
2. National Institute of Mental Health, online at www.nimh.nih.gov.
3. Ibid.
4. Ibid.
5. Stephen M. Edelson, "Autism, Puberty, and the Possibility of Seizures," online at www.autism.org/seizures.html, accessed August 15, 2004.
6. American Academy of Child and Adolescent Psychiatry, online at www.aacap.org.
7. Child and Adolescent Bipolar Foundation, online at www.bpkids.org. Also, "About Early Onset Bipolar Disorder," Child and Adolescent Bipolar Foundation, 2000. Reprinted with permission.
8. Tourette Syndrome Association, Inc., online at www.tsa-usa.org.
9. David C. Geary, "Mathematical Disabilities: What We Know and Don't Know," online at www.ldonline.org/ld_indepth/math_skills/geary_math_dis.html.
10. Facts about dyslexia from the International Dyslexia Association, online at interdys.org.
11. Learning Disabilities Association of America (LDA) fact sheet "Dyslexia," Learning Disabilities Association of America (LDA), available online at www.ldanatl.org/.
12. Adapted and reprinted with permission from Pamela B. Tanguay, "Nonverbal Learning Disabilities: What to Look For," in *Nonverbal Learning Disabilities at Home: A Parent's Guide* (London and Philadelphia: Jessica Kingsley Publishers, 2001).

13. Roger Pierangelo and George A. Giuliani, *Assessment in Special Education: A Practical Approach* (Boston: Allyn & Bacon, 2002), p. 159.

Chapter 6. Options and Interventions

1. For a more detailed discussion, see Fred R. Volkmar and Ami Klin, "Diagnostic Issues in Asperger Syndrome," in Ami Klin, Fred R. Volkmar, and Sara S. Sparrow, eds., *Asperger Syndrome* (New York: Guilford Press, 2000), pp. 25–71.

2. The exception here would be medication, which should never be stopped suddenly without first consulting the prescribing physician. Discontinuing medication without the doctor's supervision can have serious, sometimes even fatal, consequences.

3. Mitzi Waltz, *Pervasive Developmental Disorders: Finding a Diagnosis and Getting Help* (Sebastopol, CA: O'Reilly, 1999), p. 241.

4. Adapted from "Health Insurance," Autism Society of America Web site, www.autism-society.org, accessed 2001.

5. In 1987, Dr. Lovaas published a study that documented the progress of nineteen autistic children who received forty hours a week of one-on-one ABA therapy. The results were dramatic: the average gain in IQ was 20 points, and nine of the children (47 percent) successfully completed first grade in mainstream schools. When these children were tested again in 1993 (average age, thirteen years old), eight of the nine were still enrolled successfully in regular classrooms and had lost none of their skills. Subsequent studies have shown similar levels of improvement for children with autistic disorder who are not mentally retarded. The substantial gains in IQ scores following ABA suggests that the oft-cited statistic that 50 percent of persons with autistic disorder are also mentally retarded may be more a reflection of the shortcomings of diagnostic instruments in assessing these children accurately than the subjects' true abilities. Intensive ABA therapy has been shown to be one of the most successful interventions for children with autistic disorder.

6. Catherine Maurice, "ABA and Us: One Parent's Reflection on Partnership and Persuasion," address to the Cambridge Center for Behavioral Studies (CCBS), Annual Board Meeting, Palm Beach, FL, November 5, 1999, at www.behavior.org, accessed May 22, 2004.

7. Early in Dr. Lovaas's work with autistic children, undesirable behaviors resulted in consequences that included physical punishment or aversives. This is no longer the case. You may find on the Internet a site or two describing practitioners who use such approaches for individuals whose self-injurious behaviors are life-threatening, but this involves a literal handful of extreme cases and such intervention is highly regulated.

Nonetheless, the misconception that ABA may involve physical punishment persists in some quarters.

8. Dr. Vincent Carbone, a psychologist and certified behavior analyst who has made important contributions in terms of promoting, teaching, and disseminating information about VBA, has stated publicly that there is no such thing as a "Carbone" method and that AVB is ABA.

9. If this strikes you as odd, it's probably because the prevailing view of how we acquire and use language is influenced by cognitive psychology. Linguists such as Noam Chomsky argued against Skinner and the behaviorists, claiming that the ability to learn and use language is universal and innate, not something learned through "training by reward and penalty over time," as Skinner saw it. The arguments here really are the epitome of what we mean when we say "academic," so we will stop here. Even leading practitioners of VB will confess that Skinner's *Verbal Behavior* is a difficult read.

10. You can learn about more terms in "What Is Applied Verbal Behavior?" at www.christinabrukaba.com/AVB.htm.

11. Author unknown, "CAPD Handout for Parents and Teachers," 22 February 1996, online at www.homeschooljournal.bizland.com/CAPD%20 HANDOUT%20FOR%20PARENTS%20AND%20TEACHERS and several other Web sites.

12. Carol Gray, *Comic Strip Conversations: Colorful, Illustrated Interactions with Students with Autism and Related Disorders* (Arlington, TX: Future Horizons, 1994), p. 1.

13. Carol Gray, *The Original Social Story Book* (Arlington, TX: Future Horizons, 1993), pp. 2–3.

14. See Diane Twachtman-Cullen, *How to Be a Para Pro: A Comprehensive Training Manual for Paraprofessionals* (Higganum, CT: Starfish Specialty Press, 2000), p. 11.

15. Richard Lavoie, "Ask Rick," monthly column, online at LD Online, www.ldonline.org.

Chapter 7. Medication

1. Andrés Martin, David K. Patzer, and Fred R. Volkmar, "Psychopharmacological Treatment of Higher-Functioning Pervasive Developmental Disorders," in Ami Klin, Fred R. Volkmar, and Sara S. Sparrow, eds., *Asperger Syndrome* (New York: Guilford Press, 2000), p. 214, table 7.1, "Subjects Taking Psychotropic Medications on Date of Survey."

2. "Medications," NIH publication no. 95-3929, revised 1995.

3. "Treatment of Children with Mental Disorders," NIH publication no. 00-4702, September 2000. See also Howard Chua-Eoan, "Escaping from Darkness," *Time,* 31 May 1999, pp. 44–49.

4. Pharmaceutical Research and Manufacturers of America, "New Analysis Shows Prescription Medicines Are Significantly Under-insured Compared to Hospital and Physician Costs," March 5, 2004, accessed April 11, 2004 at www.pharma.org/actions/printFriendlyPage.cfm?t=46&r=917.

5. "Controversy Over Stimulant Use Among Children," Reuters News, Yahoo! January 2000.

6. See Betsy Bates, "Psychotropic Drug Scripts Way Up in Preschoolers," *Pediatric News* 34 (4) (2000), pp. 1, 5. According to a study published in the *Journal of the American Medical Association* 283 (8) (2000), pp. 1025–30, prescriptions for stimulants and other psychotropic medications written for children between the ages of two and four increased 50 percent between 1991 and 1995.

7. U.S. Food and Drug Administration, "Public Health Advisory Subject: Worsening Depression and Suicidality in Patients Being Treated with Antidepressant Medications," March 22, 2002, accessed April 11, 2004, at www.fda.gov./cder/drug/antidepressants/AntidepressantsPHA.htm.

8. Jeff Nesmith, "90 Million Americans Are 'Health Illiterate,'" New York Times Syndicate, April 8, 2004, accessed April 11, 2004, from MedlinePlus at www.nlm.nih.gov/medlineplus/print/news/fullstory_17059.html.

9. Luke Y. Tsai, *Taking the Mystery Out of Medications in Autism/Asperger Syndrome* (Arlington, TX: Future Horizons, 2001), p. xi.

10. See Alexis Jetter, "Trying to End Guesswork in Dosing Children: A Conversation with Dianne Murphy," *New York Times,* 12 September 2000, p. F7.

11. Other excellent sources are *The PDR Family Guide to Prescription Drugs*, 9th ed. (New York: Three Rivers Press, 2002) and *The PDR Pocket Guide to Prescription Drugs*, 6th ed. (New York: Pocket Books, 2004).

12. "Recognizing Psychiatric Disorders in Adolescents and Young Adults: A Guide for Prescribers of Accutane (isotretinoin)," CDER Drug Information, April 9, 2002, online at www.fda.gov/cder/drug/infopage/accutane/accutane_psychdisorders.htm, accessed August 15, 2004.

13. Despite the appeal of purchasing prescriptions from pharmacies outside the United States, the FDA warns that it cannot regulate or guarantee the safety and quality of these medications. There have been cases of consumers receiving medications that, despite arriving in what appeared to be legitimate packaging, turned out to be counterfeit, containing less than or none of the stated active ingredient. In addition, some medications can lose their potency or become dangerous to use if not shipped, stored, and handled according to manufacturer's instructions. If you have problems paying for prescriptions, visit the PhRMA (Pharmaceutical Research and Manufacturers Association) Web site for information on obtaining medications at reduced costs from manufacturers: www.pharm.org.

14. Tsai, p. 63.

15. See Nancy Rappaport and Peter Chubinsky, "The Meaning of Psychotropic Medications for Children, Adolescents, and Their Families," *Journal of the American Academy of Child and Adolescent Psychiatry* 39 (9) (September 2000), pp. 1198–1200.

16. Timothy E. Wilens, *Straight Talk About Psychiatric Medications for Kids* (New York: Guilford Press, 1999), p. 181.

17. Joyce Howard Price, "Antidepressant Use by Preschoolers Rising," *Washington Times,* April 3, 2004, online at www.washtimes.com/national/20040402-115946-9170r.html.

18. E. Hollander, A. Kaplan, C. Cartwright, and D. Reichman, "Venlafaxine in Children, Adolescents, and Young Adults with Autism Spectrum Disorders: An Open Retrospective Clinical Report," *Journal of Child Neurology* 15 (2) (February 2000), pp. 132–35.

19. Yael Waknine, "Medscape Alert: Antidepressants May Cause Depression and Suicidality," Medscape Medical News, March 22, 2004, online at www.medscape.com/viewarticle/4726364?mpid=26585, accessed April 2, 2004.

20. FDA Talk Paper, "FDA Issues Public Health Advisory on Cautions for Use of Antidepressants in Children and Adults," March 22, 2004, online at www.fda.gov/bbs/topics/ANSWERS/2004/ANS01283.html, accessed April 10, 2004.

21. Rob Waters, "FDA Was Urged to Limit Kids' Antidepressants," *San Francisco Chronicle,* April 16, 2004, online at http://sfgate.com/cgi-bin/article.cgi?file=c/a/2004/04/16/MNGQN668FL1.DTL, accessed April 16, 2004.

22. FDA Talk Paper, "FDA Issues Public Health Advisory on Cautions for Use of Antidepressants in Children and Adults."

23. Tsai, p. 142.

24. Jessica A. Hellings, "Treatment of Comorbid Disorders in Autism," *Medscape Mental Health* 5 (1) (2000).

25. Donna A. Wirshing, William C. Wirshing, Stephen R. Marder, C. Scott Sauncers, Elizabeth H. Rosotto, and Stephen Erhart, "Atypical Antipsychotics: A Practical Review," *Medscape Mental Health* 2 (10) (1997).

26. Hellings, "Treatment of Comorbid Disorders in Autism."

Chapter 8. Special Education Basics

1. There are many other types of services a student might receive, depending on establishment of need and interpretation of federal, state, and local requirements. For example, in some school districts music therapy, auditory integration training, or special programs such as the Lindamood-Bell reading program may be provided as related services,

but in other school districts they may not. If you have reason to believe that a service may benefit your child and you can demonstrate a need, pursue the matter with your school district.

2. Individuals with Disabilities Education Act, 20 U.S.C. §1401(25)(A) and (B).

3. For more on the history of special education law, see the one book on special education law that belongs on every parent's bookshelf: Peter W. D. Wright and Pamela Darr Wright, *Wrightslaw: Special Education Law* (Hartfield, VA: Harbor House Law Press, 1999), pp. 7–9.

4. Wright and Wright, *Wrightslaw: Special Education Law,* p. 9.

5. Individuals with Disabilities Education Act, 20 U.S.C. §1400(c)(3) and (4).

6. University of the State of New York and the State Education Department, March 2000, Regulations of the Commissioner of Education, 200.13(6)(d).

7. Individuals with Disabilities Education Act, 20 U.S.C. §1400(a)(4).

8. See Peter W. D. Wright and Pamela Darr Wright, "Tests and Measurements for the Parent, Teacher, Advocate & Attorney," online at www.wrightslaw.com/advoc/articles/tests_measurements.html, accessed August 15, 2004.

9. See Lawrence M. Siegel, *The Complete IEP Guide: How to Advocate for Your Special Ed Child* (Berkeley, CA: Nolo, 1999), p. 6/4.

10. Individuals with Disabilities Education Act, 20 U.S.C. §1401(3).

11. Individuals with Disabilities Education Act, 20 U.S.C. §1401(3)(B).

12. Individuals with Disabilities Education Act, 20 U.S.C. §1401(26).

13. Rehabilitation Act of 1973, 29 U.S.C., Chapter 16, Section 701 (B)(1).

14. The Rehabilitation Act of 1973 defines an individual with a disability as "any person who (i) has a physical or mental impairment which substantially limits one or more of such person's major life activities; (ii) has a record of such an impairment; or (iii) is regarded as having such an impairment."

15. Wright and Wright, *Wrightslaw: Special Education Law,* p. 261.

16. This information can be found in the LDA pamphlet "How to Participate Effectively in the IEP Process." Copies are available online at http://www.ldanatl.org/pamphlets/iep.shtml.

17. National Council on Disability, "Back to School on Civil Rights," Executive Summary, "Findings," January 25, 2000, online at www.ncd.gov/newsroom/publications/backtoschool_1.html.

18. According to special education attorney and author Lawrence M. Siegel, "The U.S. Department of Education, Office of Special Education Programs has issued several statements reinforcing the right of parents to tape record IEP meetings." Siegel, *The Complete IEP Guide,* pp. 10–17.

Chapter 9. Your Child's Emotional Life

1. Patricia Howlin, Simon Baron-Cohen, and Julie Hadwin, *Teaching Children with Autism to Mind-Read: A Practical Guide for Teachers and Parents* (Chichester, England: John Wiley & Sons, 1999), pp. 9–12.
2. Val Cumine, Julia Leach, and Gill Stevenson, *Asperger Syndrome: A Practical Guide for Teachers* (London: David Fulton, 1998), p. 25.
3. Sally Ozonoff and Elizabeth McMahon Griffith, "Neuropsychological Function and the External Validity of Asperger Syndrome," in Ami Klin, Fred R. Volkmar, and Sara S. Sparrow, eds., *Asperger Syndrome* (New York: Guilford Press, 2000), p. 86.
4. F. Fösterling, *Attribution Theory in Clinical Psychology* (New York: John Wiley & Sons, 1988), p. 11.
5. G. Barnhill, T. Hagiwara, B. S. Myles, R. L. Simpson, M. L. Brick, and D. Greenwald, "Parent, Teacher, and Self-Report of Problem and Adaptive Behaviors of Children and Adolescents with Asperger Syndrome," *Diagnostique* 25 (2), 2000, pp. 147–167.
6. Ibid.
7. From the essential book on the subject, by Lynn E. Clanahan and Patricia J. Krantz, *Activity Schedules for Children with Autism* (Bethesda, MD: Woodbine House, 1999), p. 3. This book is also essential for its discussion of graduated guidance, which can be applied to teaching children with AS an incredibly broad range of skills.
8. Brenda Smith Myles and Jack Southwick, *Asperger Syndrome and Difficult Moments* (formerly titled *Asperger Syndrome and Rage: Practical Solutions for a Difficult Moment*) (Shawnee Mission, KS: Autism Asperger Publishing, 1999), p. 93.

Chapter 10. Your Child in the Social Realm

1. Tony Attwood and Carol Gray, "Understanding and Teaching Friendship Skills," online at www.tonyattwood.com/paper3.htm.
2. Carol Gray, "Gray's Guide to Bullying" in *The Morning News* (Jenison, MI: Jenison Public Schools, 2000).
3. Tony Attwood and Carol Gray, "The Discovery of 'Aspie' Criteria," *The Morning News* (1999). Also available on Tony Attwood's Web site, www.tonyattwood.com.

Chapter 11. Your Child in School

1. See chapter 8. Contrary to what your school district may try to tell you, intellectual ability or giftedness does not make your child ineligible for accommodations under Section 504 or special education and related ser-

vices under IDEA. There is no such thing as being "too smart" to receive special help, if needed.

2. William L. Heward, *Exceptional Chidren: An Introduction to Special Education* (Upper Saddle River, NJ: Merrill, 2000), pp. 538–39.

3. Steven G. Zecker, "Underachievement and Learning Disabilities in Children Who Are Gifted," available online at www.nldline.com/gifted_and_ld.htm.

4. Maureen Neihart, "Gifted Children with Attention Deficit Hyperactivity Disorder (ADHD)," Eric EC Digest #E649, October 2003, available online at www.tourettesyndrome.net.

5. Stephanie S. Tolan, "Giftedness as Asynchronous Development," Tip Network News, spring 1994, and the eye-opening "Is It a Cheetah?" along with other writings on giftedness available online at her Web site www.stephanietolan.com.

6. Johns Hopkins University, Center for Talented Youth, "What We Know About Academically Talented Students: A Sample of Our Findings," 2004, online at www.cty.jhu.edu/research/whatweknow.html.

7. Diane Toroian, "Thomas' Struggles to Cope with a Pair of Complex Disorders in a Cruel and Provoking Teenage World," *St. Louis Post-Dispatch,* 29 August 1999, online edition, accessed 2001.

8. All second-edition additions from the authors. Based on a chart in the original edition, which was adapted from numerous sources, including *Teaching Students with Autism: A Guide for Educators,* by the Special Education Unit of the Government of Saskatchewan, 1998, online at www.sasked.gov.sk.ca, which is adapted from the work of Attwood (1998), Donnelly and Levy (1995), Grandin (1998), Moreno and O'Neal (1997), Myles and Simpson (1998), and Williams (1995). Other references used: "Asperger's Syndrome Guide for Teachers," OASIS Asperger Syndrome Forum, compiled and edited by Elly Tucker; Val Cumine, Julia Leach, and Gill Stevenson, *Asperger Syndrome: A Practical Guide for Teachers* (London: David Fulton, 1998); Diane Twachtman-Cullen, *How to Be a Para Pro* (Higganum, CT: Starfish Specialty Press, 2000); Beth Fouse, *Creating a "Win-Win IEP" for Students with Autism* (Arlington, TX: Future Horizons, 1999).

9. The Individuals with Disabilities Education Act, 20 U.S.C. §1401(30).

10. The Individuals with Disabilities Education Act, 34 C.F.R., §300.347 (b)(1).

Chapter 12. Growing Up

1. Liane Holliday Willey, *Pretending to Be Normal* (London: Jessica Kingsley Publishers, 1999), p. 117.

ACKNOWLEDGMENTS

This book began in 1998 when the two of us "met" at OASIS. We would like to jointly thank the following people for their support and encouragement in making a project so close to our hearts a reality.

First, we would like to thank the countless families, adults with Asperger Syndrome, educators, and other professionals who have visited OASIS and participated in the forums and lists. While Barb may have provided the venue by offering to share support and information, each of you is responsible for making the world a better place for those touched by Asperger Syndrome. Thanks to your participation in OASIS, never again will an individual with AS or his or her parent feel alone. Your often-voiced support for our book inspired us to do the best possible job, and your enthusiastic participation in the OASIS surveys at Zoomerang.com made possible the first look at many AS-related issues that tend to "fly under the radar" of most research. Thank you for being there for one another and thank you for being there for the two of us.

We would like to express our appreciation to the University of Delaware for its generous donation of server space for OASIS and the original AS list. While UD has no official ties to OASIS, its continued generosity helps keep OASIS up and running.

For nurturing our enthusiasm and for being her usual wise and witty self, thanks go to our agent, Sarah Lazin. Our original editor at Crown, Betsy Rapoport, believed in us from the start. Stephanie Higgs saw us through the time between editions. Shana Drehs, who came on board for this revised edition, has been an enthusiastic supporter. We would also like to thank the whole team at Crown, including Steve Ross, for making this experience such a pleasure.

Dr. Tony Attwood's classic book, *Asperger's Syndrome: A Guide for Parents and Professionals,* was a cornerstone for us and for many other parents we know. We were delighted and honored when he agreed to write the foreword for the first edition. We thank him for taking the time to read and comment on this manuscript and for allowing us to reprint the Australian Scale for Asperger Syndrome. This time out, we would like to thank Dr. Simon Baron-Cohen for a new foreword. We are again honored that someone whose contributions to our understanding of autism and Asperger Syndrome have literally changed the world for children like ours has graced our book.

It is amazing to realize that, just fifteen years ago, AS was a "rare" and largely unknown disorder. Throughout this book, we refer to parents who are pioneers, but here we wish to acknowledge some of the trailblazers who, through their commitment to our children, cleared away darkness so that the light of hope for all persons with autism spectrum disorders could shine through. We were honored that they took time to speak with us (both formally and informally), offered advice and guidance, and in some cases permitted the use of their materials. Thank you, Jeanne Angus, Dr. Simon Baron-Cohen, Dr. James Gilliam, Carol Gray, Dr. Carol Huettig, Dr. Ami Klin, Dr. Arline Lowenthal, Dr. Bobby Newman, Dr. Brenda Smith Myles, Dr. Diane Twachtman-Cullen, and Dr. Fred R. Volkmar. We would like to especially thank Dr. James Snyder for reviewing the chapter on medication. Also consulted in the preparation of this manuscript were others who have made significant contributions in related areas. Our special thanks to Diane Adreon, Lisa Cohen, Dennis Debbaudt, Shelley L. Francis, Dr. Liane Holliday Willey, Sheri Taylor-Mearhoff (who kindly reviewed chapter 8 in the original edition), Kalen Molton, Dr. Cathy Pratt, Pamela Tanguay, and Elly Tucker.

In addition, there are a number of professionals and experts whose work has informed our own. Although they had no direct involvement with this book, we wish to acknowledge what we have learned from Dr. Andrew Adesman, Dr. Teresa Bolick, Dr. Kenneth Bonnet, Mike Darcy, Dr. Herman Davidowicz, Dr. Patricia Elvir, Dr. Catherine Faherty, Dr. Uta Frith, Dr. Christopher Gillberg, Dr. Patricia Howlin, Dr. Eric London, Dr. O. Ivar Lovaas, Dr. Gary B. Mesibov, Susan Moreno, Jerry Newport, Dr. Sally Ozonoff, Dr. John Pomeroy, Dr. Michael Powers, Dr. Cathy Pratt, Dr. Nicholas Putnam, Dr. Bernard Rimland, Dr. Eric Schopler, Dr. Rachelle K. Sheely, Dr. Stephen Shore, Dr. Byrna Siegel, Dr. Digby Tantum, and Dr. Lorna Wing.

Barb's Acknowledgments

First and foremost, I would like to thank my coauthor, Patty Romanowski Bashe. Simply put, without her vision and her talent this book would never have happened. While I stand in awe of her researching, writing, and editing talents, what I admire and respect most are her passion, dedication, and unstoppable determination that the world will become a better place for children and adults diagnosed with Asperger Syndrome. As a first-time author, I could not have asked for a better experience—she encouraged me, she taught me, and along the way, she became my friend.

I would like to thank Dr. Larry Burd for being the first professional who truly listened to me when I described my son. This small act of kindness planted the seed that grew into OASIS. And I wish to acknowledge Dr. Stephen Bauer, who, in the early days, generously shared his paper on AS and, for parents, became the first "Dear Abby" of Asperger Syndrome. I would also especially like to thank Audrey McMahon for her part in bringing knowledge of Asperger Syndrome to the forefront.

I wish to acknowledge and thank three of my son's former teachers: Kate Kerrane, Marilynn Carver Magnani, and Heather Suchanec. They truly made a difference in his life, and I am forever grateful for their caring, understanding, and ability to enjoy what is most wonderful about my son.

I would also like to express my appreciation to my son's guidance counselor, Sharon Bryant, who on many occasions went out of her way to make sure what needed to happen actually *did* happen.

I would especially like to thank Jeanine Carlson for her friendship and for volunteering her time to help provide information to new OASIS forum members.

On a personal level, I would like to thank those people who are dearest to my heart. Jill Itzkowitz, who has been my best friend for thirty-one years, advised me to take a chance and accept the offer to coauthor this book, and assured me (more than once) that I was capable of doing it. She stood by me during the worst and best of times, and because she cares about my family, she made it her business to learn about and understand Asperger Syndrome. Her friendship is very precious to me.

Thank you to my husband, Kirby, for his unwavering love and faith in me. I am grateful that he is my partner, my friend, and a wonderful father to our children. Words cannot begin to express how much he means to me. Without his understanding and support, OASIS would not exist, nor would this book.

Our three wonderful sons, Josh, Nick, and Ben, bring so much joy to my life. I am so proud of them, and I feel privileged to be their mother and watch them grow into young men. Their patience, understanding, and willingness to once again eat pancakes for supper allowed me to spend the time I needed to work on the book and keep OASIS running. The answer to their often-asked question "Are you done with those revisions yet?" is "Yes, I'm done with those revisions."

Patty's Acknowledgments

As before, I first want to thank Barb for more things than I can name. Over these past seven years, she has grown into my sharpest, brightest, funniest, most trusted, and favorite friend. When I decided to "turn pro," Barb alone had the audacity—and the heart—to pop my grad school bubble with her sharp, wry wit and insight. I suspect she knew long before I did that my heart would sometimes break on the shores I've raced to reach these past four years. I'm softer but stronger because of her. I would like to again thank her entire family, but particularly Josh, without whose support this book could not exist.

Speaking of books and friends, thank you just isn't enough for my close friend, mentor, agent, and ex-boss (in that order), Sarah Lazin. More than anyone outside my home, Sarah made me a writer. Twenty-four years ago, she opened a door for me that changed my life, and she's been with me every step since.

Closer to home, thank you to Paul Aden, Jeanne Angus, Dr. Herman Davidowicz, Sue and Jack DeMasi, John Edward, Robert Emery, Shelley L. Francis, Tali Gerasi, Katie and Robert Hansen, Deidre Higgins, Mack Hopkins, Nancy Inglis, Bonnie Januszewski-Ytuarte, Barbara Kipp, Dr. Jill Leavens-Maurer, Rhona Leff, Karen Mackler, Sharon Mor, Elizabeth Morelli, Dr. Waverlyn Peters, Pat and Jim Pons, Ronna Ross, Cathy Russ, Roxana Satir, Mitch Schneider, Regina Skyer, Dr. James Snyder, Barbara Tynan, and Erin Walsh. Also, thank you to everyone at The David Center—especially Lorraine Shea, John and Amy Beyer, Joan Mazzu, and Anna Dragone, and the rest of the board—for their ongoing support and inspiration, and for my dream job.

The wonderful classmates and teachers I had in the C. W. Post/Long Island University Competencies in Autism for Special Educators (CASE) graduate program deserve special mention. First, my classmates—all wonderful teachers—deserve a nod for their friendship and encouragement. I've never felt so young—or so old. Or more like being a rock critic again than when confronted with the realization that some of them like Journey. (My attempts to modify *that* behavior failed utterly.) I would like to thank especially Dr. Douglas Dreilinger and Dr. Nancy Shamow. I owe an infinite debt of gratitude to Nancy. Not only is she an inspiring teacher, but she also gave me the opportunity to train and to teach at her school, Ascent: A School for Individuals with Autism, certainly one of the finest ABA schools in the world. There I worked with incredible teachers and some truly wonderful kids and their families.

I came to accept my son's having AS a bit more quickly than I might have because someone taught me how to see the dignity before the disability and the spirit inside the struggle, to truly believe in love. Thank you, Teddy Pendergrass.

To our wonderful, supportive, and loving family: my in-laws Rochelle and Robert Bashe; Donna, Dmitriy, and Rick Romanowski; and Mary and Douglas Vitro. I love you guys for about a million reasons. Your love and support of us, and your understanding of Justin, make you all the blessings of our lives. For their support and acceptance, I also wish to acknowledge

Michelle Assoian and Alex, Katie, and Adam; Patty Barconey; Jackie and the late Harold Bashe; Danielle Karmel and Patrick Dill; and Evelyn and David Napolin.

My husband, Philip Bashe, is fantastic in every way. He would be a great dad for any kid, but God surely made him special for his Beatles-loving, politically minded (and definitely Democrat), and opinionated, irreverent, and very funny son. I thank him for his support, encouragement, tolerance, and love, especially during the past three years. It is his belief in me that carries me through everything meaningful I do. I thank him for everything, but especially for Justin. And to my son: Thank you for choosing me and reminding me how you did it. You told me that in the years before you were born, you followed me around the garden "like a little bug." I had a feeling that was you. Welcome home.

INDEX

diagnosis *(continued)*:
sharing with your child, 116–22
starting the process, 94, 96–97
unclear, 111–12
understanding, 118
use of term, 66
warning signs and, 91–93
Diagnostic and Statistical Manual of Mental Disorders, Fourth Edition (DSM-IV), 2, 10, 18, 28–30, 189
diagnostic substitution, 20
diagnostic technology, 98
diets, 226–27, 228, 230
difference, awareness of, 116–17, 118, 337
dimethylglycine (DMG), 230
diminishing returns, point of, 171
disability, legal definitions, 290–91, 294
discrete trial teaching, 183–84
disinhibition, 262–63, 275
documentation, 145–46, 173, 317, 400
drugs and alcohol, 461–63
dyscalculia, 78, 216
dysgraphia, 76–78
dyslexia, 78–79
dyspraxia, 206

early interventions, 179, 291–93
Earobics, 192
echolalia, 22–23, 81
Edelson, Stephen M., 70
education, *see* school; school district
Effexor (venlafaxine), 263–64
Elavil (amitriptyline), 265–66
emergency contacts, 253, 351–54, 450
emotional awareness, 355–59
emotional disabilities, 80–81
emotional lability, 50–51
emotions, 331–59
belief-based, 334–35
classroom strategies, 419
crisis of, 351–54
factors in, 332–40
intense, 46–47
meltdown of, 344
neurotransmitters and, 239
parental help with, 344–46, 357–58
emotion scale, 355–57
empathy, lack of, 45–46
employment, preparation for, 437, 467–68
Endep (amitriptyline), 265–66
escape plans, 348–49, 388–90
Eskalith (lithium carbonate), 272–73
estate planning, 469
evaluation, 65, 93
child described in, 108
of children under 3, 292
confidentiality concerns in, 102–3
and diagnosis, *see* diagnosis
instruments listed in, 108
medical tests listed in, 108

narrative report of, 108–9
neuropsychological, 99
paperwork in preparation for, 100–102
preparing the child for, 103–5
private, 90
results and recommendations, 108–9
by school district, 94–96
scores interpreted in, 109–10
by a specialist, 96–97
tests administered in, 105–7, 216
understanding results of, 112–13
executive function (EF), 56, 333, 337
eye contact, 24, 55
eye control, 193

facial expression, 43, 45
family members
and adolescents, 450
autism in, 21
broader autistic phenotype (BAP), 87–88
burnout of, 170–71
confidentiality concerns of, 102–3
and diagnosis, 87–88
embarrassment felt by, 137–38
in emotional scenes, 350–51
feeling cheated, 138
and genetic studies, 16–17
harassment of, 374
and medication, 252
not getting enough attention, 133, 137
nurturing relationships with, 138
progress reports by, 171
shadow syndrome of, 139
sharing diagnosis with, 120, 121
stress for, 137–39
teasing by, 372
Tourette's syndrome and tics in, 73
family practitioners, 97–98
family therapists, 100, 224
Fast ForWord, 192
FDA
drug approvals by, 241–42, 243–44, 245
drug information from, 260, 265
on generic drugs, 246
warnings about drugs, 237, 247, 264, 272
Feingold diet, 228
females, AS diagnosed in, 12–15
financial matters, 139, 172–74, 236
see also health insurance
foundation for success, 143–60
advocate and ambassador, 159–60
building for the future, 160
daily management, 156–58
detective work, 152–55
disagreement of parents and professionals, 147–49
expert knowledge in, 145–46
information sources in, 155
inventory of concerns, 152–53
keeping a journal, 154–55

parent as bridge, 143
parents as teachers, 158–59
protectiveness, 156–58
seeing the other side, 149–50
setting priorities, 151–52
setting the agenda, 150–51
support for parents, 144–45
team for, 146–47
friendship, 220–21, 331, 361–62, 364,
374–75, 382, 392, 457–58
Frith, Uta, 9, 27
Frombonne, Eric, 20
frustration tolerance, low, 333
future
hope for, 63, 160, 329–30
without parents, 468–69

Gabitril (tiagabine), 272–74
gaze avoidance, 24, 43
generalization, 57, 80, 181, 358
generalized anxiety disorder (GAD), 69
general phobias, 70
Geodon (ziprasidone), 261, 270
gifted students, 111, 395–98
gluten-free diet, 226–27, 228, 230
Grandin, Temple, 245, 387
gravitational insecurity, 193, 210–11
Gray, Carol, 118, 198, 200, 202–3, 205, 322,
361, 373, 374, 377, 378
grief, stages of, 130–32
gustatory system (taste), 209, 210

Haldol (haloperidol), 269, 271
handwriting, 76–78, 80, 206
harassment, 371–74, 446
health insurance
appeals, 174
coverage by, 94, 96, 139, 172–74, 222
documentation for, 145–46, 173
legal assistance with, 174
and medication, 236, 246
mental health benefits of, 172–73
other payment sources, 174
state regulation of, 173, 174
steps for dealing with, 173–74
universal diagnostic code number for, 21
hearing
auditory system of, 209, 210
and listening, 193, 194
and noise, 52–54, 81–82, 192
Holliday Willey, Liane, 13, 443, 470
hope, reasons for, 63, 140–41
hygiene and grooming, 15, 453–54
hyperactivity, see attention-deficit/hyperac-
tivity disorder
hyperlexia, 81

independence
as goal, 61–62, 132, 151, 164, 332–33,
343, 358

as learnable skill, 62, 158–59
self-advocacy, 455–56
Individualized Education Programs (IEPs),
281, 282, 286, 295, 305–7, 319, 373,
400, 437, 450–51, 454–55
Individuals with Disabilities Education Act
(IDEA)
autism classified under, 20, 94
on documentation, 317
on evaluation, 107, 216
IEPs in, 305–6, 400, 437, 454–55
mandate of, 94–96
on occupational therapy, 212
on older students, 436–37
and special education, 94–96, 283–86, 287,
291, 293, 294–306, 311, 455
on speech and language therapy, 216, 217
on transition services, 437
inheritance laws, 469
insurance
state commission on, 173, 174
see also health insurance
intelligence quotient (IQ), 26–28, 79, 106,
110–11, 290
intelligence tests, 106, 110–11
International Classification of Diseases (WHO),
29
Internet, access to, 144
intervention burnout, 170–71
interventions, 175–231
alternative therapies, 228–30
applied behavior analysis (ABA), 175–88
auditory integration training (AIT),
191–98
choosing, 230–31
Comic Strip Conversations, 198–99,
202–5
costs of, 172–74
delayed benefits of, 162
diets, 226–27
early, 179, 291–93
generalizations about, 164–65
length of treatment, 167–68
limitations of, 166–67
note-taking about, 167
occupational therapy (OT), 205–14
point of diminishing returns in, 171
psychotherapy, 224–26
questions to ask about, 166–69
ranking of, 165
research behind, 166–67
social skills training, 218–23
Social Stories, 198–202
speech and language therapy, 214–18
therapy rebellion from, 171–72
verbal behavior analysis (VBA), 188–91
inventory of problems and concerns, 152–55

jargon, 167
journal, 154–55

ABOUT THE AUTHORS

PATRICIA ROMANOWSKI BASHE, M.S.Ed., co-owner of OASIS, is an award-winning author and editor. She has coauthored twenty-four books, including four national bestsellers. She is the executive director of The David Center, a Long Island–based not-for-profit that provides information, services, and support to individuals with autism spectrum disorders and their families. A certified special education teacher and early intervention provider, she speaks frequently on issues concerning Asperger Syndrome and related disorders. Her writing credits include cowriting the autobiographies of Donny Osmond, Teddy Pendergrass, Annette Funicello, Mary Wilson, La Toya Jackson, and Otis Williams's *Temptations*—on which the Emmy-winning 1998 miniseries was based. She also cowrote, with Joel Martin, the New Age classic George Anderson trilogy and *Love Beyond Life: The Healing Power of After-Death Communication*. As a coeditor and contributor, she received the ASCAP–Deems Taylor Special Recognition Award for *The New Rolling Stone Encyclopedia of Rock & Roll*. She lives on Long Island with her husband, the author Philip Bashe, and their son, Justin.

BARBARA L. KIRBY is the founder and co-owner of the award-winning OASIS (Online Asperger Syndrome Information and Support) Web page, located at http://www.aspergersyndrome.org or http://www.udel.edu/bkirby/asperger/. She started the first support list for families of children with AS and HFA and currently moderates several OASIS message board and chat room support forums. She was a founding member and former vice president of ASC-U.S., Inc. She has been providing information and support to the AS community since 1994. She lives in Newark, Delaware, with her husband, Jim ("Kirby"); her three sons, Joshua, Benjamin, and Nicholas; and their Labradoodle, Obie.